Eda Kılınç İşleyen
Editor

Health Promotion and Prevention

School-Age Children

nova
science publishers
www.novapublishers.com

DOI: https://doi.org/10.52305/GICF1015

NOTICE TO THE READER

Library of Congress Cataloging-in-Publication Data

Library of Congress Control Number: 2025945263

ISBN: 979-8-89530-758-8 (Hardcover)
ISBN: 979-8-89530-840-0 (eBook)

Published by Nova Science Publishers, Inc. † New York

Contents

Preface v

Chapter 1 **The Importance of Health Promotion and Prevention in the School Community** 1
Sabahat Coşkun

Chapter 2 **Nutrition and Physical Activity in School-Age Children** 15
İrem Nur Özdemir

Chapter 3 **Hygiene, Excretion, and Sleep in School-Age Children** 27
Ecem Çiçek Gümüş

Chapter 4 **Sexual Health in School-Age Children** 41
Bilgin Kıray Vural

Chapter 5 **Mental Health in School-Age Children** 55
İlknur Mizrahi

Chapter 6 **Anger Management in School-Age Children** 69
Özden Erdem

Chapter 7 **Preventing Violence, Bullying, Discrimination and Stigma in Schools** 81
Betül Kaplan and Metin Yıldız

Chapter 8 **Infection Control in Schools** 93
Zahide Aksoy

Chapter 9 **A Safe and Healthy School Environment** 101
Sultan Kayan

Chapter 10 **Immunizations in School-Age Children and Adolescents** 115
Gülbahar Korkmaz Aslan and Ebru Öztürk Çopur

Chapter 11 **Preventing Accidents and Injuries at School** 129
Adem Sümen and Selma Öncel

Chapter 12 **Sun Protection in School-Age Children** 141
Özüm Erkin and Ebru Konal Korkmaz

Chapter 13 **The Fundamentals and Features of Health Education in Schools** 151
Ayla Tuzcu İnce and Habibe Ozcelik

Chapter 14 **Health Promotion Theories and Models in School Health** 161
Aslı Kalkım and Zuhal Emlek Sert

Chapter 15 **Health Promotion Programs in Schools** 179
Yasemin Demir Avcı

Chapter 16 **Health Literacy in School-Age Children** 189
Adile Tümer and Fehime Nida Kürklüoğlu

Chapter 17 **The Assessment of Health in School-Age Children** 199
Asiye Kartal and Edanur Özkaya Bozkurt

Chapter 18 **School Health Screenings** 213
Eda Kılınç İşleyen and Edanur Özkaya Bozkurt

Chapter 19 **The Management of Chronic Diseases in Schools** 225
Leyla Muslu

Chapter 20 **The Management of Children with Special Needs in Schools** 239
Kamer Gür and Bahar Doğan

Chapter 21 **The Management of Neglect and Abuse in School-Age Children** 253
Aysun Erdal and Naile Bilgili

Chapter 22 **The Management of Childhood Infectious Diseases in Schools** 269
Renginar Öztürk Dönmez and Gülengül Mermer

Chapter 23 **The Management of Emergency Situations in Schools** 283
Özlem Sinan

Chapter 24 **Basic First Aid Practices in Schools** 295
Bennur Koca

Chapter 25 **Pandemic (Epidemic Diseases) and Management in Schools** 321
Ebru Öztürk Çopur and Fatma Karasu

Index 333

Preface

Schools play a pivotal role in public health, serving as environments where students can assume responsibility for their own well-being and develop lifelong health-promoting attitudes and behaviors. Academic success and the health of school-age children are closely related. The primary purpose of school health services is to ensure school-age children and young people are in a state of complete physical, spiritual, and social well-being and are able to maintain this state of well-being. In school health services carried out by a team, the school nurse plays a vital role in protecting and improving the health of students. The National Association of School Nursing (NASN) defines school nursing as a professional branch of nursing that works to improve students' health, increase their school success, and maintain a healthy lifestyle. School nurses promote a healthy environment for students and staff, coordinate school health education programs, intervene in current and potential health problems, provide case management services, and collaborate with families to increase students' self-management of their health.

The responsibilities of school nurses in promoting and safeguarding student health encompass a broad range of activities. These include, supporting healthy nutrition, encouraging physical activity, prevention smoking, alcohol, and substance abuse, promoting mental health, prevention violence, approach to child abuse, accident prevention, raising disaster awareness, providing first aid, managing chronic conditions, preventing infectious diseases, and fostering intersectoral collaboration. In the public health nursing approach, three levels of prevention (primary, secondary, and tertiary) have always been part of health care in schools. Primary prevention involves providing health promotion and education to prevent health problems in children. Secondary prevention includes screening children for various diseases, monitoring their growth and development, and providing them with emergency health care when they become sick or injured. Tertiary prevention in schools includes education at the community level as well as ongoing care and treatment to prevent complications in students who need health services on a long-term basis. Therefore, this book was designed to establish public health according to these three levels of prevention, to help the school nurse plan interventions, and to bring together high-evidence research. The book, to which 35 scientists contributed 25 chapters, is a scientific publication that attracts attention with its many topics. This book serves as a guide for school nurses to plan evidence-based practice for health promotion and prevention of school-age children.

I would like to express my endless gratitude to the chapter authors and everyone who played a role in the development of this book.

Chapter 1

The Importance of Health Promotion and Prevention in the School Community

Sabahat Coşkun*, **PhD**
Bilecik Şeyh Edebali University Faculty of Health Sciences, Health Management, Bilecik, Türkiye

Abstract

Schools have an essential position in health promotion and prevention of community, as they include families, school staff, and school-age children. The school environment is the significant environmental factor affecting the physical, cognitive, psychological, and social development of school-age children, especially after their homes. Implementing protective measures during school ensures acquired health behaviors have a lasting impact throughout life. These protective measures are detailed within the school health program. These programs include components such as acquiring healthy lifestyle habits, providing preventive health services, creating a safe school environment, supporting mental health, and increasing health literacy. Providing these programs in schools is crucial for ensuring that children who may not otherwise have access to healthcare can receive the support they need. These services are provided not only to students but also to a wide group of people called the "school community," including families and school personnel. To transform educational institutions into "health-promoting schools," it is anticipated that the essential preventive and developmental health services needed for the school community will primarily be delivered by school nurses. The school nurse's primary health strategy consists of health education, promoting healthy lifestyle behaviors, providing guidance and consultancy, and organizing healthy school policies. The school nurse plans health education programs to provide health-related information as well as to create healthy and permanent behavioral changes in the school community. The school nurse, who has a key role in health promotion and prevention for the school community, should be employed in every school.

Keywords: school health, health prevention and promotion, school nurse

---

* Corresponding Author's Email: sabahat.coskun@bilecik.edu.tr

In: Health Promotion and Prevention
Editor: Eda Kılınç İşleyen
ISBN: 979-8-89530-758-8

Introduction

Health is a fundamental determinant for people's well-being and quality of life (Junior et al., 2023). Since education and well-being are intertwined concepts, a primary objective of the education system is to ensure that students are healthy and able to learn (Pulimeno et al., 2020). Responsibility for health-related practices has traditionally been attributed to healthcare institutions such as hospitals. However, a growing body of evidence emphasizes the importance of initiating health promotion and prevention strategies in early childhood within educational and community settings (Junior et al., 2023). Since the school community encompasses a large part of the population, including students, their families, teachers, and other staff, the role of the school health promotion is critical (Okuyan and Alkaya, 2018; Junior et al., 2023).

School-age children spend a considerable portion of their time at school; therefore, health promotion and prevention behaviors must be effectively taught within the school setting. Implementing protective measures during this period allows ensure that acquired health behaviors have a lasting impact throughout life (Pekcan 2012). For children, school is the first environment where they spend substantial time away from home. For this reason, schools play a direct role in shaping the health of school-age children in terms of their physical and mental (Kurt, 2020; (Pulimeno et al., 2020).

Through mental well-being programs in schools, students can learn skills to manage stress, cope with negative emotions, and build mental resilience. The emotional support provided by the school promotes students' mental well-being and, therefore, improves academic performance by creating a safe environment (Junior et al., 2023). Students can prepare for life by learning in this environment while also safeguarding their mental health, especially against stress and pressure in competitive and challenging situations (Pekcan, 2012).

Additionally, students can develop a sense of responsibility for health from an early age through socio-cognitive learning at school. This responsibility can enhance their ability to maintain a healthy lifestyle and foster the development of self-efficacy (Pulimeno et al., 2020).

While schools have a positive impact on students' development, they also present various risks to students. Infectious diseases are the most common of these risks. The close interaction of students in schools settings may facilitate the transmission and spread of infectious diseases. However, infectious diseases can be effectively controlled through protective measures implemented in schools, such as health education, hygiene practices, vaccination, and close observation (Pekcan, 2012). The spread of infectious diseases within the school environment compromises students' health and disrupts the educational process (Wang et al., 2023).

The COVID-19 (Coronavirus Disease 2019) pandemic has particularly negatively impacted school-age children. The closure of schools and the shift to distance education during the COVID-19 pandemic deprived students of the health prevention and promotion services provided by schools. These health services include physical activity and nutrition programs, health education, general health monitoring, immunization, detection of neglect and abuse (Viner et al., 2022). As school health services were disrupted during the COVID-19 pandemic, students faced numerous health risks, such as obesity (reduced physical activity and unhealthy eating habits), visual impairment (due to prolonged screen time in online learning). It has also been reported that the COVID-19 pandemic has had short- and long-term negative psychosocial effects (symptoms such as anxiety, depression, lethargy, impaired social interaction, and decreased appetite) in students (Jiao et al., 2020). Education systems can be affected by various crises, including epidemics. However, it should not be forgotten that education and health are the inalienable rights of all children under all circumstances. The closure of schools and the transition to distance education during the pandemic have further highlighted the critical role of schools in health prevention and promotion of students health (Kurt, 2020; Pulimeno et al., 2020).

School health programs are a comprehensive approach implemented in the school environment to prevent and promote the physical, mental and social health of students (Junior et al., 2020). These programs include components such as acquiring healthy lifestyle habits, providing preventive health services, creating a safe school environment, supporting mental health, and increasing health literacy. They also aim to increase the level of social health in the long term by raising awareness of students, teachers, and families about health (IUHPE, 2010). School nurses and school staff are primarily responsible for implementing school health programs. The school nurse plans health education programs to provide health-related information as well as to create healthy and permanent behavioral changes in the school community. This education can be given to both students and school staff. The education topics that can be given to students are health nutrition, physical activity, sleep, hygiene, the harm of screen addiction, the harm of smoking and substance use, bullying, coping with stress, etc. (COSH, 2016; Akgül and Ergün, 2021). The school nurse, who has a key role in health promotion and prevention of the school community, should be employed in every school.

School Health Program

School Health Programs include components such as acquiring healthy lifestyle habits, providing preventive health services, creating a safe school environment, supporting mental health, and increasing health literacy. They also aim to increase the level of social health in the long term by raising awareness of students, teachers, and families about health (IUHPE, 2010). In Türkiye, after 1990, successful projects to improve health in schools were implemented with the implementation of the Health Promoting Schools Network Project. However, the studies could not be spread throughout the country. For this reason, as a result of the cooperation between the Ministry of Health and the Ministry of National Education, important projects and programs have been prepared to improve health in schools in our country (Table 1) (Meydanlıoğlu and Gözüm, 2019).

Table 1. Programs/projects carried out within the scope of school health

Oral and Dental Health Education and Preventive Oral Health Studies	Diabetes Education Program in Schools
Nutrition-Friendly School Program	School Milk Program
White Flag Project	Studies to Prevent Violence in Schools
Growth Development Monitoring Program	HIV/AIDS Prevention Studies,
Physical Activity Fitness Report Card	Program for Improving Health Awareness of Adolescents
Vaccinations of School-Age Children	Adolescence Change Project
Hearing Screening Program for School-Age Children	Turkey Addiction Fighting Training Program
Health Protection and Promotion Program at School	Nutrition Recommendations and Menu Programs for Preschool and School-Age Children

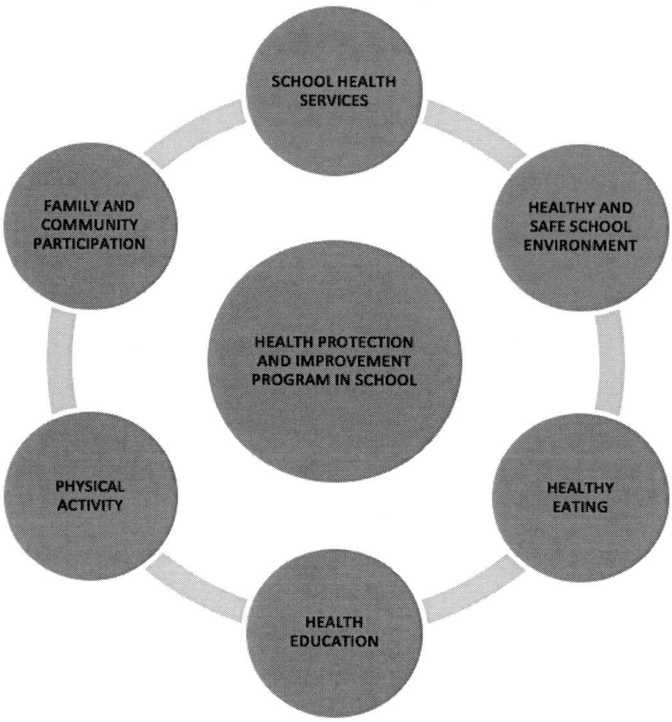
SCHOOL HEALTH SERVICES
HEALTHY AND SAFE SCHOOL ENVIRONMENT
HEALTHY EATING
HEALTH EDUCATION
PHYSICAL ACTIVITY
FAMILY AND COMMUNITY PARTICIPATION
HEALTH PROTECTION AND IMPROVEMENT PROGRAM IN SCHOOL

Figure 1. Components of the Health Prevention and Promotion Program at School.

The framework of all programs and projects carried out or to be initiated within the scope of school health in schools has been created with the "Program for the Prevention and Promotion of Health at School," which was launched in 2017. This program aims to conduct annual health screenings and periodic follow-ups for all school-age children under the supervision of family physicians (Ministry of Health, 2017). Within the scope of the program, six key areas of focus have been identified; these are shown in Figure 1.

School Health Services

School health services encompass measures aimed at prevention and promotion the health of the school community throughout the period. The purpose of school health services is to ensure and maintain the school community's best possible physical, mental, and social health (Okuyan and Alkaya, 2018).

The services provided under the scope of school health services are as follows:

School Enrollment Examination

School-age children undergo a health examination prior to the commencement of school. By obtaining a student's history, physical, psychological, social, and familial factors that may affect the student's success are assessed. Additionally, the student's general health status is evaluated through an examination of their language, motor and social development, as well as their immunization status (Kurt, 2020).

Periodic Health Examination

The purpose of periodic physical health examinations is to diagnose and treat physical and mental health conditions at an early stage by assessing the age-appropriateness of the child's ongoing growth and development (Pekcan, 2012).

Health Screenings

The purpose of school health screenings is to diagnose diseases early stage and ensure treatment. The scope of health screenings is determined by evaluating societal needs, the capabilities of school health services, the frequency of provision, and the methods employed in evaluation process (Dığrak et al., 2020).

Common health screenings for school-age children include Body Mass Index (BMI) measurement, vision and hearing screening, oral and dental health screening, scoliosis screening, blood pressure screening, and head lice screening (Dığrak et al., 2020; Özsoy et al., 2019) (See Chapter 18).

The literature highlights the importance and necessity of school health screenings, citing benefits such as the ability to reach many students simultaneously, early diagnosis and treatment of health issues, and the reduction of healthcare costs (Akgün and Ergün 2021).

Protection from Infectious Diseases

Infectious diseases can spread quickly and be easily transmitted when students are together in large groups. This can pose significant risks to their health and well-being, leading to frequent illness, school absenteeism, or even mortality. However, it is possible to protect against many infectious diseases by following basic hygiene rules and effective vaccination methods. Therefore, there is a significant need for school health services to combat infectious diseases in the school environment. Teaching students' personal hygiene habits and ensuring their continuity through school-family cooperation and preventive health education is important in protecting the school community from infectious diseases (Maughan et al., 2018; Akçay, 2017). It has been reported that health education intervention on infectious diseases significantly improved the infectious disease-related health behaviors of students (Wang et al., 2023).

Various programs have been developed for the control of infectious diseases in Türkiye, and these programs are as follows: (Maughan et al., 2018; Pekcan, 2012; Akçay, 2017).

1. Vaccinations: Vaccines provide protection against diseases that are especially common among school-age children and contribute to building community immunity.
2. Hand hygiene: Regular hand washing or disinfecting is a crucial precaution to prevent the spread of infectious diseases in schools. Hands should be washed, particularly after using the toilet, before meals, and after sharing items between students.
3. Cleaning and hygienic environments: Regular cleaning and disinfection of school environments are essential in preventing the spread of infectious diseases. Common areas such as classrooms, toilets, dining halls, and playgrounds should be cleaned and disinfected regularly.
4. Sick students staying at home: It is important that sick students refrain from attending school to prevent the spread of infectious diseases. School administration and parents should ensure that children stay home if they exhibit symptoms. It is important to note that in the case of an epidemic within the school, the school should remain open rather

than closed. Students exhibiting signs of infectious diseases should be closely monitored by the school nurse

5. Education and awareness: It is important to educate and raise awareness among the school community about the symptoms of infectious diseases, ways of spreading them, and prevention methods. These measures help prevent the spread of infectious diseases in schools and play a crucial role in protecting students' health.

Accident Prevention and First Aid

Accidents are a serious problem in medical, social, and economic terms. Injuries and deaths that occur after accidents cannot be ignored as they affect the health of students and, therefore, public health. It is stated that students have a high rate of accidents and accident-related injuries at school (Kartal and Kılınç, 2020). A study conducted in Türkiye found that 55.4% of students had experienced an accident at school. School accidents can be prevented by having school nurses with first-aid knowledge presents in the school environment. However, only a few schools in Türkiye have school nurses and other health professional (Akçay and Yıldırımlar, 2018). To ensure continuous school health services, there is a need for school nurses, who play a crucial role in health prevention and promotion activities. Research indicates that nurses have a significant impact on injury prevention and first aid (Kim et al., 2017; Kılınç and Gür, 2020) (See Chapter 10 and Chapter 24).

Mental Health Services

School mental health services support students' cognitive, emotional, and behavioral development by addressing their psychological needs through collaboration with the school's mental health team and families (Kaynak and Işık, 2019). In the literature, school mental health services are stated to be carried out effectively with the cooperation of school psychological counselors, school nurses, school employees (teachers, school administrators), student families, and external stakeholders (such as the media) (Çokamay et al., 2017).

The role of the school mental health team is to assess at an early stage whether students' psychosocial development is age-appropriate and to provide necessary interventions. In this way, students who require support can receive appropriate interventions and monitored through a team-based approach. If necessary, students can be referred to a healthcare institution for diagnosis and treatment. Additionally, programs can be implemented to address peer bullying and violence, which are among the most common issues during the school period (Kaynak and Işık, 2019; Çokamay et al., 2017) (See Chapter 5).

Early Diagnosis, Treatment, and Follow-Up of Students with Acute and Chronic Diseases

Although chronic diseases seem to be a problem of old age, they also affect school-age children. It is stated that 24.6% of school-age children have a chronic disease (Barnett et al., 2018). School-age children with chronic diseases are stated to be at risk for learning difficulties, academic failure, and school absences. For this reason, chronic health problems are an issue that needs to be carefully addressed in the health services provided in schools for students. Health services provided at school include practices such as early detection of diseases, treatment, monitoring, compliance with treatment, disease management, counseling, and rehabilitation services for students and their families. With these services, students can help them manage their chronic diseases, reduce their absenteeism, and increase their academic success (Akçan et al., 2023) (See Chapter 19).

Healthy and Safe School Environment

School-age children need a safe and supportive school environment to maintain their physical, emotional, and social health, and achieve academic success. A healthy school environment includes the school's physical and aesthetic features, as well as its cultural and psychosocial climate. A healthy and safe school environment is a place where education and learning continue uninterrupted, there is no violence, drugs, bullying, and the necessary physical and social environment are provided (Georgiev et al., 2015) (See Chapter 9).

Health Education

In order for school-age children to be healthy, happy, and productive individuals, they should be provided with the necessary basic knowledge and skills through health education. Education is important for school-age children to develop health prevention and promotion behaviors. The health problems observed in school-age children stem from unhealthy behaviors and social/environmental factors. Behaviors that negatively impact students' health include poor eating habits, lack of physical activity, insufficient sleep, excessive screen time, smoking, alcohol use, and challenges in managing stress (Baltag et al., 2025; Nalbani, 2021). These unhealthy behaviors often form in early childhood, persist throughout adulthood, and can lead to interrelated poor health, educational, and social outcomes, increasing the risks of disease and death. Health education programs offered in schools today are of vital importance in terms of early intervention before the health and social problems of the school community turn into insurmountable problems (Pulimeno et al., 2020). The purpose of health education is to provide the school community with the necessary and accurate information to protect and improve health, teach the necessary behaviors, increase the level of health literacy, and gain the behavioral changes necessary for a healthy life (Akgül and Ergün, 2021). Health education practices should go beyond the academic achievements expected from students and provide the basis for students' self-actualization, helping them grow as self-confident students and health-responsible citizens (Pulimeno et al., 2020).

Students who receive health education are more likely to form healthy and responsible friendships, adopt healthy eating habits, accept their physical appearance, recognize the importance of dental health, prioritize sleep and exercise, reduce the risk of violent tendencies, and engage in positive behaviors such as following safety rules (Lee et al., 2023; Coşgun and Kara, 2015). Additionally, students who receive health education develop the skills to resist and say confidently "no" when faced with choices between healthy and unhealthy behaviors.

Healthy Eating

School-age children's physiological, psychological, and social development are rapid. It is significant that children have adequate and balanced nutrition to support growth and development in this period, to develop their immune systems, and to maintain psychosocial well-being (Küçükkaraca Zakkour and Yıldıran, 2022). Schools offer an appropriate environment for promoting healthy eating habits. Teaching school-age children about healthy nutrition behaviors at school plays a crucial role in preventing many possible nutrition-related diseases in the future. Nutritional problems commonly seen in school-age children include inadequate and unbalanced nutrition, high consumption of fast food and processed foods, low intake of fruits and vegetables, excessive sugar and salt consumption, skipping breakfast, and insufficient water intake. The incidence of obesity increases in school-age children who eat this way (Salman and Günay, 2023).

It is stated that obesity is a health problem in the school community, especially among students, and increases morbidity and mortality rates at older ages. Schools are an important part of the nationwide fight to prevent chronic diseases such as obesity, coronary heart disease, diabetes, and cancer in the school community. Additionally, nutrition programs implemented in schools not only improve students' health but also enhance their learning, attention, perception, and cognitive abilities, increase academic success, and ensure school attendance (Okuyan and Alkaya, 2018). School-based nutrition education programs should be given national priority to ensure a healthy future for school-age children. Studies conducted on school-age children emphasize that children's nutritional knowledge, attitudes, and behaviors increase significantly after nutrition education, but family participation is important to ensure continuity (Küçükkaraca Zakkour and Yıldıran, 2022). School nutrition programs should be supported and maintained with the participation of governments, community leaders, doctors, dieticians, nurses, teachers, and families (Okuyan and Alkaya, 2018).

Physical Activity

Regular physical activity during the school period is significant to health problems in later years. Therefore, physical activity is of great importance in school health practices. Schools are in a unique position to provide students with the opportunity to engage in at least 60 minutes of moderate to vigorous physical activity each day (Cornett et al., 2023). Regular physical activity that starts in childhood also has positive effects on mental health, such as reducing the risk of chronic diseases such as type 2 diabetes, hypertension, obesity, cardiovascular diseases, and colon cancer, protecting body mass index and musculoskeletal health, feeling team spirit, the virtue of accepting the success of others and improving self-esteem. In addition, the activity in question allows school-age children to contribute to motor skills, hand-eye coordination, long-term attention and concentration, and academic success (Akhter and Ahmed, 2021; Cornett et al., 2023).

Family/Community Participation

Active participation and collaboration within the school staff, parents, local businesses, and non-governmental organizations are crucial health-promoting school practices. This participation and collaboration strengthen both the school and society in terms of health, and well-being (WHO, 2020).

Encouraging family participation in school health education helps improve the health and well-being of school-age children. This approach enables children to achieve desired behavioral changes both at school and at home in a safe and controlled manner. In this process, the school nurse, teachers, school administration, and families should work together in cooperation (Küçükkaraca Zakkour and Yıldıran, 2022).

In the literature, the benefits of teachers and parents observing children and actively participating in children's education and school activities are mentioned. The gains in question promote the health and well-being of children (healthy nutrition, regular exercise, adequate sleep, avoiding smoking, alcohol, and substance use, etc.), increase the possibility of participation and access to preventive health services (vaccinations, health screenings, etc.), help students' emotional well-being (confidence, sense of belonging, and support, etc.) and increase their academic success (WHO, 2020; Küçükkaraca Zakkour and Yıldıran, 2022; Şahinöz et al., 2017). For this reason, necessary partnerships (school, family, local and national governments, non-governmental organizations, etc.) should be established for all health-promoting practices for the school community (student, school staff, family, etc.).

The Role of the School Nurse

Health promotion and prevention of the school community is the primary responsibility of the school nurse. In this regard, the school nurse aims to raise awareness in the school community and develop the responsibility of stakeholders to improve and maintain their health levels (COSH, 2016). School nursing has emerged as a branch of public health nursing and carries out programs closely related to the developments in public health nursing. It is stated that the first nurses to serve as school nurses were public health nurses. With the home visits and school screenings made by the school nurse, the health problems of the students were resolved, and significant successes were achieved in health prevention. School nurses evaluate all students in the environment in which they live, recognize the needs of their families, provide health education, and ensure necessary care through cooperation with relevant institutions (Tokur Kesgin and Çağlar, 2019).

The National Association of School Nurses (NASN) defines school nursing as "a specialized practice of professional nursing that improves the well-being and academic success of students and ensures their continued lifelong." To this end, school nurses help students adapt to the normal developmental process, promote health and safety, treat existing and potential health problems, provide case management services, and collaborate effectively with other members of the school community to develop students' and families' capacity for adaptation, self-advocacy, and learning (COSH, 2016).

School nurses have certain roles and responsibilities in the provision of school health services. The school nurse promotes health in the school community by preventing illness, disability, and injury from occurring, as well as strengthening their strategies for coping with health risks. The school nurse's primary health strategy consists of health education, promoting healthy lifestyle behaviors, providing guidance and consultancy, and organizing healthy school policies (Akgül and Ergün, 2021). The school nurse plans health education programs to provide health-related information as well as to create healthy and permanent behavioral changes in the school community. This education can be given to both students and school staff. The education topics that can be given to students are health nutrition, physical activity, sleep, hygiene, the harms of screen addiction, the harms of smoking and substance use, bullying, coping with stress, etc. (COSH, 2016; Akgül and Ergün, 2021).

School nurses can fight against many contagious infections by protecting the health of the school community and organizing immunization services, which are effective, cost-effective, and safe methods. In addition, the school nurse promotes a healthy school environment by assessing the school and its surroundings for safety risks (such as playgrounds hazards, indoor air quality, school violence and abuse, injuries, bullying, and disasters) that may negatively affect the health of the school community. The school nurse takes prevention measures and helps develop school policies aimed at protecting and improving health, such as increasing access to healthy foods in canteens and expanding physical activity areas (COSH 2016, Akgül and Ergün, 2021).

The school nurse conducts health screenings for school-aged children and refers them to healthcare providers when necessary. Thus, existing health problems are diagnosed and treated early, the progression of the disease is prevented, mortality rates and health expenses are reduced, the negative effects of health problems on education are reduced, and a positive contribution is made to academic success (Akgül and Ergün, 2021). It is important that health screening programs are conducted by the school nurse for diseases that are common in schools and affect a large part of the school community. Early intervention and effective treatment of diseases detected by these screening programs should be implemented. In a study, 15.4% of the students were found to be obese, 72.6% had decayed teeth, 8% had possible visual impairment, and 5.1% had possible scoliosis. For this reason, health screenings should be performed regularly; priority should be given to vision, hearing, dental health, growth, and development screenings. As a result of not detecting these problems in the early period in students, health problems may progress and cause more serious health consequences (Özsoy et al., 2019).

The school nurse evaluates the student's health status, identifies health problems that may interfere with educational progress, and develops a health care plan to manage these problems in the school environment. Furthermore, the school nurses collaborate in the development and implementation of this plan with the full participation of the students, family, and other members of the school community, including the pediatrician. Thus, the school nurse helps students with chronic diseases and disabilities to increase their self-care power and reach the highest level of life skills possible, compliance with treatment, and management of disease symptoms (COSH, 2016; Çakır and Altay, 2021). The school nurse also shares the results of their studies on issues such as crisis/disaster management, mental health protection and intervention, emergency medical situation management, acute disease management, infectious disease prevention, and management to the development of school health policies (Kurt, 2020).

Many studies have shown that school nurses make significant contributions to health promotion and prevention of the school community in line with their responsibilities (Cheng et al., 2021; WHO, 2021; Banfield et al., 2015). However, the continuity of school health services provided in schools cannot be ensured without employing a nurse in each school. Important organizations in this regard emphasize the importance of having a full-time school nurse who has important responsibilities in health promotion and prevention of the school community. It is stated that there should be one nurse for every 750 students in schools and one nurse for every 225 students with special education needs (COSH, 2016). However, the employment problem of school nurses in schools still continues (COSH, 2016; Özsoy et al., 2019; Tokur Kesgin and Çağlar). The school nurse, who has a key role in health promotion and prevention of the school community, should be employed in every school.

Conclusion

The health promotion and prevention program at school is an indispensable condition to create a healthier and more productive school society. The findings of the research show that various factors affecting the health of the school community (obesity, addiction, sedentary life, diabetes, chronic and infectious diseases, school climate and environment, etc.) have a significant impact on academic success, physical and emotional well-being, and social relations. Implementation of programs and policies focused on the health promotion and prevention at school supports the physical, mental, and spiritual health of the school community, especially students. Such programs address issues such as improving eating habits, encouraging physical activity, and improving stress-coping skills. However, for these programs to be effective, a school nurse is needed in every school. The school nurse has a critical role in identifying the health needs of the school community, providing preventive health services, and providing health education.

Consequently, health promoting and prevention at school significantly impacts the general well-being of the school community and requires the active participation of the school nurse. Therefore, schools need to adopt and implement health-oriented policies. Additionally, all stakeholders (school nurses, school administration, teachers, students, parents, local government, etc.) need to work collaboratively to support the health and well-being of the school community.

Disclaimer

None.

References

Akçan, A., Meydanlıoğlu, A. and Yalçın, E. (2023). Determination of chronic illnesses in school children in a province in Turkey. *The Journal of Effective Nursing*, 16(3), 340-354.

Akçay, D. (2017). The role of the school nurse of school environment protection from infectious diseases. *Cumhuriyet Nurs J*, 5(2), 84-94.

Akçay, D. and Yıldırımlar, A. (2018). Investigation of children's school accident and behavior of their parents safety measures. *DEUHFED,* 11(1), 48-55.

Akgül, E. and Ergün, A. (2021). School Health Nursing in Promotion Public Health. *Journal Of Public Health Nursing,* 3(2): *141-153.*

Akhter, S. and Ahmed, A. (2021). Need and importance of physical education for school students. *International Journal of Physiology, Nutrition and Physical Education*, *6*(1), 352-355.

Akoğlu, G. and Karaaslan, B. T. (2020). *Possible psychosocial effects of the COVID-19 and isolation process on children. İKÇÜSBFD*, 5(2), 99-103.

Baltag, V., Pachyna, A. and Hall, J. (2015). Global overview of school health services: Data from 102 countries. *Health Behavior and Policy Review*, 2(4): 268–283.

Banfield, M., McGorm, K. and Sargent, G. (2015). Health promotion in schools: A multi-method evaluation of an Australian school youth health nurse program. *BMC Nursing*, 14(1): 1–11.

Barnett, T., Giallo, R., Kelaher, M., Goldfeld, S. and Quach, J. (2018). Predictors of learning outcomes for children with and without chronic illness: an Australian longitudinal study. *Child Care Health Dev,* 44, 832–840.

Cheng, H., George, C., Dunham, M., Whitehead, L. And Denney-Wilson, E. (2021). Nurse-led interventions in the prevention and treatment of overweight and obesity in infants, children and adolescents: A scoping review. *International Journal of Nursing Studies*. 121:104008, 1-15.

Cornett, K., Murfay, K. and Fulton, JE.(2023). Physical activity interventions during the school day: reviewing policies, practices, and benefits. *J Sch Health*. 93: 778-787.

Coşgun, M. and Kara, F. (2015). Evaluation of the impact of health education given to students on knowledge and attitudes. *STED*, 24(2):55-63.

Council On School Health (COSH). (2016). Role of the school nurse in providing school health services. *Pediatrics,* 137(6), 1052-1057.

Çakır, G. and Altay, N. (2021). Duties and responsibilities of school nurses in care of children with chronic disease. *DEUHFED,* 14(1), 55-61.

Çalık, T., Kurt, T. and Çalık, C. (2016). School climate in creating safe school: A conceptual analysis. *Pegem Education and Instruction Journal,* 1(4), 73-84.

Çokamay, G., Kapçı, E. G. and Sever, M. (2017). Problems encountered on school mental health services: School psychological counselors' Opinions. *Elementary Education Online*, 16(4), 1395-1406.

Dığrak, E., Eyimaya, Öztürk, A., Zengin, H. and Tezel, A. (2020). Evaluation of health screening results of two public primary school students. *TJFMPC,*14 (2): 289-298.

Georgiev, S., Kamburova, M. S., and Un, M. (2015). A Healthy School Environment As A Precondition For The Welfare Of Students And Staff. *International Journal of Health Administration and Education Congress (Sanitas Magisterium), (2)*, 31-43.

International Union for Health Promotion and Education (IUHPE) (2010). Promoting health in schools *from evidence to action.* https://healtheducationresources.unesco.org/library/documents/promoting-health-schools-evidence-action

Jiao, W. Y., Wang, L. N., Liu, J., Fang, S. F., Jiao, F. Y,. Mantovani, P. M. and Somekh E. (2020). Behavioral and Emotional Disorders in Children during the COVID-19 Epidemic. *The Journal of Pediatrics.* 221, 264-266.

Junior, L. G. L., Rocha K. J, Rocha K., Silva, L. M., Lira, M. M., Silva, K. S. A., Oliveira, M. M. A., Machado, R. O. A., Marinho, E. S. and Silva, K. A. (2023). Health in the school environment: Some reflections about. In book: *Pathways to Knowledge: Exploring The Horizons of Education*, Chapter 79. 1-12.

Kartal, A., and Kılınç, E. School based training programs for preventing injuries: systematic review. *ESTÜDAM Public Health Journal*, *5*(1), 131-141.

Kaynak, Ü., and Işık, Ş. (2019). Views of school counselors on social interest in school mental health services. *School Counseling Journal*, 2(1), 1-28.

Kılınç, E., Gür, K. (2020). Behaviours of adolescents towards safety measures at school and in traffic and their health beliefs for injuries. *International journal of nursing practice*, *26*(5), e12861.

Kim, S. J., Baek, S. S., and Kang, K. A. (2017). Development and exploratory testing of a school-based educational program for healthy life behaviors among fifth grade children in South Korea. *Japan Journal of Nursing Science*, 14 (1), 13-26.

Kurt A. (2020). Developing school health services evaluation scale for students, İzmir Kâtip Çelebi University, Master's Thesis, İzmir.

Kurt, G. and Özcan, C. (2024). The past, present and future of school health. 5. International Mediterranean Congress 1314-1319.

Küçükkaraca Zakkour, H., and Yıldıran, H. (2022). The effect of parent's nutrition education on nutrition education of school-age children. *Gazi Journal of Health Sciences*, 7(3), 135-148.

Lee, S. M., Szucs, L. E., Young, E. and Fahrenbruch, M. (2023). Using health education to address student physical activity and nutrition: Evidence and implications to advance practice. *J Sch Health*, 93, 788-798.

Maughan, E. D., Cowell, J., Engelke, M. K., McCarthy, A. M., Bergren, M. D., Murphy, M. K., Barry, C., Krause-Parello, C. A., Luthy, K. B., Kintner, E. K. and Vessey, J. A. (2018). The vital role of school nurses in ensuring the health of our nation's youth. *Nursing Outlook*, 66(1), 94–96.

Meydanlıoğlu, A., and Gözüm, S. (2019). Practices and programs developing school health in Turkey. *Türkiye Klinikleri Public Health Nursing-Special Topics,* 5(1), 16-23.

Nallbani, G. (2021). Importance of health promotion and education to young people in educational institutions (schools). *European Journal Of Medicine And Natural Sciences*. 4(2), 60-70.

Okuyan, C. B. and Alkaya, S. A. (2018). The role of school-based programs in protection and development of school health. *J Comm Pub Health Nurs*, 4(2), 1-5.

Özsoy, S., Kalkım, A., and Emlek, Sert, Z. (2019). Identification of the state of health and health risks in primary school children. *Balıkesir Health Sciences Journal,* 8(3), 135-142.

Pulimeno, M., Piscitelli, P., Colazzo, S., Colao, A. and Miani, A. (2020). School as ideal setting to promote health and wellbeing among young people. *Health Promot Perspect,*10(4), 316-324.

Salman, D. D. and Günay, T. (2023). School Nutrition Programs in the World and in Türkiye. *The Journal of Public Health Research and Practice*, *1*(1),17–26.

NASN (2014). Overweight and obesity in youth in schools-The role of the school nurse. *NASN School Nurse.* 1-4.

Şahinöz, T., Şahinöz, S., and Kıvanç, A. (2017). The easiest way to promote health: School health. *Gümüşhane University Journal of Health Sciences*, 6(4), 303-312.

Ministry of Health. (2017). *School health protection and promotion program implementation guide.* https://hsgm.saglik.gov.tr/depo/birimler/cocuk-ergen-sagligi-db/Programlar/Uygulama_Klavuzu.pdf.

Tokur Kesgin, M. and Çağlar, S. *The development of school nursing around the world and in Turkey.* KUHEAD, 16(4):343-352.

Viner, R., Russell, S., Saulle, R., Croker, H., Stansfield, C., Packer, J., ... & Minozzi, S. (2022). School closures during social lockdown and mental health, health behaviors, and well-being among children and adolescents during the first COVID-19 wave: a systematic review. *JAMA pediatrics*, *176*(4), 400-409.

Wang, X., Liu, J., Wu, Y. Su, B., Chen, M., Ma, O., Ma, T., Chen, L., Zhang, Y., Dong, Y., Song, Y. and Ma, J. *(2023).* Enhancing the effectiveness of infectious disease health education for children and adolescents in China: a national multicenter school-based trial. *BMC Public Health*, 23 (1161), 1-11.

World Health Organization (WHO) (2021). *Web annex e. Systematic reviews of the effectiveness and acceptability of comprehensive school health services: evidence summaries.* https://iris.who.int/bitstream/handle/10665/343760/9789240030701 ng.pdf?sequence=1.

World Health Organization (WHO). (2020). Global standards and indicators for health promoting schools https://cdn.who.int/media/docs/default-source/mca-documents/adolescents-and-youth/hps-global-standards-draft3-sept2020-final-ss-changes-accepted6c9038a66e454da989.

Chapter 2

Nutrition and Physical Activity in School-Age Children

İrem Nur Özdemir*, **PhD**
Health Sciences University, Hamidiye Faculty of Nursing, Department of Public Health Nursing, İstanbul, Türkiye

Abstract

For the healthy growth and development of school-age children, nutrition and physical activity are of great importance. Adopting healthy lifestyle behaviors is essential for children to maintain their health and well-being throughout their lives. School nurses play a critical role in ensuring that children have a healthy lifestyle. School nurses are responsible for assessing children's nutritional and physical activity habits, encouraging them, raising awareness through health education, and finding solutions to their nutritional and physical activity-related problems. School nurses also play an active role in the development of school and community resources and in the implementation of support programs. These responsibilities not only support the growth, development, and cognitive functions of children but also play a critical role in preventing chronic diseases such as obesity and diabetes. Therefore, the supportive roles of school nurses in nutrition and physical activity are crucial for both children to have a healthy future and for the overall health of the community in the long term.

Keywords: nutrition, physical activity, school-age children

Introduction

For the healthy growth and development of school-age children, nutrition and physical activity are of great importance. Adopting healthy lifestyle behaviors is essential for children to maintain their health and well-being throughout their lives (WHO, 2022; Physical Activity Guidelines Advisory Committee, 2018). The rapid rise in sedentary lifestyles and unhealthy behaviors, such as poor dietary habits commonly seen in many children and adolescents, contributes to the prevalence of lifestyle-related diseases, including obesity.

---

* Corresponding Author's Email: iremozdemir92@gmail.com

In: Health Promotion and Prevention
Editor: Eda Kılınç İşleyen
ISBN: 979-8-89530-758-8

Developing physical activity and healthy eating habits from childhood increases the likelihood of continuing these habits into adulthood, which can have a lasting impact on an individual's health. Therefore, school nurses can support healthy growth and development by promoting nutrition and physical activity in school-aged children. School nurses should focus on developing strategies that encourage healthy lifestyle behaviors and aim to identify potential risk factors (Bonde Høstgaard et al., 2014; Khan et al., 2020; Mendonca et al., 2014; Moberg et al., 2021). In conclusion, school nurses play significant roles in nutrition and physical activity management for school-aged children, contributing to their overall health, development, and academic achievements. School nurses collaborate with school administrators, staff, and community partners to implement nutrition education programs, promote access to healthy food options, and create supportive environments that encourage healthy eating behaviors (NASN, 2020; Muckian et al., 2017).

Nutrition in School-Age Children

The importance of nutrition cannot be overlooked as it plays a fundamental role in the physical health, cognitive development, academic performance, and well-being of school-age children. Adequate and balanced nutrition provides essential nutrients that support physical growth, cognitive function, and immune system functions during this critical period of children's growth and development (Roberts et al., 2022; Corkins et al., 2016; Maggini et al., 2018; Munteanu and Schwartz, 2022). Furthermore, proper nutrition ensures that children have the energy and nutrients they need to actively participate in school activities, concentrate in class, and enhance their academic achievements (Baldridge et al., 2019). Adequate nutrition also helps prevent various health problems such as obesity, diabetes, and cardiovascular diseases (Reedy et al., 2014). Establishing healthy eating habits during childhood, an early stage of life, can lead to lifelong sustainable behaviors that promote optimal health and well-being (Ding et al., 2020). Therefore, promoting healthy eating behaviors in the early stages of life can contribute to nutrition habits that reduce the risk of chronic diseases in the later years (Mikkilä et al., 2004). Moreover, prioritizing nutrition in school-age children is of great importance for their current and future health outcomes.

The socioeconomic status of families is one of the most significant factors affecting children's food choices and their participation in healthy behaviors, influencing children's nutrition (Darmon and Drewnowski, 2015). Lower socioeconomic status of the family is associated with limited access to nutritious foods, food insecurity, and increased consumption of energy-dense but nutrient-poor foods (Gundersen and Ziliak, 2015; Darmon and Drewnowski, 2015; Larson et al., 2009). Lower socioeconomic status reduces a child's ability to access nutrient-rich foods, leading to both inadequate nutrition and laying the groundwork for overweight or obesity (World Health Organization-WHO 2017). Childhood obesity is one of the most serious public health issues of the twenty-first century (WHO 2018; WHO 2020).

Another factor influencing children's nutrition is the influence of parents. Parents play a significant role in shaping children's eating habits and food choices. Parental modeling, feeding practices, and the meal environment at home influence children's eating behaviors. Additionally, the increase in refined, packaged, and processed foods has led to the increased consumption of lower-nutrient foods. In modern lifestyles, urbanization, increased working hours for parents, and the overconsumption of convenience foods have significantly impacted children's eating habits. The rise in globalization and inequalities in food access make it challenging for many to access safe and nutritious food (Haddad et al., 2016; Kickbusch et al., 2016; Monteiro et al., 2019; Seto and Ramankutty, 2016; Mills et al., 2017).

School nutrition programs, food policies, the presence of healthy food options, and nutrition education programs significantly influence children's eating behaviors and nutrient intake (Bergman and Gordon, 2010; Briefel et al., 2009; Mozaffarian et al., 2010). Numerous calls to action have been made to maintain, promote, and support healthy eating in schools. Schools play a crucial role in the promotion of healthy nutrition and can create an environment conducive to healthy eating for children. Schools play an important role in the promotion of nutrition at different socioeconomic levels. A child who eats healthily performs better in school, and good education provides a foundation for the child's future, contributing to the economic and social development of societies (Second International Conference on Nutrition, 2014; WHO 2018).

School nutrition programs, food policies, the presence of healthy food options, and nutrition education programs significantly influence children's eating behaviors and nutrient intake (Bergman and Gordon, 2010; Briefel et al., 2009; Mozaffarian et al., 2010). Numerous calls to action have been made to maintain, promote, and support healthy eating in schools. Schools play a crucial role in promoting healthy nutrition and can create an environment conducive to healthy eating for children. Schools play an important role in promoting nutrition across different socioeconomic levels. A child who eats healthily performs better in school, and good education provides a foundation for the child's future, contributing to the economic and social development of societies (Second International Conference on Nutrition, 2014; World Health Organization, 2018).

The literature provides strong evidence supporting the importance of nutrition in supporting optimal health, cognitive development, academic performance, and long-term well-being in school-age children. In a systematic review conducted by Eilander et al., (2010), which examined the effects of specific nutrients such as omega-3 fatty acids, vitamins, and minerals on cognitive function and academic performance in children, it was revealed that adequate intake of nutrients is necessary for optimal brain development, learning, and memory, highlighting the critical role of nutrition in supporting cognitive function during childhood and adolescence. Micha et al., (2017) found in their study investigating the impact of dietary patterns on cardiometabolic health outcomes in children and adolescents that a healthy eating pattern characterized by a high intake of fruits, vegetables, whole grains, and lean protein was associated with a reduced risk of obesity, diabetes, and cardiovascular disease in school-age children. These findings underscore the need for comprehensive strategies and interventions aimed at improving nutrition in school environments to support children's health and development. The WHO initiated the Nutrition-Friendly Schools Initiative to promote healthy eating in school-aged children. The Nutrition-Friendly Schools Initiative (NFSI) has identified 26 key criteria under 5 broad components (WHO 2018) (Table 1).

These recommendations aim to promote nutrition management among school-aged children, contributing to their overall health and well-being. Nutrition management plays a significant role in the health and well-being of school-aged children, affecting their growth, development, and academic performance. School nurses, as key members of the health team, are uniquely positioned to contribute significantly to nutrition management in school-aged children. Through their expertise in health promotion and development, education, and intervention, school nurses play an important role in meeting the nutritional needs of school-aged children and promoting healthy eating behaviors.

School nurses' roles in nutrition management encompass various aspects, including assessing nutrition status, developing personalized nutrition plans, implementing interventions, and evaluating outcomes. School nurses play a crucial role in conducting nutrition assessments of school-aged children to identify inadequate nutrition and associated risk factors (Hockenberry and Wilson, 2019). Through comprehensive assessments, school nurses can identify children at risk for inadequate nutrition and develop interventions to meet their specific nutrition needs.

School nurses' expertise in health education is effective in promoting healthy eating habits and empowering school-aged children to make informed food choices. Through nutrition education programs and counseling roles, school nurses provide valuable information about the importance of balanced nutrition, food groups, portion control, and meal planning strategies (Australian College of Nursing, 2024; Rabbitt and Coyne, 2012; Ben-Sefer et al., 2009).

Table 1. Nutrition friendly schools intervention

1. Have a written nutrition-friendly school policy 1.1. Developing a written nutrition-friendly school policy that addresses all five points outlined in this framework 1.2. Rationale 1.3. Objectives 1.4. Action plan 1.5. Monitoring and evaluation plan
2. Raising awareness and capacity building of the school community 2.1. Dissemination of a nutrition-friendly school policy 2.2. Activities for families and the community, community participation, and outreach on nutrition and health-related issues 2.3. Training of school staff on nutrition and health-related issues
3. Develop a school curriculum that promotes nutrition and health promotion 3.1. Culturally appropriate and effective nutrition education 3.2. Physical education curriculum appropriate to age, gender, and culture 3.3. Healthy living and life skills training curriculum 3.4. Regular monitoring of school curriculum relevant to the Nutrition Friendly School Initiative, and evaluation of impact of how well the education meets the objectives
4. Creating a supportive school environment 4.1. School lunches, food vendors, and snack bars, if available, promote healthy eating 4.2. Positive messages about nutrition and active living 4.3. Lack of food and beverage marketing at school 4.4. Access to adequate dining facilities if the school provides food or drink to children 4.5. Adequate school cooking facilities 4.6. Access to safe drinking water 4.7. Promotion of safe hygiene and sanitation 4.8. Availability of clean and separate toilets for boys and girls 4.9. Opportunity for all age groups to access school sports facilities and space for physical activity within the curriculum 4.10. Attitudes towards bullying, stigma, and discrimination 4.11. School staff as role models in the promotion of healthy eating and healthy lifestyles
5. Providing supportive school nutrition and health services 5.1. Regular monitoring of children's growth and development 5.2. Effective feedback system for parents and children on regular monitoring findings 5.3. Supportive school health service, including referral system

In addition to health education, school nurses play a critical role in implementing and monitoring nutrition interventions in school settings. They monitor nutrition interventions and outcomes, tracking children's nutrition status, eating behaviors, and health outcomes over time (Ashton et al., 2017). School nurses evaluate the effectiveness of interventions and ensure that children receive continuous support for their nutritional needs by making necessary adjustments when necessary.

School nurses collaborate with educators, policymakers, and community stakeholders to advocate for policies and initiatives that promote healthy eating in school environments. They aim to create supportive environments for children's nutritional well-being (NASN, 2020; Muckian et al., 2017; National Academies Press, 2021). Serving as advocates for child health and nutrition, nurses ensure that their voices are heard in discussions related to nutrition policies and programs.

In conclusion, school nurses play significant roles in nutrition management for school-aged children, contributing to their overall health, development, and academic achievements. School nurses assess nutrition routines, identify children at risk by pinpointing nutritional deficiencies, and provide targeted interventions to enhance nutrition programs. Additionally, school nurses collaborate with school administrators, staff, and community partners to implement nutrition education programs, promote access to healthy food options, and create supportive environments that encourage healthy eating behaviors.

Physical Activity in School-Age Children

Insufficient physical activity is the fourth leading risk factor for mortality worldwide (Available from: https://www.who.int/data/gho/indicator-metadata-registry/imr-details/3416). Regular physical activity is known to improve both mental and physical health in people of all ages. However, today, 81% of adolescents do not meet the physical activity levels recommended by the WHO (WHO, 2022). Despite being more inclined towards active play and entertainment during adolescence, it is observed that young people are increasingly inactive. The latest global data reveal that 81% of children aged 11-17 engage in less than 1 hour of moderate to vigorous-intensity physical activity per day, with girls being less active than boys in most countries (Guthold et al., 2020).

Regular physical activity is crucial to improve the health and well-being of school-aged children. Physical activity in children and adolescents;

1. Supports healthy growth and development. Regular exercise helps children develop strong muscles and bones, improve coordination and balance, and maintain a healthy weight (Pearson et al., 2014; Physical Activity Guidelines Advisory Committee, 2018).
2. Improves cardiovascular health. Engaging in regular physical activity is important for maintaining cardiovascular health in school-aged children. Positive associations are observed with cardio-metabolic health outcomes, including improved blood pressure, lipid balance, glucose control, and insulin resistance (WHO, 2022; Physical Activity Guidelines Advisory Committee, 2018). Exercise strengthens the heart and improves blood circulation, thereby reducing the risk of heart disease in later life (Poitras et al.,

2016). Evidence in the literature suggests that school-based physical activity programs, high-intensity interval training, and resistance training interventions are associated with better cardio-metabolic outcomes (Pozuelo-Carrascosa et al., 2018; Eddolls et al., 2017; Bea et al., 2017).

3. Improves mental health. Physical activity has positive effects on the mental health of school-age children. Exercise can reduce symptoms of anxiety and depression, improve mood, and enhance self-esteem. Physical activity also has positive effects on cognitive functions, academic outcomes, and school performance in children and adolescents. A systematic review by Lubans et al., (2016) found that participation in physical activity programs was associated with better psychosocial outcomes and quality of life in children and adolescents (WHO, 2022; Lubans et al., 2016; Physical Activity Guidelines Advisory Committee, 2018).

The World Health Organization provides recommendations for physical activity to improve the health and well-being of school-aged children. The World Health Organization's physical activity recommendations for school-age children include:

Moderate to Vigorous Physical Activity

The WHO recommends that children and adolescents aged 5-17 engage in at least 60 minutes of moderate to vigorous physical activity daily (WHO, 2022). Additionally, it suggests including vigorous-intensity aerobic activities and muscle-strengthening activities at least 3 days per week. This updated guideline aligns with the physical activity recommendations of countries such as Canada, Australia, the United States, and the United Kingdom (WHO, 2022; Tremblay et al., 2016; Australian Government Department of Health, 2019; U.S. Department of Health and Human Services, 2018; Chief Medical Officers, United Kingdom, 2019).

Limiting Sedentary Behaviour

In children and adolescents, sedentary behaviour is associated with poor health indicators such as increased adiposity, weaker cardio-metabolic health, fitness, behavioral issues, and reduced sleep duration. The WHO advises limiting sedentary behaviors in children and adolescents, such as prolonged sitting, screen time (watching TV, playing video games), and excessive use of electronic devices. Guidelines from some countries recommend limiting screen-based sedentary time to no more than 2 hours per day and taking breaks from prolonged sitting as frequently as possible (Tremblay et al., 2016; Australian Government Department of Health, 2019; Chief Medical Officers, United Kingdom, 2019). However, there is currently insufficient evidence regarding the duration of screen time for entertainment purposes. Minimizing sedentary behavior is important for overall health and well-being.

The World Health Organization's "Global Action Plan on Physical Activity (2018–2030)" has emphasized the need to strengthen the development and implementation of behavioral public health interventions targeting women and disadvantaged populations that assess and increase opportunities for physical activity (WHO, 2018). The school environment is well recognized as a potential setting to enhance physical activity behavior among adolescents (Hills et al., 2015). School health services play a critical role in the promotion and improvement of health (WHO, 2019). School nurses hold a significant position in empowering children with healthy lifestyle choices that will impact them throughout their lives, by collaborating with families, school administrators, and the community to help foster healthy eating and physical activity behaviors in children through the interventions they carry out (Robbins et al., 2012). Roles of school nurses in supporting and enhancing physical activity in school-aged children:

1. Health Education and Health Promotion:

School nurses play a crucial role in providing health education to support physical activity in school-aged children. They can offer evidence-based interventions and educational programs to promote the importance of regular physical activity and its health benefits.

2. Individualized Assessment and Counseling:

School nurses can conduct individualized assessments to evaluate the physical activity levels of school-aged children, identify barriers to participation, and provide personalized counseling and guidance. This personalized approach can assist children and their families in setting realistic goals and developing strategies to increase physical activity.

3. Collaboration with School Staff and Community Partners:

School nurses can collaborate with school staff and community partners to develop and implement physical activity programs and initiatives. This interdisciplinary approach can help create supportive environments that promote physical activity among school-aged children (Bonde Høstgaard et al., 2014; Khan et al., 2020; Mendonca et al., 2014; Moberg et al., 2021).

Physical activity is a significant component of the health of school-aged children. By understanding the importance of physical activity and implementing evidence-based strategies, we can strive to create environments that support and encourage regular physical activity participation among school-aged children. School nurses empower children and their families to adopt healthy lifestyle behaviors and incorporate regular physical activity into their daily lives through personal assessments, counseling, and health education. Additionally, school nurses collaborate with school staff, community, and policymakers to create supportive environments that facilitate children's participation in physical activity. Through their dedication, expertise, and advocacy efforts, school nurses make a substantial contribution to improving the health and well-being of school-aged children, laying the foundation for them to remain healthy throughout their lives.

Conclusion

While the diverse health benefits of physical activity are widely recognized, the majority of children and adolescents are not sufficiently active. The rapid rise in sedentary lifestyles and unhealthy behaviors, such as poor dietary habits commonly seen in many children and adolescents, contributes to the prevalence of lifestyle-related diseases, including obesity.

Developing physical activity and healthy eating habits from childhood increases the likelihood of continuing these habits into adulthood, which can have a lasting impact on an individual's health. Therefore, school nurses can support healthy growth and development by promoting nutrition and physical activity in school-aged children. School nurses should focus on developing strategies that encourage healthy lifestyle behaviors and aim to identify potential risk factors.

Disclaimer

None.

References

Ashton, J. J., Kammermeier, J., Spray, C., Russell, R. K., & Hansen, R. (2017). Nutritional management of children with Crohn's disease: a practical guide. *Drugs*, 77(14), 1559-1570.

Australian College of Nursing (ACN). 2024, '*The effectiveness of nurse-led interventions in the assessment and management of overweight and obese children and young people – Position Statement*,' ACN, Canberra.

Australian Government Department of Health. Australian 24-Hour Movement Guidelines for Children (5–12 years) and Young People (13–17 years): An Integration of Physical Activity, Sedentary Behaviour, and Sleep; 2019. p. 148. Available from: https://www.health.gov.au/internet/main/publishing.nsf/Content/ti-5-17years.

Baldridge, A. S., Huffman, M. D., Taylor, F., Xavier, D., Bright, B., Van Horn, L. V., ... & Dunford, E. (2019). The healthfulness of the US packaged food and beverage supply: a cross-sectional study. *Nutrients*, *11*(8), 1704.

Bea, J. W., Blew, R. M., Howe, C., Hetherington-Rauth, M., & Going, S. B. (2017). Resistance Training Effects on Metabolic Function among Youth: A Systematic Review. *Pediatric exercise science*, *29*(3), 297–315. https://doi.org/10.1123/pes.2016-0143.

Ben-Sefer, E., Ben-Natan, M., & Ehrenfeld, M. (2009). Childhood obesity: current literature, policy and implications for practice. *International nursing review*, *56*(2), 166–173. https://doi.org/10.1111/j.1466-7657.2008.00708.x.

Bergman, E. A., Gordon, R. W., & American Dietetic Association (2010). Position of the American Dietetic Association: local support for nutrition integrity in schools. *Journal of the American Dietetic Association*, *110*(8), 1244–1254. https://doi.org/10.1016/j.jada.2010.06.014.

Bonde Høstgaard, A., Bentsen, P., & Hindhede Lykke, A. (2014). School nurses' experiences with motivational interviewing for preventing childhood obesity. *Journal of School Nursing*, 30(6), 448–455. https://doi.org/10.1177/1059840514521240.

Briefel, R. R., Wilson, A., & Gleason, P. M. (2009). Consumption of low-nutrient, energy-dense foods and beverages at school, home, and other locations among school lunch participants and nonparticipants. *Journal of the American Dietetic Association*, *109*(2 Suppl), S79–S90. https://doi.org/10.1016/j.jada.2008.10.064.

Chief Medical Officers, United Kingdom (2019). Physical activity guidelines: UK Chief Medical Officers' report [Online]. Available from: http://publichealthwell.ie/node/1278661.

Second International Conference on Nutrition. (2014). Conference outcome document: a framework for action. Rome.

Corkins, M. R., Daniels, S. R., de Ferranti, S. D., Golden, N. H., Kim, J. H., Magge, S. N., & Schwarzenberg, S. J. (2016). *Nutrition in Children and Adolescents. Medical Clinics of North America, 100(6), 1217–1235.*doi:10.1016/j.mcna.2016.06.005.

Darmon, N., & Drewnowski, A. (2015). Contribution of food prices and diet cost to socioeconomic disparities in diet quality and health: a systematic review and analysis. *Nutrition reviews*, *73*(10), 643–660. https://doi.org/10.1093/nutrit/nuv027.

Ding, Z., Lange, T., & McLanahan, S. (2020). *Maternal education and child health: A life course perspective. Demography*, 57(5), 1653-1678.

Eddolls, W. T. B., McNarry, M. A., Stratton, G., Winn, C. O. N., & Mackintosh, K. A. (2017). High-Intensity Interval Training Interventions in Children and Adolescents: A Systematic Review. *Sports medicine (Auckland, N.Z.)*, *47*(11), 2363–2374. https://doi.org/10.1007/s40279-017-0753-8.

Eilander, A., Gera, T., Sachdev, H. S., Transler, C., van der Knaap, H. C., Kok, F. J., & Osendarp, S. J. (2010). Multiple micronutrient supplementation for improving cognitive performance in children: systematic review of randomized controlled trials. *The American journal of clinical nutrition*, *91*(1), 115-130.

World Health Organization. (2022). Global status report on physical activity. Geneva: Licence: CC BY-NC-SA 3.0 IGO.

Golley, R. K., Maher, C. A., Matricciani, L., & Olds, T. S. (2013). Sleep duration or bedtime? Exploring the association between sleep timing behaviour, diet and BMI in children and adolescents. *International journal of obesity (2005)*, *37*(4), 546–551. https://doi.org/10.1038/ijo.2012.212.

Gundersen, C., & Ziliak, J. P. (2015). Food Insecurity And Health Outcomes. *Health affairs (Project Hope)*, *34*(11), 1830–1839. https://doi.org/10.1377/hlthaff.2015.0645.

Guthold R., Stevens G. A., Riley L. M., Bull F. C. (2020). Global trends in insufficient physical activity among adolescents: a pooled analysis of 298 population-based surveys with 1.6 million participants. *Lancet Child Adolesc Health*; 4(1):23–35.

Haddad L., Hawkes C., Waage J., Webb P., Godfray C., Toulmin C. *Food Systems and Diets: Facing the Challenges of the 21st Century*. Global Panel on Agriculture and Food Systems for Nutrition; London, UK: 2016.

Hills, A. P., Dengel, D. R., & Lubans, D. R. (2015). Supporting public health priorities: recommendations for physical education and physical activity promotion in schools. *Progress in cardiovascular diseases*, *57*(4), 368–374. https://doi.org/10.1016/j.pcad.2014.09.010.

Khan, S. R., Uddin, R., Khan, A., & Mandic, S. (2020). Parental and peer support are associated with physical activity in adoles- cents: Evidence from 74 countries. International Journal of Environmental Research and Public Health, 17(12), 1–11. https://doi.org/10.3390/ijerph17124435.

Kickbusch, I., Allen L., Franz C. The commercial determinants of health. *Lancet Glob. Health.* 2016;4:e895–e896. doi: 10.1016/S2214-109X(16)30217-0.

Larson, N. I., Story, M. T., & Nelson, M. C. (2009). Neighborhood environments: disparities in access to healthy foods in the U.S. *American journal of preventive medicine*, *36*(1), 74–81. https://doi.org/10.1016/j.amepre.2008.09.025.

Lubans, D., Richards, J., Hillman, C., Faulkner, G., Beauchamp, M., Nilsson, M., Kelly, P., Smith, J., Raine, L., & Biddle, S. (2016). Physical Activity for Cognitive and Mental Health in Youth: A Systematic Review of Mechanisms. *Pediatrics*, *138*(3), e20161642. https://doi.org/10.1542/peds.2016-1642.

Maggini, S., Pierre, A., & Calder, P. C. (2018). Immune Function and Micronutrient Requirements Change over the Life Course. *Nutrients*, *10*(10), 1531. https://doi.org/10.3390/nu10101531.

Mendonca, G., Cheng, L. A., Nunes Mélo, E., & Cazuza de Farias Júnior, J. (2014). Physical activity and social support in adoles- cents: A systematic review. *Health Education Research*, 29(5), 822–839. https://doi.org/10.1093/her/cyu017.

Micha, R., Peñalvo, J. L., Cudhea, F., Imamura, F., Rehm, C. D., & Mozaffarian, D. (2017). Association Between Dietary Factors and Mortality From Heart Disease, Stroke, and Type 2 Diabetes in the United States. *JAMA*, *317*(9), 912–924. https://doi.org/10.1001/jama.2017.0947.

Mikkilä, V., Räsänen, L., Raitakari, O. T., Pietinen, P., & Viikari, J. (2004). Longitudinal changes in diet from childhood into adulthood with respect to risk of cardiovascular diseases: The Cardiovascular Risk in Young Finns Study. *European journal of clinical nutrition*, *58*(7), 1038–1045. https://doi.org/10.1038/sj.ejcn.1601929.

Mills, S., White, M., Brown, H., Wrieden, W., Kwasnicka, D., Halligan, J., Robalino, S., & Adams, J. (2017). Health and social determinants and outcomes of home cooking: A systematic review of observational studies. *Appetite*, *111*, 116–134. https://doi.org/10.1016/j.appet.2016.12.022.

Moberg, M., Golsäter, M., & Norman, Å. (2021). Parents' thoughts regarding their normal-weight children's food and physical activity as expressed during health conversations with the school nurse: A qualitative analysis informing health-promoting practices. *The Journal of School Nursing*, 1–11. https://doi.org/10.1177/10598405211025440.

Monteiro C. A., Cannon G., Lawrence M., Louzada M. d. C., Machado P. P. *Ultra-Processed Foods, Diet Quality, and Health Using the NOVA Classification System.* Volume 48 FAO; Rome, Italy: 2019.

Mozaffarian, R. S., Wiecha, J. L., Roth, B. A., Nelson, T. F., Lee, R. M., & Gortmaker, S. L. (2010). Impact of an organizational intervention designed to improve snack and beverage quality in YMCA after-school programs. *American journal of public health*, *100*(5), 925–932. https://doi.org/10.2105/AJPH.2008.158907.

Muckian, J., Snethen, J., & Buseh, A. (2017). School Nurses' Experiences and Perceptions of Healthy Eating School Environments. *Journal of pediatric nursing*, *35*, 10–15. https://doi.org/10.1016/j.pedn.2017.02.001.

Munteanu, C., & Schwartz, B. (2022). The relationship between nutrition and the immune system. *Frontiers in nutrition*, *9*, 1082500. https://doi.org/10.3389/fnut.2022.1082500.

National Academies Press (US); 2021 May 11. 5, The Role of Nurses in Improving Health Equity. Available from: https://www.ncbi.nlm.nih.gov/books/NBK573898/.

National Association of School Nurses (NASN), School Wellness (2020). Available from: https://www.nasn.org/nasn-resources/resources-by-topic/school-wellness.

World Health Organization. (2020). Nutrition action in schools: a review of evidence related to the Nutrition-Friendly Schools Initiative. Geneva. Licence: CC BY-NC-SA 3.0 IGO. Available from: https://iris.who.int/bitstream/handle/10665/338781/9789241516969-eng.pdf?sequence=1.

Pearson, N., Braithwaite, R. E., Biddle, S. J., van Sluijs, E. M., & Atkin, A. J. (2014). Associations between sedentary behaviour and physical activity in children and adolescents: a meta-analysis. *Obesity reviews : an official journal of the International Association for the Study of Obesity*, *15*(8), 666–675. https://doi.org/10.1111/obr.12188.

Physical Activity Guidelines Advisory Committee. 2018 Physical Activity Guidelines Advisory Committee Scientific Report. Washington, DC: US Department of Health and Human Services; 2018.

Poitras, V. J., Gray, C. E., Borghese, M. M., Carson, V., Chaput, J. P., Janssen, I., Katzmarzyk, P. T., Pate, R. R., Connor Gorber, S., Kho, M. E., Sampson, M., & Tremblay, M. S. (2016). Systematic review of the relationships between objectively measured physical activity and health indicators in school-aged children and youth. *Applied physiology, nutrition, and metabolism = Physiologie appliquee, nutrition et metabolisme*, *41*(6 Suppl 3), S197–S239. https://doi.org/10.1139/apnm-2015-0663.

Pozuelo-Carrascosa, D. P., Cavero-Redondo, I., Herráiz-Adillo, Á., Díez-Fernández, A., Sánchez-López, M., & Martínez-Vizcaíno, V. (2018). School-Based Exercise Programs and Cardiometabolic Risk Factors: A Meta-analysis. *Pediatrics*, *142*(5), e20181033. https://doi.org/10.1542/peds.2018-1033.

Rabbitt, A., & Coyne, I. (2012). Childhood obesity: nurses' role in addressing the epidemic. *British journal of nursing (Mark Allen Publishing)*, *21*(12), 731–735. https://doi.org/10.12968/bjon.2012.21.12.731.

Reedy, J., Krebs-Smith, S. M., Miller, P. E., Liese, A. D., Kahle, L. L., Park, Y., & Subar, A. F. (2014). Higher diet quality is associated with decreased risk of all-cause, cardiovascular disease, and cancer mortality among older adults. *The Journal of nutrition*, *144*(6), 881-889.

Robbins, L. B., Pfeiffer, K. A., Maier, K. S., Lo, Y. J., & Wesolek Ladrig, S. M. (2012). Pilot intervention to increase physical activity among sedentary urban middle school girls: a two-group pretest-posttest quasi-experimental design. *The Journal of school nursing : the official publication of the National Association of School Nurses*, *28*(4), 302–315. https://doi.org/10.1177/1059840512438777.

Roberts, M., Tolar-Peterson, T., Reynolds, A., Wall, C., Reeder, N., & Rico Mendez, G. (2022). The Effects of Nutritional Interventions on the Cognitive Development of Preschool-Age Children: A Systematic Review. *Nutrients*, *14*(3), 532. https://doi.org/10.3390/nu14030532.

Scarallo, L., & Lionetti, P. (2021). Dietary Management in Pediatric Patients with Crohn's Disease. *Nutrients*, *13*(5), 1611. https://doi.org/10.3390/nu13051611.

Seto K.C., Ramankutty N. Hidden linkages between urbanization and food systems. *Science.* (2016) 352:943–945. doi: 10.1126/science.aaf7439.

Tremblay, M. S., Carson, V., Chaput, J. P., Connor Gorber, S., Dinh, T., Duggan, M., Faulkner, G., Gray, C. E., Gruber, R., Janson, K., Janssen, I., Katzmarzyk, P. T., Kho, M. E., Latimer-Cheung, A. E., LeBlanc, C., Okely, A. D., Olds, T., Pate, R. R., Phillips, A., Poitras, V. J., ... Zehr, L. (2016). Canadian 24-Hour Movement Guidelines for Children and Youth: An Integration of Physical Activity, Sedentary Behaviour, and Sleep. *Applied physiology, nutrition, and metabolism = Physiologie appliquee, nutrition et metabolisme*, *41*(6 Suppl 3), S311–S327. https://doi.org/10.1139/apnm-2016-0151.

U.S. Department of Health and Human Services. (2018). *Physical Activity Guidelines for Americans*. 2nd ed. Washington, DC: U.S. Department of Health and Human Services.

World Health Organization (WHO). 2017. *The double burden of malnutrition.* Policy brief. Geneva: WHO. Available from: https://apps.who.int/iris/bitstream/handle/10665/255413/WHO-NMH-NHD-17.3-eng.pdf?ua = 1.

World Health Organization (WHO) 2018. *Global action plan on physical activity 2018–2030: more active people for a healthier world.* Geneva: World Health Organization; 2018b. Available from: http://apps.who.int/iris/bitstream/handle/10665/272722/9789241514187-eng.pdf.

World Health Organization. (WHO) (2019). *School Health Services Guideline: Guideline on school-based or school-linked health services provided by a health worker.* Available from: https://www.who.int/maternal_child_adolescent/guidelines/development/schoolinterventions-child-adolescent-health/en/.

World Health Organization. (2020). *Nutrition in schools: A framework for action.* Available from https://www.who.int/publications/i/item/9789240015111.

Chapter 3

Hygiene, Excretion, and Sleep in School-Age Children

Ecem Çiçek Gümüş*, **PhD**
Department of Public Health Nursing, Bartın University Faculty of Health Science, Bartın, Türkiye

Abstract

The early years of childhood shape the foundation of lifelong habits and behaviors. In this context, school-age children transition from parental supervision to entering a whole new environment. This transition affects not only their hygiene habits but also their excretion and sleep patterns. The school environment, the attitudes of peers, the family structure, socioeconomic factors, and many other parameters contribute to the reshaping of a healthy lifestyle for school-age children. During this period, one of the most critical aspects of development is establishing a healthy lifestyle. Hygiene lies at the foundation of the conditions for a healthy life. As individuals and as a society, the path to preserving and enhancing human health, ensuring the prolonged and efficient continuation of life at a healthy level, involves the synthesis and application of health-related knowledge, and hygiene serves as a cornerstone. Instilling hygiene habits is one of the essential steps in developing healthy living behaviors in children and fostering societal participation. In the context of education, imparting clean and healthy living behaviors to school children entails consistently adopting hygienic practices both within and outside the classroom. Hygienic practices in school-age children have a profound impact on them in many aspects. Hygiene not only brings about the control of infectious diseases, the continuity of school attendance, the fulfillment of excretory needs, healthy nutrition, and quality sleep but also affects social adaptation and academic success of schoolchildren due to its broad scope of influence involving various parameters. The inadequacy of school hygiene and children's hygiene leads to adverse effects on oral and dental health, nutrition, the desire to use the toilet, and, consequently, excretion. Situations such as children refraining from drinking fluids or postponing defecation emerge when they do not want to go to the toilet. One of the key points in maintaining the healthy lives of schoolchildren is that they have sufficient quality sleep. Establishing a healthy lifestyle in school-age children is crucial to their overall well-being and development. Giving priority to sleep hygiene, which is among the healthy lifestyle behaviors, is included in fundamental strategies to promote optimal health and academic success in school-age children. Hygiene, excretion, and sleep in school-age children are interconnected factors that directly influence each other. In this context, considering these concepts is important for effectively monitoring school-age children in

* Corresponding Author's Email: egumus@bartın.edu.tr

In: Health Promotion and Prevention
Editor: Eda Kılınç İşleyen
ISBN: 979-8-89530-758-8

light of these contexts, thereby identifying and addressing potential issues at an earlier stage and supporting a healthy adulthood process.

Keywords: school-age, children, hygiene, excretion, sleep

Introduction

Childhood forms lifelong habits, emphasizing the importance of teaching school-age children consistent hygiene practices. Proper personal hygiene safeguards their health and education by preventing infectious diseases. So far, 2.3 billion people lack basic handwashing facilities, underscoring the need for accessible sanitation services, especially for adolescents (UNICEF, 2021). The WHO estimates that 2.2 million, mainly children, die annually in poorer countries due to poor sanitation and unsafe water. However, improving access to safe water, waste disposal systems, and sanitation services can reduce diarrheal deaths by up to 65% and related diseases by 26% (WHO, 2018).

In developing nations, respiratory and gastrointestinal infections are prevalent. The school entry age is pivotal for learning healthy habits. Interventions should foster hygiene awareness and behavior change among school-age children (Joshi, 2019). Hygiene and health initiatives cover homes, workplaces, public areas, and healthcare settings. Promoting proper personal hygiene practices enhances health outcomes, starting with regular handwashing with soap in schools (Nuraini et al., 2019). Oral and dental hygiene, hand, foot, facial hygiene (including eyes, ears, and nose), body and skin hygiene, hair hygiene, toilet hygiene, clothing hygiene, food hygiene, and environmental cleanliness are all areas related to hygiene that are important for preserving and promoting health. Primary school-age is pivotal for instilling cleanliness and hygiene habits. Initially cultivated within families, awareness of hygiene evolves throughout the school years. School-age children merge home and school hygiene knowledge, shaping their behavior.

Hygiene behaviors directly influence children's excretion and sleep habits. Adequate and quality sleep is essential for children to maintain healthy growth, complete physical and emotional capabilities, and avoid various problems associated with insufficient or poor-quality sleep, such as attention, learning, academic, and cognitive impairments (Matricciani et al., 2012). School processes such as increased workload and social factors disrupt their sleep routines (Paruthi et al., 2016). School-aged children's sleep habits are influenced by various factors, including biological, psychological, cultural, social, environmental, academic changes, familial factors, and extracurricular activities (Bahammam et al., 2006). In addition, obesity, dietary habits, fast-food consumption, high-calorie beverages, sleep routines (İnci et al., 2020), and screen time on television, computers, or smartphones also influence the sleep habits of school-aged children (Matricciani et al., 2012). Due to technological advancements, screen exposure, especially close to bedtime, among school-aged children affects bedtime, shortening sleep duration and impacting sleep quality (Tambalis et al., 2018). School nurses should assess children's sleep patterns diligently and inform parents about sleep issues. Developing educational programs for parents on positive and negative parenting practices can enhance children's sleep health awareness (Koç & Kadiroğlu, 2021).

Hygiene Practices in School-Age Children

Hygiene is the science of teaching healthy living conditions and synthesizing health-related information to protect and improve individual and community health. Personal hygiene involves self-care practices to maintain health (Balaban, 2011). Maintaining good hygiene is crucial for preventing the spread of infectious diseases and ensuring children's overall well-being, enabling them to thrive academically by reducing absenteeism. However, adopting essential hygiene practices proves challenging without proper knowledge, skills, community support, and the belief in the efficacy of personal actions. Numerous school-age children worldwide face obstacles in upholding good hygiene, particularly in environments characterized by dirt floors in homes, schools, and health facilities, limited access to handwashing water, and cohabitation with domestic animals. Furthermore, the responsibility for practicing good hygiene is often unfairly placed on women, exacerbating their caregiving responsibilities (UNICEF, 2023). School-age children, as well as adults, are concerned about access to clean water, sanitary conditions, and cleanliness in developing or impoverished nations. Children become sick, their health deteriorates, and they contract numerous diseases as a result of inadequate water, sanitation, and hygiene facilities in schools. Poor handwashing habits are also widespread, which worsens health and education by facilitating the transmission of infectious diseases (UNICEF, 2021). Oral and dental hygiene, hand, foot, facial hygiene (including eyes, ears, and nose), body and skin hygiene, hair hygiene, toilet hygiene, clothing hygiene, food hygiene, and environmental cleanliness are all areas related to hygiene that are important for preserving and promoting health (Balaban, 2011).

Primary school-age is pivotal for instilling cleanliness and hygiene habits. Initially cultivated within families, awareness of hygiene evolves throughout the school years. School-age children merge home and school hygiene knowledge, shaping their behavior (Ayhan et al., 2015). The "Health-Promoting Schools in Europe (HPSE) Project" and initiatives like "Making every school a health-promoting school" by WHO and UNESCO aim to enhance school health globally. However, only a few countries have effectively integrated health promotion into their educational systems on a large scale (WHO, 2021).

Factors Influencing Hygiene Behaviors in Children and Their Impact on Children's Lives and Health

Studies have revealed various parameters affecting children's hygiene, highlighting deficiencies in hygiene practices across multiple areas that adversely impact children's lives and lead to various health issues:

Hand hygiene plays a critical role in preventing infectious diseases. However, according to UNICEF, schools and health facilities worldwide lack adequate handwashing facilities, impacting approximately 802 million school-age children (UNICEF, 2021). Clean toilets are necessary, but handwashing is critical to health, minimizing germ transmission, and avoiding illnesses such as diarrhea. Handwashing is essential for children, caregivers, instructors, and food handlers. Thus, health education initiatives stressing hand cleanliness are essential. Initiatives encouraging personal cleanliness and clean living in schools could act as a starting point, dramatically improving health outcomes via basic yet effective activities such as hand washing (Sardar & Behera, 2024). In societies, education and health are vital institutions that influence each other. The impact of education on health is undeniable. Hygiene education is critical for children to learn hygiene habits from an early age and grow into healthy individuals within society (Balaban, 2011).

Oral hygiene in children is crucial for overall public health, especially among school-aged children who face higher risks. Dental problems such as cavities can impact their well-being, leading to issues such as low self-esteem and academic performance. Family background, particularly socioeconomic status, influences oral hygiene, with lower-income families experiencing more dental issues. In the study by Yigit and Kucukesmen (2020), efforts to prevent dental caries in children from low socioeconomic backgrounds were observed to be less effective compared to those from higher socioeconomic backgrounds. Therefore, the role of parents as role models in shaping children's habits is crucial. Oğuzöncül et al., (2020) studied 173 students aged 6-15 in 13 villages in Elazığ to assess their nutrition and hygiene habits. Findings showed inadequate hygiene practices, with less than half of the children regularly brushing their teeth and only 23.1% washing their hands after key activities. Another study also highlighted insufficient hygiene among school-age children, influenced by parental education and economic status. The short-term effectiveness of hygiene education calls for a reconsideration of its content and delivery (Seçilmiş Çetinçakmak, 2022). Joshi (2019) examined the personal hygiene knowledge and attitudes of primary school children in both public and private schools. The study revealed a significant increase in knowledge and attitudes among students in public schools, while students in private schools generally exhibited good knowledge and attitudes.

Çelik (2018) conducted a study examining the cleanliness and hygiene practices of 1300 secondary school students in Kars province. The results showed high levels of cleanliness and hygiene among the students, with increased habits associated with higher parental education levels. Another study found that the students' knowledge and skills regarding personal hygiene, cleanliness, and handwashing were below the desired level. Therefore, it emphasized the need for further education to improve students' personal hygiene practices. It was concluded that providing education in schools to instill proper hygiene habits could address this issue (Oğuzöncül et al., 2020). According to a study, the promotion of soap-based handwashing among older youths reduces disease transmission, but the lack of consistent financial backing hinders the effective implementation of hygiene interventions targeting this group (Watson et al., 2023). The lack of cooperation within and between sectors hinders handwashing programs for youngsters.

Increased personal hygiene and practice levels among students enhance academic performance and reduce absenteeism due to illness. Proper personal hygiene knowledge and application play a critical role in avoiding contagious diseases, benefiting children's healthy living and school attendance (Joshi, 2019). Ödek (2018) found in their study on hygiene habits among primary school students in grades 6-8 that as students' positive hygiene habits increased, their academic success also improved.

Education Interventions in Promoting Hygiene Behavior

Research conducted in randomized controlled trials (RCTs) has shown that educational interventions given to children are effective in promoting hygiene behavior. The results indicate that the Hygiene Habit Formation Education Program implemented in the preschool period is effective in improving children's hygiene behaviors at school (Balaban, 2011). It is crucial to explore different methods that capture their attention and interest to enhance hygiene habits among school children. For instance, research has found that implementing storytelling methods to improve handwashing knowledge and attitudes among school-aged children has a significant impact (Srinatania et al., 2022). In school settings, educational interventions on handwashing enhance both knowledge and awareness of proper hand hygiene and improve adherence to handwashing habits. Yumru and Koç (2021) assessed the effect of Hand Hygiene Education using the Role-Playing Method on primary school students' handwashing knowledge and skills. They found a significant improvement in students' hand hygiene knowledge and skills after the education compared to before.

Hygiene conditions, particularly in school toilets, significantly affect children's toileting habits. Access to clean and functional toilets is essential in learning environments to meet children's physiological and psychosocial needs. Research in impoverished urban areas found that inadequate and poorly maintained toilets negatively impact children's access and usage, correlating with health and psychosocial risks due to irregular toilet visits (Linet Imbosa Muhati-Nyakundi, 2022).

Excretion in School-Age Children and Associated Factors

Bladder control develops around 2-2.5 years, bowel control develops around 2.5-3 years, and nighttime bladder control and full bowel control is typically established by 4-5 years of age. Children exhibit varying bowel habits, which are considered normal by different studies. At 2 years old, bowel movements average twice a day; these decrease to once after age 4. With age, this decrease is attributed to reduced transit time and colonic motility. The average gastrointestinal transit time is 8.5 hours at 1-3 months, 16 hours at 4-24 months, 26 hours between 3-13 years, and 30-48 hours post-puberty (Afzal et al., 2011).

Urine problems in school-age children include nocturia, urine incontinence, urgency, and an increased and decreased frequency of urination (Austin et al., 2016). Fecal issues can also include hemorrhoids, encopresis, constipation, functional constipation, and trouble training oneself to use the bathroom (Zhaksylyk et al., 2021). Functional constipation in school-aged children is often not caused by an underlying pathology. It primarily results from stool withholding, leading to prolonged retention and increased density in the colon. Other factors include a low-fiber diet, inadequate fluid intake, stress, uncomfortable toilet conditions, and activities encouraging stool withholding (Benninga et al., 2004). Commonly observed in school-aged children (estimated prevalence of 15-20%), bladder and bowel dysfunction (BBD) manifests itself with symptoms such as functional constipation, fecal incontinence (FI), daytime incontinence (DI), and nocturnal enuresis (NE) (Heron et al., 2017). These conditions are associated with disruptions in normal bowel and bladder function and can adversely affect the self-esteem and psychosocial development of affected children. However, these children are often not taken seriously, hindering appropriate diagnosis and treatment processes. The socioeconomic impacts of urinary incontinence (UI) are significant (Jørgensen et al., 2021). Bedwetting, or NE, can cause emotional distress and worry for both children and their parents. It often leads to psychological effects such as diminished self-esteem in children and reduced academic performance. Research findings suggest that age, male gender, parental history of enuresis, and siblings' history of enuresis are significant predictive factors for bedwetting. Moreover, many parents show insufficient concern for their enuretic children, leaving a large proportion untreated (Sarici et al., 2016).

A study aimed at estimating the prevalence of voiding dysfunctions among school-age children in Turkey examined 907 participants. The results indicated that 19.2% of the children experienced voiding dysfunctions, 16.8% reported daytime urinary incontinence, and 14.5% reported nocturnal enuresis. Significant correlations were found between voiding dysfunctions and daytime/nighttime urinary incontinence and fecal incontinence. The prevalence of voiding dysfunctions decreased with age and was associated with a positive family history. It was concluded that these dysfunctions significantly impacted the children's quality of life (Kaplan et al., 2021). In a study, a total of 1515 mothers completed the questionnaire, with 368 providing information about children aged 0-3 years and 1147 for children aged 4-18 years. According to Rome IV criteria, 25.0% of children and adolescents aged 4-18 were found to have a functional gastrointestinal disorder (FGD) by meeting symptom-based criteria, with functional constipation being the most common disorder in children and adolescents (14.1%). It was revealed that the quality of life decreased in pediatric patients with FGDs, and children whose parents had an FGD were found to have a higher likelihood (Robin et al., 2018).

The Impact of Elimination Habits on School-Age Children's Health and Well-Being: Understanding Influential Factors

Inappropriate urine and bowel habits can lead to bladder and bowel issues. School-age children receiving therapy for these disorders frequently fail to attend regular bathroom trips at school, citing bad opinions about school restrooms as a cause. When it came to utilizing campus bathrooms, students emphasized cleanliness. The visual assessment of the general cleanliness of the restrooms had the greatest influence on students' decisions to use them.

An intervention study focused on improving elementary students' toilet experience revealed that 90% of the comments cited a lack of privacy due to poor student behavior. Focus group discussions highlighted toilet avoidance due to poor conditions and student behavior, leading to privacy concerns. Involving students in renovations increased usage and decreased vandalism, but more intervention is needed to address behavior issues (Senior, 2014). In a study exploring the experiences of 9-16-year-old elementary school students regarding toilet usage and the importance of school rules, it was found that teachers employ rules to maintain classroom order. However, these rules were deemed inadequate for children's physical and developmental needs. Students found it challenging to adhere to these rules, particularly during short breaks when privacy concerns were high. Having to disclose the need to use the toilet in front of classmates was cited as the most uncomfortable aspect, potentially affecting their willingness to use school toilets and consequently impacting their health during school hours (Lundblad et al., 2010). In research done in Denmark, online data was collected from 19,577 pupils from 252 schools. One-quarter of the youngsters (28% of females, 23% of boys) said they avoided school restrooms, with unhappiness being the most common reason. This discontent is closely linked to symptoms of Bladder and Bowel Dysfunction (BBD). Access to adequate bathroom facilities at school is critical for children's well-being owing to the quantity of time spent there (Jørgensen et al.,2021). The perceptions of school toilets significantly influence the urinary and bowel habits of schoolchildren aged 6 to 16. Negative perceptions, particularly among older children (aged 13 to 16), lead to avoidance of using school toilets. Factors such as appearance, odor, and feelings of insecurity contribute to this avoidance behavior. As a result, a significant portion of older children reported never using the school toilet for urination and refraining from using it for defecation. This avoidance behavior poses challenges for children experiencing urinary tract or intestinal problems due to the lack of regular toilet visits during the day (Lundblad & Hellström, 2005).

An experimental study involving 60 children diagnosed with enuresis, aged 7-12, attending a urology clinic aimed to evaluate the effectiveness of a nursing-led educational program to improve their quality of life. Implementation of targeted nursing interventions aimed to reduce the negative impact of enuresis on various aspects of children's lives, including psychosocial well-being, self-esteem, and overall quality of life. It was concluded that a detailed explanation of the condition positively influenced the child's quality of life (Yilmaz & Büyük, 2021). Children diagnosed with enuresis experience low-level depression and moderate-level social anxiety, with depression increasing as social anxiety worsens. A significant proportion of children aged 7-12 with enuresis expressed feeling bad about themselves due to bedwetting, especially when their peers are aware of it. Enuresis causes psychosocial difficulties for children, highlighting the importance of addressing both the affected child and their families comprehensively during treatment to achieve faster and more positive responses, both physically and psychosocially (Yılmaz Oztorun et al., 2022).

Urinary incontinence (UI) is widespread among school-aged children, and it has a substantial influence on their overall health and way of life. There are adjustable risk factors for UI in children. A study found that the prevalence of Stress UI was 22.95%, preceding Urge UI at 19.34% and Nocturnal Enuresis (NE) at 3.93% (Shrestha et al., 2021). Findings from surveys analyzing over 130,000 children indicate a significant impact of NE on children and adolescents, but it remains inadequately assessed. The study revealed a 7.1% prevalence rate of NE, with only 25% experiencing Monosymptomatic Nocturnal Enuresis (MNE) (Ferrara et al., 2020). Children diagnosed with recurrent urinary tract infections (UTIs) often experience frequent hospital visits, leading to school absenteeism. Regular voiding is crucial in preventing bladder infections. Incomplete bladder emptying increases the risk of UTIs. Studies have shown a higher incidence of UTIs in children with urinary retention habits compared to those without. Despite aiming to urinate less frequently, many of these children exhibit urinary retention behavior, even when their bladder functions normally (Çetin & Kavaz Tufan, 2022). It has been reported that children delay urination due to reasons such as engaging in play, watching television, or avoiding the school toilet, and as a result, they employ various maneuvers such as crossing their legs, squatting, or applying pressure to the perineum, leading to an increase in the frequency of functional daytime incontinence (Nieuwhof-Leppink et al., 2019).

In a study designed for primary school on the prevalence of constipation and functional abdominal pain (FAP), it was discovered that children kept their feces, resulting in abdominal pain, because of unfavorable toilet circumstances and a low inclination to use them. Among individuals who avoided using toilets, there were notable increases in the prevalence of constipation and abdominal pain, and this tendency continued a year after school started (Laffolie et al., 2020). A systematic review reveals a significant link between psychological stress and constipation in children, categorized into family, school, and other stress factors. Stress and burden are associated with constipation, emphasizing the need for collaboration among parents, children, and healthcare professionals (Gozali et al., 2023).

Constipation resulting from organic, systemic, and intestinal disorders is rare and often stems from deliberate fecal withholding. Despite adequate hygiene knowledge, students exhibit reluctance to use school toilets due to their uncleanliness and peers' poor hygiene habits, as revealed by responses indicating a preference against frequent toilet use (79.7%) due to these reasons. Additionally, the short duration of recess leads students to prioritize play over restroom breaks (Klar et al., 2022). Among children experiencing health issues, a family history of constipation, abnormal oral habits, and insufficient regular physical activity were more prevalent in constipated children compared to others ($p < 0.05$). Logistic regression analysis identified never using school toilets and experiencing difficulty controlling the bowels after age two as primary risk factors for constipation among school-age children aged 7-12. Childhood constipation risk factors can be genetic, psychological, or organic. Bowel functions can be influenced by dietary habits. Parents, health, and education professionals should pay special attention to childhood constipation (Inan et al., 2007). Additionally, findings suggest that school children resort to fluid restriction to avoid using school toilets. Despite having access to water, they delay their toilet needs due to the conditions of the toilets, leading to various bowel and bladder issues (Michels et al., 2019). Family socioeconomic status and family history were found to be associated with bedwetting. Rates of bedwetting were higher among those with a family history and lower income levels (Pandey et al., 2019).

Sleep in School-Age Children

Sleep, a fundamental need, emerges through the interaction of anatomical and neurochemical regions within the central nervous system, enhancing growth, development, and learning abilities while allowing individuals to rest throughout the day, contributing to their mental and physical health. It significantly influences children's brain development, behavior regulation, and learning. Adequate and quality sleep is essential for children to maintain healthy growth, complete physical and emotional capabilities, and avoid various problems associated with insufficient or poor-quality sleep, such as attention, learning, academic, and cognitive impairments (Matricciani et al., 2012).

Various studies indicate that approximately 25-50% of preschool children experience various sleep problems, while around 20-30% of school-age children and adolescents are reported to have significant sleep disturbances (Tekeoğlu, 2024). In their study, İnci et al., (2020) found a sleep disorder rate of 71.2% among 1876 students aged 6-11 years old. Experiencing sleep problems can significantly impact various aspects of mental and social development, including brain development, learning, memory, growth, behavior, and emotion regulation, albeit at different levels of severity (Tekeoğlu, 2024). Adequate sleep is vital to regulate metabolism, psychology, and hormones in children and adolescents. Shortened sleep affects hormone secretion, leading to insulin resistance and glucose intolerance. It increases appetite and promotes the consumption of high-calorie foods, influencing dietary choices adversely (Lee & Cho, 2022).

Understanding Sleep Needs by Age

Sleep is crucial for healthy growth and development in children and adolescents. While individual sleep needs vary, newborns sleep 16-18 hours daily, and preschoolers sleep 11-12 hours. Studies suggest ideal sleep durations: approximately 7-8 hours for adults and 10 hours for school-aged children and adolescents, ensuring sufficient rest without accumulating sleep debt or experiencing daytime sleepiness (Mayda Domaç et al., 2020). According to the American Academy of Sleep Medicine, school-aged children (6-12 years) need 9-12 hours of sleep, while adolescents (13-18 years) require 8-10 hours for healthy growth and development (Paruthi et al., 2016).

Factors Associated with Sleep Habits in School-Aged Children

Healthy sleep habits are crucial for children, and awareness of factors that can negatively affect their sleep habits should be prioritized. School-aged children's sleep habits are influenced by various factors, including biological, psychological, cultural, social, environmental, academic changes, familial factors, and extracurricular activities (Bahammam et al., 2006). In addition, obesity, dietary habits, fast-food consumption, high-calorie beverages, sleep routines (İnci et al., 2020), and screen time on television, computers, or smartphones also influence the sleep habits of school-aged children (Matricciani et al., 2012). Due to technological advancements, screen exposure, especially close to bedtime, among school-aged children affects bedtime, shortening sleep duration and impacting sleep quality (Tambalis et al., 2018).

Family factors play a significant role in determining sleep habits. A study highlighted various findings indicating that school-aged children's sleep habits are influenced by factors such as parental education level, age, income status, and the child's health condition (Koç and Kadiroğlu, 2021). The presence of domestic violence, parental alcohol use, crowded households, and excessive electronic devices in the bedroom increase the frequency of sleep problems (Matricciani et al., 2012). Research indicates that parental education level significantly influences children's sleep habits, with lower-educated parents showing resistance to bedtime routines and their children experiencing more sleep issues (Koç and Kadiroğlu, 2021). Another study found statistically significant differences in children's sleep habits based on variables such as parental education, family structure, income, screen time, and dietary habits (İnci et al., 2020).

Research suggests that negative parenting practices can adversely affect children's sleep quality, while positive parenting behaviors positively influence sleep health. Children in supportive family environments with positive parent-child relationships tend to have a higher quality of sleep, indicating the positive impact of positive parenting practices (Yang et al., 2020; Chary et al., 2020). Higher income relative to expenses is associated with lower sleep anxiety in parents, indicating the influence of socioeconomic status on children's sleep habits. Chronic illness in children affects sleep patterns, with difficulties in falling asleep noted, influenced by changes in habits during illness for both children and parents (Koç ve Kadiroğlu, 2021; İnci et al., 2020). Both internal and external factors influencing sleep patterns affect sleep quality. Considering cortisol's role in preparing for the next day during sleep, regulating sleep patterns is crucial for overall health (Kurt & Erol, 2024).

The Effects of Sleep Problems on the Health of School-Age Children

Sleep significantly influences an individual's quality of life and well-being. Good sleep fosters resistance against illnesses, prevents injuries, enhances mental clarity, and stabilizes mood (Paruthi et al., 2016). Various studies indicate that sleep problems impact children's healthy lifestyle behaviors:

Another study examining the relationship between sleep disorder symptoms and healthy lifestyle behaviors in school children highlighted the impact of sleep on various health behaviors such as nutrition and physical activity (Bildirici et al., 2023). Insufficient sleep has been observed to negatively affect dietary habits, leading to increased consumption of unhealthy foods (Kurt & Erol, 2024). In a study by Golley et al., (2013), it was noted that individuals with similar sleep durations but later bedtimes had higher BMI compared to those with earlier bedtimes. This observation reflects the significant impact of sleep patterns on BMI. Deng et al., (2021) conducted a meta-analysis indicating that short sleep duration increases BMI and is associated with obesity. This finding aligns with a broad literature on the impact of sleep duration on obesity risk. Studies emphasize the importance of sleep patterns in maintaining a healthy BMI. Additionally, a published report highlights a relationship between sleep patterns and the immune system, indicating mutual influence. Sleep problems weaken the immune system, leading to disease, while the weakening of the immune system can also cause sleep problems (Mayda Domaç et al., 2020).

Adequate sleep and stress management strategies in school-age children are vital components of a healthy lifestyle, safeguarding against the negative effects of chronic stress and sleep deprivation on health and academic performance (Kalandarova, 2024). Studies emphasize the significant influence of family in developing and maintaining healthy behaviors such as hygiene and sleep in school-age children (Devi et al., 2023). Thus, ensuring parental involvement is crucial in achieving sustainable outcomes in interventions for children and promoting a healthy lifestyle for future adults. Childhood behaviors can persist into adulthood, impacting health outcomes. School nurses should assess children's sleep patterns diligently and inform parents about sleep issues. Developing educational programs for parents on positive and negative parenting practices can enhance children's sleep health awareness (Koç & Kadiroğlu, 2021).

Conclusion

As a result, addressing toilet training challenges with appropriate methods promotes consistent personality development. Effective maternal facilitation of toilet training highlights the importance of health education. Positive traits influence health issues related to toilet habits. Mothers' characteristics are crucial in both training and child development. Teachers note that subpar toilet conditions in schools affect voiding patterns. Awareness is the key for children, parents, teachers, and medical professionals. Education and health are intertwined, stressing hygiene in school-aged children. Schools promote well-being and educational success. Research shows inadequate hygiene habits among school-age children. Recommendations include educational interventions involving parents and educators. Addressing urinary incontinence in children is vital for long-term health and academic success. Involving parents and educators is crucial to effective management. Community campaigns foster understanding and reduce stigma around urinary incontinence.

The research findings underscore the significance of parents' use of positive parenting practices in reducing children's sleep problems. Therefore, fostering positive relationships and supportive family environments is crucial. Parents should support their children's sleep routines, ensure consistent practices, and establish household rules related to sleep to promote positive sleep characteristics in children. Elevating hygiene, excretion, and sleep to optimal levels in schoolchildren can be achieved through collaboration among schools, families, and children. Future studies should focus on interactive educational programs targeting school-age children, particularly involving families, regarding hygiene, excretion, and sleep.

Disclaimer

None.

References

Afzal, N. A., Tighe, M. P., & Thomson, M. A. (2011). Constipation in children. *Italian Journal of Pediatrics*, *37*, 28. https://doi.org/10.1186/1824-7288-37-28.

Austin, P. F., Bauer, S. B., Bower, W., Chase, J., Franco, I., Hoebeke, P., et al., (2016). The standardization of terminology of lower urinary tract function in children and adolescents: Update report from the standardization committee of the International Children's Continence Society. *Neurourology and Urodynamics*, *35*(4), 471-481. https://doi.org/10.1002/nau.22751.

Ayhan, E., Gökler, M. E., Işıklı, B., Önsüz, F. M., Özay, Ö., Aydın, E., Durmaz, G., & Kalyoncu, C. (2015). Hand hygiene knowledge and practice in primary school students in rural Eskişehir: An intervention study. *STED*, *24*(3), 99-108.

Bahammam, A., Alfaris, E., Shaikh, S., & Bin Saeed, A. (2006). Prevalence of sleep problems and habits in a sample of Saudi primary school children. *Annals of Saudi Medicine*, *26*, 7-13.

Balaban, M. (2011). *The effect of a hygiene education program in preschool period on children's hygiene behaviors.* Master's thesis, Institute of Social Sciences.

Benninga, M. A., Voskuijl, W. P., & Taminiau, J. A. J. M. (2004). Childhood constipation: Is there new light in the tunnel? *Journal of Pediatric Gastroenterology and Nutrition, 39*(5), 448-464.

Bildirici, Y., Sungur, S., Muz, F. N. O., Bal, M., Akkoca, Z., & Metintaş, S. (2023). The relationship between sleep disorder symptoms and health-promoting lifestyle habits in school-aged children. *Osmangazi Journal of Medicine*, *45*(5), 732-746. https://doi.org/10.20515/otd.1344793.

Çelik, H., Başer Baykal, N., & Kılıç Memur, H. N. (2020). Qualitative data analysis and basic principles. *Eğitimde Nitel Araştırmalar Dergisi* [*Journal of Qualitative Research in Education*], *8*(1), 379-406. https://doi.org/10.14689/issn.2148-2624.1.8c.1s.16m.

Çetin, N., & Kavaz Tufan, A. (2022). Evaluation of toilet habits in children with recurrent urinary tract infections and investigation of risk factors in the development of kidney damage. *Abant Medical Journal*, *11*(2), 243-249. https://doi.org/10.47493/abantmedj.1094312.

Chary, M., McQuillan, M. E., Bates, J. E., & Deater-Deckard, K. (2020). Maternal executive function and sleep interact in the prediction of negative parenting. *Behavioral Sleep Medicine*, *18*, 203-216.

Deng, X., He, M., He, D., Zhu, Y., Zhang, Z., & Niu, W. (2021). Sleep duration and obesity in children and adolescents: Evidence from an updated and dose–response meta-analysis. *Sleep Medicine*, *78*, 169-181.

Devi, H. M., Putri, R. M., & Rosdiana, Y. (2023). The role of family healthcare in the social development of vulnerable school-aged children groups. *Healthcare in Low-Resource Settings*, *11*(2). https://doi.org/10.4081/hls.2023.11798.

Dewi, R. K., & Sumarni, S. (2023). Parenting style and family empowerment for children's growth and development: A systematic review. *Journal of Public Health Africa, 14*, 2582.

Ferrara, P., Franceschini, G., Bianchi Di Castelbianco, F., Bombace, R., Villani, A., & Corsello, G. (2020). Epidemiology of enuresis: A large number of children at risk of low regard. *Italian Journal of Pediatrics, 46*(1), 128. https://doi.org/10.1186/s13052-020-00896-3.

Golley, R. K., Maher, C. A., Matricciani, L., & Olds, T. S. (2013). Sleep duration or bedtime? Exploring the association between sleep timing behavior, diet, and BMI in children and adolescents. *International Journal of Obesity, 37*(4), 546-551.

Gozali, F. S., Febiana, B., Putra, I. G. N. S., Karyana, I. P. G., & Hegar, B. (2023). Relationship between psychological stress with functional constipation in children: A systematic review. *Pan African Medical Journal, 46*, 8. https://doi.org/10.11604/pamj.2023.46.8.41130.

Heron, J., Grzeda, M. T., von Gontard, A., Wright, A., & Joinson, C. (2017). Trajectories of urinary incontinence in childhood and bladder and bowel symptoms in adolescence: A prospective cohort study. *BMJ Open, 7*(3), e014238. https://doi.org/10.1136/bmjopen-2016-014238.

Inan, M., Aydiner, C. Y., Tokuc, B., Aksu, B., Ayvaz, S., Ayhan, S., Ceylan, T., & Basaran, U. N. (2007). Factors associated with childhood constipation. *Journal of Paediatrics and Child Health, 43*(10), 700-706. https://doi.org/10.1111/j.1440-1754.2007.01165.x.

İnci, F. H., Kostu, N., Cinar, I. O., Aslan, G. K., & Kartal, A. (2020). Sleep habits and affecting factors in primary school children. *Journal of Turkish Sleep Medicine, 7*, 91-96. https://doi.org/10.4274/jtsm.galenos.2020.19483.

Jørgensen, C. S., Breinbjerg, A. S., & Rittig, S. (2021). Dissatisfaction with school toilets is associated with bladder and bowel dysfunction. *European Journal of Pediatrics, 180*, 3317-3324. https://doi.org/10.1007/s00431-021-04111-1.

Joshi, K. B. (2019). Effectiveness of school-based educational program on knowledge and attitude regarding personal hygiene among primary school-going children of selected govt. and private school. *International Journal of Aesthetic Health Rejuvenation, 2*(3), 40-44.

Kalandarova, G. D. (2024). The benefits of forming a healthy lifestyle in school-age children. *Galaxy International Interdisciplinary Research Journal, 12*(2), 242-244. https://giirj.com/index.php/giirj/article/view/6418.

Kaplan, F., Tabel, Y., & Elmas, A. T. (2021). Prevalence estimates of voiding disorders in Turkish school-age children. *Lower Urinary Tract Symptoms, 13*, 244-248. https://doi.org/10.1111/luts.12358.

Klar, K., Knaack, D., Kampmeier, S., Hein, A. K., Görlich, D., Steltenkamp, S., Weyland, U., & Becker, K. (2022). Knowledge about hand hygiene and related infectious disease awareness among primary school children in Germany. *Children, 9*(2), 190. https://doi.org/10.3390/children9020190.

Laffolie, J., Ibrahimi, G., & Zimmer, K. P. (2020). Poor perception of school toilets and increase of functional constipation. *Klinische Pädiatrie* [Clinical Pediatrics], *233*(01), 5-9. https://doi.org/10.1055/a-1263-0747.

Lee, J. H., & Cho, J. (2022). Sleep and obesity. *Sleep Medicine Clinics, 17*, 111-116.

Linet Imbosa, M. N. (2022). Teachers' perceptions of children's access to toilets in urban ECDE institutions, and the psychosocial consequences. *Global Public Health, 17*(12), 3785-3801. https://doi.org/10.1080/17441692.2022.2059693.

Lundblad, B., & Hellström, A. L. (2005). Perceptions of school toilets as a cause for irregular toilet habits among schoolchildren aged 6 to 16 years. *Journal of School Health, 75*, 125-128. https://doi.org/10.1111/j.1746-1561.2005.tb06656.x.

Lundblad, B., Hellström, A. L., & Berg, M. (2010). Children's experiences of attitudes and rules for going to the toilet in school. *Scandinavian Journal of Caring Sciences, 24*(2), 219-223. https://doi.org/10.1111/j.1471-6712.2009.00707.x.

Matricciani, L., Olds, T., & Petkov, J. (2012). In search of lost sleep: Secular trends in the sleep time of school-aged children and adolescents. *Sleep Medicine Reviews, 16*, 203-211.

Mayda Domaç, F., Uludüz, D., & Özge, A. (2020). Immunity nutrition and lifestyle report: Sleep and the immune system. Turkish Academy of Sciences Publications.

Michels, N., Van den Bussche, K., Vande Walle, J., & De Henauw, S. (2019). School policy on drinking and toilets: Weaknesses and relation with children's hydration status. *Journal of Nutrition Education and Behavior, 51*(1), 32-40. https://doi.org/10.1016/j.jneb.2018.07.001.

Nieuwhof-Leppink, A. J., Schroeder, R. P. J., van de Putte, E. M., de Jong, T. P. V. M., & Schappin, R. (2019). Daytime urinary incontinence in children and adolescents. *The Lancet Child & Adolescent Health, 3*(7), 492-501. https://doi.org/10.1016/S2352-4642(19)30113-0.

Nuraini, N., Riadi, A., Umanailo, M. C. B., Rusdi, M., Badu, T. K., & Suryani, S. (2019). Political policy for the development of education. *International Journal of Scientific & Technology Research, 8*(10).

Ödek, Ö. (2018). Effect of middle school talents' organization on illness situations. (Master's thesis, Yozgat Bozok University).

Oğuzöncül, A. F., Bulut, İ., Pirinçci, E., Yurt, N., & Deveci, S. E. (2020). Evaluation of hygiene and nutrition behaviors of primary school-aged children living in rural areas. *ESTÜDAM Public Health Journal, 5*(1), 73-83.

Pandey, S., Oza, H. J., Shah, H., & Vankar, G. K. (2019). Rate and risk factors of nocturnal enuresis in school-going children. *Industrial Psychiatry Journal, 28*(2), 306-311. https://doi.org/10.4103/ipj.ipj_15_18.

Paruthi, S., Brooks, L. J., D'Ambrosio, C., Hall, W. A., Kotagal, S., Lloyd, R. M., et al., (2016). Consensus statement of the American Academy of Sleep Medicine on the recommended amount of sleep for healthy children: Methodology and discussion. *Journal of Clinical Sleep Medicine, 12*(11), 1549-1561.

Robin, S. G., Keller, C., Zwiener, R., Hyman, P. E., Nurko, S., Saps, M., Di Lorenzo, C., Shulman, R. J., Hyams, J. S., Palsson, O., & van Tilburg, M. A. L. (2018). Prevalence of pediatric functional gastrointestinal disorders utilizing the Rome IV criteria. *The Journal of Pediatrics, 195*, 134-139. https://doi.org/10.1016/j.jpeds.2017.12.012.

Sardar, A., & Behera, D. K. (2024). Wash practices of school-going children in South Asia. *International Research Journal of Education and Multidisciplinary Studies, 3*(1), 255-262. https://doi.org/10.56472/25835238/IRJEMS-V3I1P128.

Sarici, H., Telli, O., Ozgur, B. C., Demirbas, A., Ozgur, S., & Karagoz, M. A. (2016). Prevalence of nocturnal enuresis and its influence on quality of life in school-aged children. *Journal of Pediatric Urology, 12*(3), 159.e1-159.e1596. https://doi.org/10.1016/j.jpurol.2015.11.011.

Seçilmiş Çetinçakmak, Ö. (2022). Evaluation of hygiene behaviors of 4th-grade students based on student, parent, and teacher opinions and curricula. Master's thesis, Institute of Education Sciences.

Senior, E. (2014). We love our school toilets: Involving primary school students in improving their school toilets. *Global Health Promotion, 21*(1), 23-28. https://doi.org/10.1177/1757975913508420.

Shrestha, N., Sahukhala, S., K C, D., Sandalcidi, D., & Adhikari, S. P. (2021). Prevalence of urinary incontinence in school-going children: A cross-sectional study. *Journal of Nepal Health Research Council, 18*(4), 676-680. https://doi.org/10.33314/jnhrc.v18i4.2506.

Srinatania, D., Dahlia, L., & Perdani, A. L. (2022). The effectiveness of storytelling to improve handwashing knowledge and attitude in school-age children in Indonesia. *KnE Life Sciences*, 467-472. https://doi.org/10.18502/kls.v7i2.10343.

Tambalis, K. D., Panagiotakos, D. B., Psarra, G., & Sidossis, L. S. (2018). Insufficient sleep duration is associated with dietary habits, screen time, and obesity in children. *Journal of Clinical Sleep Medicine, 14*(10), 1689-1696.

Tekeoğlu, U. (2024). Sleep-wake disorders in children and adolescents. *Journal of Medical Clinics, 7*(1), 21-33. https://doi.org/10.52797/jmc.v7i1.13927.

UNICEF. (2021). A summary of WASH in the new UNICEF Strategic Plan 2022-2025. https://www.unicef.org/media/119056/file/WASH%20in%20the%20new%20UNICEF%20Strategic%20Plan_Summary.pdf.

UNICEF. (2023). Water, sanitation, and hygiene (WASH). https://www.unicef.org/wash.

Watson, J., Cumming, O., & Dreibelbis, R. (2023). Nongovernmental organization practitioners' perspectives on the challenges and solutions to changing handwashing behavior in older children: A qualitative study. *Global Health: Science and Practice, 11*(1), e2200231. https://doi.org/10.9745/GHSP-D-22-00231.

WHO. (2018). *The top 10 causes of death*: World Health Organization. https://www.who.int/news-room/factsheets/detail/the-top-10-causes-of-death.

WHO. (2021). *Making every school a health-promoting school*, 2020. World Health Organization. https://www.who.int/news-room/factsheets/detail/making-every-school-a-health-promoting-school.

Chapter 4

Sexual Health in School-Age Children

Bilgin Kıray Vural*, PhD

Pamukkale University, Denizli Healthcare Vocational School,
Department of Medical Services and Techniques, Dialysis Program, Denizli, Türkiye

Abstract

School years mark a transition as children venture beyond their homes into the broader world. During this period, risky sexual behaviors often emerge, leading to significant health concerns. Many of these issues stem from insufficient education and unhealthy socialization surrounding sexuality, fueled by taboo perceptions and hearsay. Sexual health education aims to address young people's need for reliable information about sexuality but also focuses on taking responsibility for their sexual behavior. Parents serve as children's initial sexual educators, while teachers and school nurses, well-educated in this area, play a crucial role in schools. A comprehensive sexual health education curriculum should encompass content and skills tailored to tackle fundamental behavioral outcomes, foster healthy sexual development, ensure medical accuracy, be relevant to the child's developmental stages and cultural nuances, and promote sustainability. School nurses oversee this education, ensuring that students receive relevant reproductive and sexual health information while also identifying and addressing potential health risks.

Keywords: Sexuality, sexual health, sexual education, school-age children, school nurse

Introduction

Sexuality is a concept that starts in the mother's womb and continues throughout one's whole life. It has biological, psychological, and cultural dimensions and is shaped by the personalities, behaviors, emotions, attitudes, values, and physical structures of individuals and the characteristics of society (Tessier et al., 2009; Yalın and Alabay, 2024). Although inherent in human history, sexuality entered the verbal discourse in the late 16th century and gained prominence in the early 19th century (Alkan-Ersoy, 2014). Various cultures have struggled to understand sexual development in different periods, and it has evolved into scientific

* Corresponding Author's Email: bvural@pau.edu.tr

In: Health Promotion and Prevention
Editor: Eda Kılınç İşleyen
ISBN: 979-8-89530-758-8

perspectives over time (Saranlı, 2020). Considered a positive force, sexuality ensures the continuation of the species and maintains the existence and socialization of the person in balance with inner and bodily desires (Evcili-Gölbaşı, 2017). It is a physiological need that exists at every stage of life (Ceylan, 2020). While children's sexuality is based on curiosity and playfulness, adult sexuality tends to be informed by knowledge and behavioral patterns. Contrary to children's innate openness, adults commonly exhibit a more reserved and discreet demeanor regarding their sexuality. Children have sensitivity and excitement, which is replaced by passion and sensuality in adults (Alkan-Ersoy, 2014). Middle childhood (ages 6-12) signifies a critical developmental phase characterized by physical, social, behavioral, and cognitive changes, influencing long-term health outcomes. It is also a phase in which children develop curiosity about reproduction and anatomy, experience the first physical changes related to sexual and reproductive development (puberty), develop basic capabilities for social relationships with the opposite sex, and sometimes have their first sexual experiences (Fantaye et al., 2020). As children venture beyond the family unit, their socialization with peers intensifies, gender-specific games emerge, and sexual interest in parents of the opposite sex develops (Çakmak and Çakmak, 2011). Freud defines these ages as the latent period. Children's curiosity about sexual matters seems to decrease, and the libido energy is not active at these times. With children attending school, their energies are directed more towards play and learning, and sexual impulses become latent. Sexual discussions become more and more common among friends of their gender (Saranlı, 2014). The subsequent genital period (12-18 years) marks the onset of puberty, characterized by heightened sexual urges and explorations as the genitals become the primary erogenous zone (Tuncer, 2023).

For school-age children and young people, engaging in non-safe sexual behaviors during this period can lead to serious health issues (DesOrmeaux, 2019). In the US, 40.0% of 9-12th grade students have reported engaging in sexual intercourse, according to the 2019 Youth Risk Behavior Surveillance System Report (CDC, 2019). Similarly, in Ireland, research shows that 25.7% of boys and 21.2% of girls aged 15 and 18 have had sexual intercourse, and the rate of first intercourse at a very early age (<14 years) is 22.8% for boys and 13.4% for girls. Furthermore, 10.5% of boys and 6.8% of girls have had unprotected sexual intercourse at their recent intimacy (Young et al., 2018). These early sexual intercourse and inadequate knowledge about sexually transmitted diseases are indicators of the sexual and reproductive health risks faced by schoolchildren, impacting their rights (Fantaye et al., 2020). Inadequate education and unhealthy sexual socialization contribute to such issues, perpetuated by the taboo nature of discussing sexuality and reliance on hearsay information (Üstgörül et al., 2020). Any precautionary measures taken during this period have an impact on children's lives (Erkin and Kılınç, 2021).

The Factors Affecting Sexuality

Biological Factors

It is a fundamental instinct. Sexual functioning is a mechanism involving the whole body, especially the central nervous system, senses, and genital organs, governed by over 30 hormones and chemicals produced by our body (Dicle, 2020).

Psychological Factors

Sexuality is influenced by complex psychological factors. The notion of ourselves as men and women and the idea of our behavior conforming to our gender, our previous life experiences, self-esteem, and personal values affect our sexual feelings and behaviors (Alkan-Ersoy, 2014).

Cultural Factors

Considering society, sexual attitudes and perceptions constitute an important part of the cultural structure (Üstgörül et al., 2020). While some societies regard sexual development as secretive or taboo, others integrate sexuality into daily life (Saranlı, 2014). Some parts of the human body (legs, shoulders, ears, etc.), body embellishments (jewelry, clothing, cosmetics, etc.), and human behaviors (kissing, hugging, etc.) have no sexual connotation in some cultures, whereas in others they are considered as sexual elements (Alkan-Ersoy, 2014).

Sexual Health Education

Sexual health is the physical, mental, and social well-being of individuals in all age groups, including their sexual attitudes and behaviors, and is defined as the possibility of having pleasant and safe sexual experiences without force, discrimination, and violence, with a positive, respectful approach to sexuality and sexual relationships (Gültürk et al., 2018; WHO, 2021).

Sexual education is about understanding physical, emotional, and sexual development, fostering a positive personality concept, acquiring a respectful perspective on human sexuality and rights, and promoting positive behavior and values (Artan, 2014). It covers topics such as violence prevention, human rights, and gender, providing age-appropriate information (UNESCO, 2018). The practice of sex education launched in the early 20th century in the world (Alkan-Ersoy, 2014). According to the Global School-Based Student Health Survey, teaching sexuality is among the priorities within the health education program (WHO, 2021). A healthy sexual education is the first step towards creating contented individuals and prosperous societies (Artan, 2014). It aims to empower individuals and societies and promote human rights, tolerance, and critical thinking. It is also tailored to different age groups and developmental stages (WHO, 2010; Alkan-Ersoy, 2014).

Children ask many questions out of curiosity to learn about sexuality. In cases where they cannot get an answer from adults, they turn to other sources and try to find an explanation. However, this might not always be the right answer, might not reflect the truth, and might contain values that adults do not believe (Alkan-Ersoy, 2014). For this reason, sexual health education content should be provided by norms, values, and practices, taking into account the needs of the young population, and should be updated as practices evolve (Bergström et al., 2018).

Education on sexual health aims to encircle young people's need for reliable information on sexuality and promote responsibility for their sexual behavior (Gürsoy and Gençalp, 2010; Bakır et al., 2019). It is seen as vital to changing negative attitudes of the individual/society

(Tasa and Namatoğlu, 2018). Access to sexual education is recognized as a fundamental human right (UNESCO, 2018). Nevertheless, it is often excluded from formal education curricula, especially in countries where it is not welcomed due to religious reasons and is considered shameful, sinful, and taboo (Ünal-Toprak and Turan, 2021). Therefore, many young people lack essential, accurate information about sexuality.

According to a study in Sweden, 49.0% of high school freshmen rely on the Internet for sexual information (Borneskog, 2021). TikTok, on the other hand, offers a new opportunity to tackle the gaps in sexual education and provide information to adolescents. To explain the utility and content of sex education on TikTok, 100 sex education-oriented videos' themes have been analyzed, revealing the most common themes, which are female anatomy, sexual pleasure, contraception, and sexual health. In this regard, the discrepancies in these videos and the training provided by health professionals in the home or school-based sexuality education may provide an opportunity to initiate conversations with young people about sexuality or to provide them with resources (Fowler et al., 2022). Borneskog's (2021) study reveals that 37.0% of the students had sexual intercourse, with a median age of 15. Furthermore, adolescents are less engaged in non-penetrative sexual intercourse and physical intimacy. Such findings call for a new approach when designing sex and relationship education and health counseling for adolescents. Sex education during pre-adolescence may foster a healthy sexual identity and provide accurate sexual health information in a supportive environment (Alkan-Ersoy, 2014). A comprehensive sexual education program should equip students with knowledge and skills to promote health and prevent human immunodeficiency virus (HIV), sexually transmitted infections (STIs), and unwanted pregnancy (CDC, 2024a).

The differences between urban-rural settlement, educational levels, and household wealth affect adolescents' sexual behaviors. Adolescent sexual and reproductive health policies and programs need to be country-specific, culturally sensitive, multi-sectoral, and comprehensive since the underlying causes of inequalities include poverty, lack of education, and gender-based violence. Gender inequalities dramatically influence sexual and reproductive health in adolescents, even as early as ages 10-14, and may affect the ability of individuals, especially girls, to fulfill their sexual and reproductive health rights (Melesse et al., 2020).

What Are the Benefits of Providing Sexual Health Education to Students?

Promoting and implementing well-designed sexual health education positively impacts student health (CDC, 2024a).

1. It increases self-esteem since it helps to develop a positive attitude towards one's sexual nature.
2. Misinformation is recognized. Accompanied by reliable knowledge, healthy attitudes lead to healthier sexual behaviors.
3. It contributes to gaining effective sexual communication skills where feelings and thoughts are shared.
4. Children learn to be tolerant of differences in sexual orientation at an early age.
5. It involves training in decision-making skills. Indecision and impulsive behavior are underdeveloped decision-making skills.

6. Sexual education includes knowledge, attitudes, and values education (Alkan-Ersoy, 2014).

Students who participate in these programs are more likely to;

- Start having sexual intercourse at older ages,
- Have fewer sexual partners,
- Have fewer unprotected sex experiences,
- Increase the use of contraception - especially condoms,
- Improve their academic performances (CDC, 2024a).

Sexual Health Education in School Programs

Sexual health education should include age-oriented physical, mental, emotional, and social dimensions of human sexuality as part of a planned and sequenced health education program. It must also be within the framework of specific content and a curriculum (CDC, 2024b). Reproductive and sexual health education in schools raises awareness of safe sexual behaviors and minimizes sexual risks (Bergström et al., 2018).

Research shows that students do not receive direct sexuality education in mainstream education institutions. Besides, the partial information acquired in different courses fails to fill the knowledge gap on this subject (Erenoğlu and Bayraktar, 2017; Üstgörül-Önür and Tekin-Önür, 2020). Students receiving sexual health education have more positive beliefs and attitudes toward sexual health care (Gürsoy and Gençalp, 2020). While some studies indicate that receiving sexual education increases students' knowledge and enables them to exhibit positive behaviors and attitudes (Özkan et al., 2020), other studies suggest that sexual health courses make little change in personal attitudes about sexuality (Ross et al., 2021). Sexual health education is considered to be significantly effective in raising awareness and improving attitudes among young people who have never talked about sexuality with family members or experts and have inadequate, sometimes inaccurate information. Hence, counseling students, whether they are sexually active or not, is recommended in schools (Bergström et al., 2018).

Schools are responsible for providing accurate information to children through sexual health education programs. Such programs may help children understand issues related to sexual health and build healthy relationships. It is recommended that schools should;

- Implement policies promoting environments supportive of sexual health education,
- Use medically accurate, developmentally appropriate, culturally inclusive, and scientifically grounded materials,
- Ensure that staff have the knowledge and skills needed to deliver sexual health education,
- Involve parents and relevant stakeholders in the process (CDC, 2024a).

A qualified sexual health education curriculum should encompass content and skills, targeting key behavioral outcomes, supporting healthy sexual development, ensuring medical accuracy, aligning with the child's developmental stages and cultural preferences, and being sustainable. Children need to be taught concepts such as anatomy, physiology, reproductive health, contraception, sexual communication, sexually transmitted diseases, sexual abuse, gender, sexual identity, sexual orientation, and recognizing personal boundaries while respecting the boundaries of others (Ceylan, 2020; Baran et al., 2020; Arslan, 2021; Gökçay and Çevirme, 2022; CDC, 2024a).

High-quality sexual health education programs share many common characteristics, and these programs require the following;

- Implement strategies relevant and appealing to all students,
- Address the well-being needs of all students identifying themselves as lesbian, gay, bisexual, transgender, transsexual, queer-undecided/undeclared and questioning, intersex, asexual (LGBTQIA+),
- Ensure that students have access to sexual and other health services at school or in the community,
- Encourage positive relationships between adolescents and adults (CDC, 2024a).

School health education programs, including a high-quality sexual health education curriculum, aim to develop students' functional knowledge and skills to encourage healthy behaviors and avoid risks. Giving students time to practice, evaluate, and reflect on the skills helps lead them toward independence, critical thinking, and problem-solving to avoid STIs, HIV, and unintended pregnancy. Effective sexual health education programs teach students to:

- Analyze the influence of family, peers, and the media on health,
- Access current and reliable health information, products, and services (e.g., STI/HIV and pregnancy tests),
- Communicate with family, peers, and teachers about issues affecting health,
- Make informed and thoughtful decisions about their health,
- Take responsibility for themselves and others to improve their health (CDC, 2024a).

To successfully deliver sexual health education, schools need supportive policies, appropriate content, trained staff, and engaged parents and communities (CDC, 2024a). The scope and sequence of topics should determine what learners need to know or do and when they should be taught. The CDC's Health Education Curriculum Analysis Tool (HECAT) offers valuable guidance for defining the health education scope and sequence. HECAT outlines desired healthy behavior outcomes, core knowledge, and skill expectations, defining each group's outcomes by standard and grade (CDC, 2024b).

Both health education instructors and school nurses are of great value in relaying reproductive health information to high school students. Nonetheless, the most effective method is the inclusion of school nurses in these programs to protect adolescents from high-risk sexual behaviors (impulse control, condom technique skills, etc.) (Borawski et al., 2015).

Sexual Health Education in Intellectually Disabled Children

Schools often fail to provide comprehensive health education to special students exposed to sexual abuse and exploitation (Treacy et al., 2018). Health education targeting intellectually disabled learners should be tailored to learners' abilities, learning styles, and maturity, as well as parents' values and beliefs (Nelson et al., 2020).

Sexual development in children with intellectual disability follows the same sequence as in normal development. Questioning about sexual development is not based on chronological age but on developmental age. Sex education begins with children becoming familiar with their bodies and recognizing the differences between male and female genitals. Masturbation is common in intellectually disabled children, but as academic activities take precedence with schooling, sexual impulses may diminish while development continues. Since these children have a limited social environment, their sources of information are also restricted (Şahin, 2014). Unfortunately, children with intellectual disabilities are at higher risk of forced sexual interaction. Most of these may be perpetrated by other people with disabilities or, more often, by caregivers or other people known to the child (Stein et al., 2018). Families need to receive appropriate professional support to prevent victimization, especially sexual abuse, due to the cognitive limitations of intellectually disabled children, their difficulty in distinguishing between reality and fantasy, the high likelihood of fulfilling the demands of others without questioning, and the tendency of especially those with a very low IQ to obtain insufficient information through sexual education. Since sexual problems concern not only the intellectually disabled individual but also their family, they both need education (Şahin, 2014; Stein et al., 2018). According to a study, parents may be hesitant to believe their children will engage in consensual or non-consensual sexual activity before the age of 18, but they still seek sex education for their children through professionals or workshops (Stein et al., 2018).

Who Should Provide Sexual Health Education?

The Role of Parents/Adults in Sexual Health Education

Adults have a significant responsibility to offer children education that is both scientifically grounded and tailored to their developmental needs. Parents serve as children's primary sexual educators, and their interactions and demonstrations of love serve as crucial role models (Alkan-Ersoy, 2014; SIECUS, 2018).

Stein et al., (2018) report that parents' sources of information include interactive websites, professionals, workshops, and books for their children's sexual development. Effective sexual education programs within families should embrace children's inquiries about sexuality, provide accurate information, and foster healthy sexual values and behaviors.

It is also recommended by the Sexuality Information and Education Council of the United States (SIECUS) that parents should be the primary guide in children's sexuality education, advocating for early and ongoing communication starting from childhood (SIECUS, 2018). Despite widespread support for sexual education, many misconceptions persist, claiming children will be stimulated and start sexual life at an early age once educated. There are also those who are convinced that without talking about such issues, there will be no problems, and these misconceptions stem from parents' fear of inadequacy (Alkan-Ersoy, 2014). Another study reveals that parents are concerned about sexual education, are afraid of misleading their children, and consider themselves inadequate (Aycan et al., 2024). They feel anxious both because they lack sufficient knowledge and because sexuality is considered a social taboo (Yalın and Alabay, 2024). Hence, during this phase of sexual development, adults may hesitate to talk to children, may not know how to talk, may condemn the child, and may not provide the necessary support (Artan, 2017). Working parents, higher education levels, and more children positively affect sexual communication, and there is a positive correlation between parents' age and sexual communication (Yalın and Alabay, 2024; Aral and Deleş, 2024). The level of anxiety felt by parents with only girls in sexual communication is significantly higher than those with boys and girls (Yalın and Alabay, 2024). Additionally, another study has found that a significant positive correlation exists between parents' sexual communication skills and gender justice levels (Yalın and Alabay, 2024).

While talking to children about sexuality,

1. Children should be encouraged to ask questions and speak up,
2. Explanations should be clear for knowledge and comprehension levels,
3. No one should fear talking about uncomfortable issues and expressing them explicitly with a touch of humor,
4. The adult should be open to sharing their values and concerns,
5. One should answer the questions with a neutral facial expression and tone of voice (Alkan-Ersoy, 2014).

Research indicates that parental involvement in school health education correlates with improved student behavior, social skills, reduced health risk behaviors, and higher academic achievement (Kolbe, 2019).

The Role of Teachers in Sexual Health Education

As children socialize, the models around them differ in their gender-related behaviors; they observe their teachers and friends at school and try out their attitudes and behaviors (Alkan-Ersoy, 2014). Teachers become both role models and sexual health educators. In this context, qualified sexual health education is required to be provided by qualified and well-trained teachers (CDC, 2024a).

According to a study, sexual education has been defined as privacy education by teachers (Aycan et al., 2023). By primary grades, the child should have developed a positive image of their body. Teachers shall teach the children that their body is precious and that they should value and be proud of it. The child should be taught to respect their and others' privacy, and their body belongs only to them, and no one has the right to touch them without permission, while the difference between sexual harassment and loving touches is clarified (Alkan-Ersoy, 2014). After all, teachers are crucial in recognizing sexual abuse (Artan, 2014).

The Role of School Nurses in Sexual Health Education

School nursing, a specialized practice in nursing, protects and improves student health, facilitates optimal development, and fosters academic success (NANS, 2024a). School nurses undertake an essential role in the field of sexual health with responsibilities that include;

- Identifying problems and needs related to sexual health and reporting them to the school administration,
- Ensuring early diagnosis of sexual health risks (adolescent pregnancy, sexually transmitted diseases, sexual abuse, etc.), planning appropriate interventions, and taking the necessary measures with school management,
- Assessing students' reproductive and sexual health, taking part in periodic examinations, and recording students' health status, as well as creating a health report after periodic examinations and notifying the school administration,
- Facilitating communication between students, teachers, and families while providing health counseling,
- Protecting the student's privacy under all medical conditions,
- Tracking HPV and Hepatitis B vaccinations of students and playing a role in educating students and families about the benefits of immunization. The HPV vaccine taken during adolescence protects against more than 90% of cancers caused by the virus. Thus, the vaccination is recommended between the ages of 9 and 12.
- Planning and conducting *Sexual Health Education* to provide students with accurate information on reproductive health and sexual health issues and to promote positive behaviors in this regard (DesOrmeaux, 2019; Erkin and Kılınç, 2021; NANS, 2024b; AAP, 2024).

To ensure excellence in school health, it is emphasized to have a school doctor in every local district and a nurse in every school (COSH, 2023). The Centers for Disease Control and Prevention's Division of Adolescent and School Health in the United States has created the "Sexual Health Toolkit" for school nurses to reduce HIV, other sexually transmitted diseases, unintended pregnancy, and behaviors that contribute to adolescent health risks. Following the identified need for an easily accessible source of information, this material has been developed especially for school nurses (NANS, 2024b).

The Importance of Sexual Health Education in Sexual Abuse

The World Health Organization defines child sexual abuse as "... the involvement of a child in sexual activity that they cannot fully comprehend, cannot give informed consent, or for which they are developmentally unprepared and unable to give consent, or that violates laws or social taboos..." (Büber et al., 2024; WHO, 2022). Not all sexual abuse cases necessarily involve oral, anal, or vaginal penetration; exposition to sexually explicit materials, and oral-genital, genital-genital, genital-anal touching, and genital fondling also count as sexual abuse (Gonzalez et al., 2023).

To prevent sexual abuse, early sexual education is crucial to raise awareness about responsible sexuality and protection against exploitation (Özüdoğru and Duran, 2023). Children are often exploited for sexual gratification by adults, elders, or individuals with developmental maturity (Artan, 2014). The diagnosis of child abuse requires a high level of suspicion (Gonzalez et al., 2023). The fact that children experiencing sexual abuse cannot perceive and express what they have undergone as a crime makes it difficult to uncover and report the abuse (Büber et al., 2024). Child sexual abuse is, unfortunately, a common problem in our country, Türkiye, and the world, characterized by complications that impair quality of life in the short and long term. Despite its prevalence, cases of child sexual abuse represent only the tip of the iceberg, often concealed either intentionally or unintentionally by children (Emül et al., 2023). Moreover, this situation paves the way for new forms of abuse and child sexual exploitation (Finkelhor, Turner, and Colburn, 2022). Particularly with the widespread use of the Internet, digital platforms are becoming a common means for children to explore sexuality with their peers (WeProtect, 2021). A study shows that there has been a significant increase in the number of children receiving sexually explicit messages on the Internet (Aslan ve Karakuş-Yılmaz, 2021). Following the six-session training delivered to fifth-grade students, it has been observed that there has been a significant positive difference in knowledge of sexual abuse prevention and self-protective behaviors (Kang et al., 2022). Considering this, it is extremely critical to implement school-based child sexual abuse prevention programs (Lu et al., 2023).

Child sexual abuse is generally a developmental and sudden traumatic stress-inducing crisis that often develops and unfolds unexpectedly for families (Yıldırım, 2016). The legal procedures for abuse victims begin upon the detection or suspicion of abuse and the reporting of the crime committed or suspected to have been committed. The report is filed directly with the security forces by the child, their family, a relative, or other persons suspecting abuse (MFSPP, 2024). Once the abuse is revealed, a planned period of change begins with the child. The expert's observations and assessments of the child's sexual health and educational information regarding the child's age are important. This assessment is also necessary to understand the child's vulnerability to abuse and to determine the scope of the activity for the child and the family (Barut-Bektaş, 2024).

Conclusion

Many parents express feelings of inadequacy when it comes to initiating sexual communication with their children. For this reason, workshops, trainings, or seminars may be organized in cooperation with universities for parents on key aspects to be considered when talking to children about sexuality. In schools, on the other hand, comprehensive sexual health education must be provided by qualified teachers and school nurses to provide children and parents with the proper information and develop the skills they need. Furthermore, educational interventions and prevention activities targeting risky sexual behaviors should be included in classroom and school programs.

School nurses are required to know and understand the signs of sexual abuse and preventive factors, gather a thorough story, and evaluate the child based on their current health status. This is necessary to stop child sexual abuse, recover from the negative consequences, and address its long-term effects. Children with intellectual disabilities are particularly at risk, as they may not be aware of or report the abuse in a negative situation.

Each school needs a professional school nurse every day to optimize the health, safety, and learning of children and their families. The school nurse protects and promotes student health, facilitates optimal development, and improves academic achievement.

Disclaimer

None.

References

Alkan-Ersoy, Ö. (2014). Cinsel gelişimle ilgili temel kavramlar ve okul öncesi dönemde cinsel eğitim [Basic concepts related to sexual development and sexual education in preschool period]. In İ. Artan (Ed.), *Her yönüyle okul öncesi eğitim-9* [*Preschool education in all aspects-9*] (1st ed., pp. 281-301). Hedef CS Basın Yayın.

American Academy of Pediatrics (AAP). (2024). *Human Papillomavirus vaccines.* https://www.aap.org/en/patient-care/immunizations/human-papillomavirus-vaccines/ Accessed 20 February 2024.

Aral, N., Deleş, B. (2024). Anne babaların çocuklarıyla kurdukları cinsel iletişim düzeyleri ile tutumları arasındaki ilişkinin incelenmesi [Investigation of the relationship between parents' sexual communication levels with their children and their attitudes]. *Hacettepe University Faculty of Health Sciences Journal*, 11(1), 73-88. https://doi.org/10.21020/husbfd.1070956.

Arslan, A. (2022). Erken çocukluk döneminde çocuğun gelişiminin desteklenmesinde aile [Family's role in supporting children's development in early childhood]. *Gümüşhane Üniversitesi Sağlık Bilimleri Dergisi Gümüşhane-University Journal of Health Sciences*, 11(4), 1676-1684.

Artan, İ. (2014). Okul öncesi dönemde cinsel sorunlar [Sexual issues in preschool period]. In İ. Artan (Ed.), *Her yönüyle okul öncesi eğitim-9* [Preschool education in all aspects-9] (1st ed., pp. 303-317). Hedef CS Basın Yayın.

Artan, İ. (2017). Cinsel gelişim ve eğitim [Sexual development and education]. In İ. Artan (Ed.), *Doğum öncesinden ergenliğe çocuk gelişimi* [Child development from prenatal to adolescence] (2nd ed., pp. 198-262). Pegem Akademi Yayıncılık.

Aslan, A., Karakuş-Yılmaz, T. (2017). Türkiye'de güvenli internet kullanımına yönelik gerçekleştirilen uygulamalar [Implementations for safe internet usage in Turkey]. *Dumlupınar University Journal of Social Science/Dumlupınar Üniversitesi Sosyal Bilimler Dergisi*, (53), 121-143.

Ministry of Family and Social Policies Publication (MFSPP). (2024). *Abuse prevention guide for personnel working in child care institutions. Ministry of Family and Social Policies Publication.* No:07. https://www.aile.gov.tr/media/2499/cocuk-bakim-kuruluslarinda-calisan-personele-yonelik-istismarla-mucadele-rehber-kitapcigi.pdf.

Aycan, İ. B., Hassamancıoğlu, U., Arslan, Z. G., Kurnaz, F. B., Ceylan, Ş., & Artan, İ. (2023). Erken çocukluk döneminde cinsel gelişimle ilgili öğretmen ve ebeveyn görüşlerinin değerlendirilmesi [Evaluation of teachers' and parents' views on sexual development in early childhood]. *Uluslararası V. Çocuk Gelişimi Kongresi* [*International 5th Child Development Congress*], Ankara. S003, 12-23.

Bakır, N., Irmak Vural, P., Demir, C. (2019). Üniversite öğrencilerinin cinsel eğitime yönelik tutumları ve toplumsal cinsiyet algılarının bazı değişkenler açısından incelenmesi [Examination of university students' attitudes towards sexual education and their gender perceptions in terms of certain variables]. *Yaşam Becerileri Psikoloji Dergisi* [*Life Skills Psychology Journal*], 3(5), 119–128. https://doi.org/10.31461/ybpd.548926.

Baran, B., Kaptanoğlu, Ş. N., Esen, E., Siyez, D. M. (2020). Reproductive system augmented reality application for sexual health classes. *International Journal of Sexual Health*, 32(4), 408–420.

Barut-Bektaş, B. (2024). Unspoken agenda of the digital age: Online child sexual abuse. *Journal of Medical Social Work*, (22), 83-106. https://doi.org/10.46218/tshd.1348555.

Bergström, A., Ugarte Guevara, W. J., Eustachio Colombo, P. (2018). Knowledge about sexual and reproductive health among school-enrolled adolescents in Tololar, Nicaragua: A cross-sectional study. *Journal of Public Health International*, 1(2), 27-38.

Borneskog, C., Häggström-Nordin, E., Stenhammar, C., Tydén, T., & Iliadis, S. I. (2021). Changes in sexual behavior among high-school students over a 40-year period. *Scientific Reports*, 11(1), 13963. https://doi.org/10.1038/s41598-021-93410-6.

Borawski, E. A., Tufts, K. A., Trapl, E. S., Hayman, L. L., Yoder, L. D., & Lovegreen, L. D. (2015). Effectiveness of health education teachers and school nurses teaching sexually transmitted infections/human immunodeficiency virus prevention knowledge and skills in high school. *Journal of School Health*, 85(3), 189-196. https://doi.org/10.1111/josh.12234.

Büber, Ö., Alsancak, F., Kara, H. Z., Oksal, H. (2024). Uygulama deneyimleri ışığında çocuk izlem merkezlerinin işlevselliği [Functionality of child monitoring centers in light of practical experiences]. *Türkiye Adalet Akademisi Dergisi* [*Turkish Justice Academy Journal*], (57), 169-196. https://doi.org/10.54049/taad.1418211.

CDC. (2024a). Sexual health education. *https://www.cdc.gov/healthyyouth/whatworks/what-works-sexual-health-education.htm* Accessed 2 February 2024.

CDC. (2024b). Developing a scope and sequence for sexual health education. *https://www.cdc.gov/healthyyouth/hecat/pdf/scope_and_sequence.pdf* Accessed 8 March 2024.

CDC. (2019). Youth Risk Behavior Surveillance System (YRBSS). *https://www.cdc.gov/healthyyouth/data/yrbs/index.htm* Accessed 8 March 2024.

Ceylan, Ş., Artan, İ., Kurnaz, F. B. (2020). Attitude scale towards sexual education: A reliability and validity study. Education for Life, 34(2), 468–490. https://doi.org/10.33308/26674874.2020342210.

Council of School Healht (COSH). (2023). COSH principles. https://www.aap.org/en/community/aap-councils/council-on-school-health/about-cosh/ Accessed 2 March 2024.

Çakmak, S., Çakmak, S. (2011). Sexual education practices for children with special needs. Vize Yayıncılık.

DesOrmeaux, C. N. (2019). School health. In M. A. Nies & M. McEwen (Eds.), *Community/public health nursing: Promoting the health of populations* (pp. 1270-1305). Elsevier.

Dicle, A. N. (2020). Cinsel etik ve cinsellikle ilgili yasal konular [Sexual ethics and legal issues related to sexuality]. In E. Kurtman H. Kumcağız (Eds.), *Cinsel sağlık eğitimi* [Sexual health education] (2nd ed.). Pegem Yayınevi.

Emül, E., Özerdoğan, N., Kiliç, K. N. (2023). Çocukluk çağı cinsel istismarının belirtileri, açığa çıkarılmasının önündeki engeller [Signs of childhood sexual abuse and barriers to disclosure]. *Selçuk Sağlık Dergisi* [Selçuk Journal of Health], 4(3), 520-538.

Erenoğlu, R., Bayraktar, E. (2017). Hemşirelik bölümü öğrencilerinin cinsel tutumları ve etki eden faktörler [Sexual attitudes and influencing factors of nursing students]. *Journal of Human Sciences*, 14(2), 1745-1756.

Erkin, Ö., Kılınç, E. (2021). School health nursing. In Ö. Erkin, A. Kalkım, & İ. Göl (Eds.), *Public health nursing.* (pp. 915-1952). Çukurova Nobel Kitapevi.

Evcili, F., Gölbaşı, Z. (2017). Sexual health knowledge test: Development, validity, and reliability. *ACU Journal of Health Sciences,* 1, 29-33.

Fantaye, A. W., Buh, A. W., Idriss-Wheeler, D., Fournier, K., Yaya, S. (2020). Effective educational interventions for the promotion of sexual and reproductive health and rights for school-age children in low- and middle-income countries: A systematic review protocol. *Systematic Reviews*, 9(1), 216. https://doi.org/10.1186/s13643-020-01464-w.

Finkelhor, D., Turner, H., Colburn, D. (2022). Prevalence of online sexual offenses against children in the US. *JAMA Network Open*, 5(10), e2234471-e2234471.

Fowler, L. R., Schoen, L., Smith, H. S., & Morain, S. R. (2022). Sex education on TikTok: A content analysis of themes. *Health Promotion Practice*, 23(5), 739-742. https://doi.org/10.1177/15248399211031536.

Gonzalez, D., Bethencourt Mirabal, A., McCall, J. D. (2023). Child abuse and neglect. In *StatPearls*. StatPearls Publishing. https://www.ncbi.nlm.nih.gov/books/NBK29083602/.

Gökçay, G., Çevirme, A. (2022). Knowledge of students at health-related departments about sexual health and related factors. *Sağlık ve Spor Bilimleri Teknolojileri Dergisi* [Journal of Health and Sport Sciences], 45, 1-19.

Gültürk, E., Akpınar, A., Şen, Ş. R., Balcı, H. (2018). Cinselliğin değerlendirilmesi: Hemşirelerin cinsellikle ilgili tutum ve inançları [Evaluation of sexuality: Nurses' attitudes and beliefs about sexuality]. *İstanbul Bilim Üniversitesi Florence Nightingale Tıp Dergisi* [Istanbul Science University Florence Nightingale Medical Journal], 4(1), 63-70.

Gürsoy, E., & Gençalp, N. S. (2010). Importance of sexual health education. *Family and Society*, 6(23), 29-36.

Kang, S. R., Kim, S. J., & Kang, K. A. (2022). Effects of child sexual abuse prevention education program using hybrid application (CSAPE-H) on fifth-grade students in South Korea. *The Journal of School Nursing*, 38(4), 368-379. https://doi.org/10.1177/1059840520940377.

Kolbe, L. J. (2019). School health as a strategy to improve both public health and education. *Annual Review of Public Health*, 40, 443–463. https://doi.org/10.1146/annurev-publhealth-040218-043727.

Lu, M., Barlow, J., Meinck, F., & Neelakantan, L. (2023). Unpacking school-based child sexual abuse prevention programs: A realist review. *Trauma, Violence & Abuse*, 24(4), 2067-2081. https://doi.org/10.1177/15248380221082153.

Melesse, D. Y., Mutua, M. K., Choudhury, A., Wado, Y. D., Faye, C. M., Neal, S., & Boerma, T. (2020). Adolescent sexual and reproductive health in sub-Saharan Africa: Who is left behind? *BMJ Global Health*, 5(1), e002231. https://doi.org/10.1136/bmjgh-2019-002231.

National Student Nurses' Association (NANS). (2024a). Strategic Plan 2022-2026, Core value. https://www.nasn.org/about-nasn/about. Accessed 5 February 2024.

NANS. (2024b). Introduction and purpose of the toolkit. *https://learn.nasn.org/courses/41997.* Accessed 6 March 2024.

Nelson, B., Odberg Pettersson, K., & Emmelin, M. (2020). Experiences of teaching sexual and reproductive health to students with intellectual disabilities. *Sex Education*, 20(4), 398-412. https://doi.org/10.1080/14681811.2019.1707652.

Özkan, H., & Üst Taşgın, Z. D. (2020). Comparison of sexual health knowledge levels of students who received and did not receive sexual education. *Journal of Midwifery and Health Sciences*, 3(1), 11-21.

Özüdoğru, B., & Duran, B. N. (2023). Violence phenomenon and solution searches from different disciplines. In B. Özüdoğru & B. Duran (Eds.), Ondokuz Mayıs University Publications, (p. 338).

Ross, M. W., Bayer, C. R., Shindel, A., & Coleman, E. (2021). Evaluating the impact of a medical school cohort sexual health course on knowledge, counseling skills, and sexual attitude change. *BMC Medical Education*, 21, 37. https://doi.org/10.1186/s12909-020-02482-x.

Saranlı, A. G. (2014). Cinsel gelişim teorileri [Theories of sexual development]. In İ. Artan (Ed.), *Her yönüyle okul öncesi eğitim-9* [Preschool education in all aspects-9] (1st ed., pp. 303-317). Hedef CS Basın Yayın.

Saranlı, A. G. (2020). Cinsel gelişim teorileri [Theories of sexual development]. In İ. Artan (Ed.), *Cinsel gelişim ve eğitim* [Sexual development and education] (pp. 31-45). Hedef CS Basın Yayın.

Sexuality Information and Education Council of the United States. (SIECUS). (2018). *Guidelines for comprehensive sexuality education* (1-3rd ed.). Fulton Press. *https://siecus.org/wp-content/uploads/2018/07/Guidelines-CSE.pdf.*

Stein, S., Kohut, T., & Dillenburger, K. (2018). The importance of sexuality education for children with and without intellectual disabilities: What parents think. *Sexuality and Disability*, 36(2), 141–148. https://doi.org/10.1007/s11195-017-9513-9.

Şahin, S. (2014). Uzman görüşü, okul öncesi dönemde cinsel sorunlar [Expert opinion on sexual issues in the preschool period]. In İ. Artan (Ed.), *Her yönüyle okul öncesi eğitim-9* [Preschool education in all aspects-9] (1st ed., pp. 347-349). Hedef CS Basın Yayın.

Tasa, H., & Namatoğu, M. (2018). Engelli bireylere yönelik tutum değişimi ve duyarlılık eğitimleri [Attitude change and sensitivity training for individuals with disabilities]. *Türkiye Klinikleri Journal of Psychology-Special Topics* [*Turkish Clinics Journal of Psychology-Special Topics*], 3(1), 1-21.

Tessier, R., Charpak, N., Giron, M., Cristo, M., de Calume, Z. F., & Ruiz-Peláez, J. G. (2009). Kangaroo mother care, home environment, and father involvement in the first year of life: A randomized controlled study. *Acta Paediatrica*, 98(9), 1444-1450. https://doi.org/10.1111/j.1651-2227.2009.01370.x.

Treacy, A., Taylor, S., & Abernathy, T. (2018). Sexual health education for individuals with disabilities: A call to action. *American Journal of Sexuality Education*, 13(1), 65-93. https://doi.org/10.1080/15546128.2017.1399492.

Tuncer, B. (2023). Sosyal gelişim [Social development]. In A. Kızılkaya-Namlı (Ed.), *Eğitimin kavramsal temelleri eğitim psikolojisi* [Conceptual foundations of education: Educational psychology] (pp. 115-132). Efe Akademik Yayıncılık.

UNESCO. (2015). *Sexuality education*. https://en.unesco.org/themes/health-education/hiv-sexuality-education. Accessed 1 February 2024.

UNESCO. (2018). *International technical guidance on sexuality education: An evidence-informed approach* (2018–260770eng.pdf). https://unesdoc.unesco.org/ark:/48223/pf0000260770. Accessed 5 February 2024.

Ünal-Toprak, & Turan, Z. (2021). The effect of sexual health courses on the level of nursing students' sexual/reproductive health knowledge and sexual myths beliefs in Turkey: A pretest-posttest control group design. *Perspectives in Psychiatric Care*, 57, 667–674.

Üstgörül, S., Önür, H., & Tekin-Önür, H. (2020). Üniversite öğrencilerinin toplumsal cinsiyet algıları ile cinsel tutumlarının incelenmesi [Examination of university students' gender perceptions and sexual attitudes]. *Al-Farabi International Journal on Social Sciences*, 5(3), 77-87. https://doi.org/10.46291/Al-Farabi.050308.

WePROTECT Global Alliance. (2021). *Global Threat Assessment. https://www.weprotect.org/global-threat-assessment-21/#report.* Accessed 10 December 2024.

World Health Organization (WHO). (2010). *Developing sexual health programmes: A framework for action. https://healtheducationresources.unesco.org/library/documents/developing-sexual-health-programmes-framework-action.* Accessed 3 February 2024.

WHO & BZgA. (2010). *Standards for sexuality education in Europe.* Federal Centre for Health Education, BZgA Cologne. *https://www.bzga-whocc.de/en/publications/standards-for-sexuality-education/* Accessed 5 February 2024.

WHO. (2021). *Global school-based student health survey (GSHS)*. https://www.who.int/teams/noncommunicable-diseases/surveillance/systems-tools/global-school-based-student-health-survey/questionnaire. Accessed 15 January 2024.

WHO. (2022). *Child maltreatment*. https://www.who.int/news-room/factsheets/detail/child-maltreatment.

Yalın, A., & Alabay, E. (2024). Examination of the relationship between parents' sexual communication skills and gender justice. *Istanbul Gelişim University Journal of Health Sciences*, (21), 1077-1096. https://doi.org/10.38079/igusabder.1323134.

Yıldırım, Ş. (2016). Crisis intervention approach in social work. *Celal Bayar University Journal of Health Sciences Institute*, 3(4), 481-486.

Young, H., Burke, L., & Nic Gabhainn, S. (2018). Sexual intercourse, age of initiation and contraception among adolescents in Ireland: Findings from the Health Behaviour in School-aged Children (HBSC) Ireland study. *BMC Public Health*, 18(1), 362. https://doi.org/10.1186/s12889-018-5217-z.

Chapter 5

Mental Health in School-Age Children

İlknur Mizrahi[*], PhD
Istanbul Medipol University, Faculty of Health Sciences, Nursing Department, İstanbul, Türkiye

Abstract

Mental health is a significant factor in the well-being of school-age children. Mental health effects go beyond academics by influencing school-age children's social connections, emotional strength, and overall quality of life. Understanding the importance of mental health as a key part of the overall well-being of school-aged children is crucial. This chapter highlights the importance of school-based health interventions, including emotional learning programs, counseling services, peer support groups, and health education integration. Additionally, it emphasizes the vital role of school nurses in advocating for mental health through their responsibilities, interventions, and contributions to creating supportive environments for school-age children. Furthermore, the chapter explores evidence-based strategies such as cognitive behavioral therapy, mindfulness programs, and peer support activities to enhance well-being in schools. As a result, mental health needs to be prioritized so that school-age children can become successful, resilient and happy individuals.

Keywords: school health, school-age children, mental health, health interventions

Introduction

Mental health is a key factor in the well-being of individuals during childhood and adolescence (Fazel et al., 2018). In recent years, the importance of mental health in school-age children has become increasingly recognized, as it affects their social interactions, well-being and overall development (Lyon et al., 2021b). Numerous studies have consistently shown the relationship between mental health and academic success, showing how emotional well-being greatly affects cognitive abilities, learning outcomes, and engagement in school activities (Lyon et al., 2021b; Klapp, Klapp, and Gustafsson, 2024). Furthermore, health effects go beyond academics by influencing school-age children's social connections, emotional strength, and overall quality

* Corresponding Author's Email: Ilknur.Yalcin@unilever.com

In: Health Promotion and Prevention
Editor: Eda Kılınç İşleyen
ISBN: 979-8-89530-758-8

of life. Addressing health issues among school-age children is crucial not only for enhancing academic achievements but also for nurturing positive socio-emotional growth and preventing long-term challenges (Fazel et al., 2018).

Moreover, overlooking the mental well-being of school-age children can have long-term negative effects on their overall health into adulthood (Rones & Hoagwood 2018). Early detection and intervention are crucial in preventing mental health issues in students (Fergusson et al., 2021). Addressing mental health issues in schools allows educators, mental health professionals, school nurses, and policymakers to create supportive environments that promote the well-being and development of school-age children (Brennan et al., 2019).

In essence, recognizing mental health as a crucial aspect of overall well-being has led to an increased focus on its importance in the lives of school-age children. Understanding and addressing mental health challenges in school-age children are vital for promoting healthy growth, improving academic achievements, and lessening long-term difficulties.

Understanding Mental Health in School-Age Children: Definition and Conceptualization of Mental Health

To understand the well-being of school-age children, it is crucial to define and outline its conceptual framework. Mental health in this context covers a range of factors, including emotions, psychology, and social connections (American Academy of Pediatrics, 2018; Patel et al., 2018). This definition highlights how different aspects of children's lives, including their emotions, thoughts, and social engagements, contribute to their mental health.

As mentioned by the American Academy of Pediatrics in 2018, mental well-being in school-age children go beyond not having identifiable mental illnesses. Mental well-being involves managing emotions, coping with challenges, and building positive relationships within the school environment. Studies that highlight the significance of resilience and coping strategies support this perspective on the mental well-being of school-age children (Shoshani and Steinmetz, 2021; Forman-Hoffman et al., 2019). Furthermore, the National Institute of Mental Health (2020) underscores that mental health plays a vital role in helping children navigate everyday complexities and engage meaningfully with others (National Institute of Mental Health, 2020). This emphasizes the need to consider both school-age children's unique characteristics and their environment when addressing health issues in school-aged children (Chang and Lengua 2018).

School-age children require a comprehensive approach to mental well-being that integrates emotional, psychological, and social factors. Teachers, mental health professionals, and nurses can develop interventions and support plans to enhance school-age children's well-being within the school setting.

Mental Health Promotion in Schools

Importance of Mental Health Promotion in School Settings

The significance of promoting well-being in school environments goes beyond addressing individual issues. It involves creating a supportive environment that promotes the overall well-being of all school-age children (Weare and Nind, 2018). Studies consistently show the effects of promoting mental health on school-age children's academic performance, behavior, and prospects (Patel et al., 2018). By giving importance to health promotion, schools can establish a strong foundation for success that reaches beyond the confines of the classroom.

Approaches to Enhancing Mental Health in Schools

Enhancing well-being within school settings requires implementing various strategies focused on fostering school-age children's social and emotional welfare. An effective method is to introduce social and emotional learning (SEL) programs designed to improve school-age children's abilities in areas such as self-awareness, self-regulation, empathy, interpersonal skills, and decision-making (Greenberg et al., 2019). Research suggests that engaging in SEL programs enhances school-age children's social and emotional skills while also reducing issues and emotional challenges (Durlak et al., 2011).

Counseling services in schools are an important way to support mental health. These services provide school-age children with a private place to address various mental health issues, such as stress, anxiety, depression, and conflicts with others (Gloppen et al., 2019). Research has shown that having access to counseling services at school is linked to academic performance, higher attendance rates, and improved emotional well-being for school-age children (Sink et al., 2015). Building peer networks is also crucial to promoting mental health within schools. Programs that provide peer support, such as mentoring or counseling, offer school-age children the opportunity to connect with their classmates, receive assistance, and develop positive relationships (Schwartz et al., 2016). Studies indicate that these peer support programs enhance school-age children' social connections, self-esteem, and mental well-being (Schwartz et al., 2016).

Moreover, incorporating health education lessons into the school curriculum can increase students' understanding of mental health issues, reduce the stigma, and encourage seeking help when necessary (Werner Seidler et al., 2017). By integrating health topics into lessons or offering dedicated mental health courses, schools can provide school-age children with support needed to navigate difficulties and prioritize their own well-being. Additionally, establishing a culture of acceptance and inclusivity in schools is crucial for advancing mental health awareness and reducing the stigma associated with mental illness (Werner Seidler et al., 2017). Teachers and nurses can create supportive environments by enforcing anti-bullying policies, advocating for diversity and equality, and conducting education sessions for school-age children on mental health-related subjects.

In summarize, promoting mental well-being in schools requires a holistic approach, including emotional intelligence development, counseling services, peer support programs, mental health education, and fostering an inclusive and accepting environment. By implementing these strategies, schools can create environments that address the mental health needs of school-age children.

The Role of School Nurses in Advocating Mental Health

School-age children face a range of challenges that can affect their mental well-being. These challenges may stem from pressures, interpersonal relationships with peers, family dynamics, or societal expectations (National Institute of Mental Health, 2020). School nurses are valuable members of the interdisciplinary team dedicated to enhancing mental well-being of school-age children (NASN, 2017; Neil and Christensen, 2019).

The role of school nurses in advocating for mental health is crucial, as they are often the first point of contact for school-age children facing emotional, behavioral, or psychological challenges. School nurses are in a unique position to identify early signs of mental health issues and provide the necessary support, whether through direct intervention, referrals, or coordination with other school staff. School nurses can recognize the physical symptoms that may indicate mental health struggles, such as headaches, stomachaches, sleep disturbances, and behavioral changes. Additionally, they can spot signs of anxiety, depression, or bullying, which makes timely intervention even more important. Below are the responsibilities of school nurses in promoting the mental health of school-age children.

Responsibilities of School Nurses

School nurses carry out a range of tasks with the goal of enhancing the mental well-being of school-aged children. These tasks include;

1. Providing health education: School nurses educate school-age children, families, and school staff on stress management, coping strategies and the importance of seeking help for mental health issues (Cameron et al., 2022).
2. Conducting screening and assessment: School nurses conduct screenings and assessments to identify school-age children at risk of mental health challenges. They use tools to evaluate students' emotional and behavioral well-being, recognize early signs of mental disorders, and facilitate prompt referrals for further assessment and support (McCarthy et al., 2020).
3. Developing individualized care plans: School nurses collaborate with school-age children, families, teachers, and mental health professionals to develop care plans for school-age children with mental health needs. These plans outline strategies for managing health concerns issues, accessing support services, and enhancing overall well-being in school settings (Watts et al., 2019).
4. Crisis management: In crisis or urgent situations, school nurses provide immediate support through counseling, crisis management, and referrals, ensuring the safety and well-being of school-age children facing mental health challenges (National Association of School Nurses, 2017).

5. Ensuring collaboration: School nurses collaborate with school staff, teachers, mental health professionals, and community organizations to advocate for policies that enhance health and well-being in school settings. School nurses collaborate in teams, attend meetings, and advocate for resources and services to meet students' mental health needs (Bradshaw et al., 2021b).

School Nurses' Interventions for Mental Health Promotion

School nurses employ a range of strategies to promote well-being and prevent mental health issues in school-age children. These strategies include;

1. Building resilience: School nurses promote resilience in school-age children by emphasizing factors such as social support, problem-solving abilities, and positive coping mechanisms. They organize activities, workshops, and groups designed to strengthen students' effectively overcome challenges.
2. Stress management techniques: School nurses educate school-age children on techniques to reduce stress, including breathing exercises, mindfulness practices, and relaxation methods. These education assist school-age children cope with stress, anxiety, and emotional challenges, and ultimately improve their health.
3. Peer support interventions: School nurses organize programs that encourage peers to support each other during times of health challenges. Through these initiatives, school-age children feel a sense of belonging, decrease isolation, and cultivate positive connections with their peers.
4. Parental involvement in mental health education: School nurses play a role in establishing positive environments within schools that promote mental health and well-being for all school-age children. School nurses actively engage parents and caregivers in mental well-being and support programs. School nurses provide support, and guidance on strengthening collaboration between families and school staff to support students' well-being (Brennan et al., 2019). Their efforts involve;

Establishing safe areas: School nurses create private areas where school-age children can discuss their mental health concerns openly, without fear of judgment or stigma. They build relationships with school-age children, acting as a supportive presence within the school community (Atkins et al., 2019).

Promoting mental health awareness: School nurses advocate for increasing awareness of health concerns and reducing stigma within the school environment. They coordinate campaigns, events, and interventions to enhance understanding, acceptance, and compassion toward individuals facing health concerns (Levitt et al., 2007).

Providing education and skill development: School nurses organize education sessions and capacity-building programs for school staff mental health promotion and intervention. They empower educators with the knowledge, skills, and tools to effectively address students' mental health needs (Greenberg et al., 2019). In summary, school nurses play a crucial role in promoting mental health and well-being among school-age children. Their roles, actions, and impact help create environments that support students' mental health and contribute to their academic success. Through collaboration with stakeholders and the use of evidence-based practices, school nurses play a key role in fostering a culture of mental health and resilience within schools.

5. The involvement of stakeholders: Promoting mental health in schools requires collaboration among various stakeholders, such as school nurses, teachers, parents, and the wider community (Lyon et al., 2019). Teachers are crucial in identifying signs of distress and providing support to school-age children, while parents can reinforce positive behaviors and facilitate open discussions about mental well-being (Bear et al., 2019). Involving the community through partnerships with health organizations and local agencies further enriches the resources available to support students' welfare (Wyman et al., 2018).

School-Based Interventions for Mental Health

Given the increasing awareness of health issues among school-aged children, various evidence-based interventions have been developed to address these concerns effectively. These interventions cover methods from specific treatments for disorders such as anxiety and depression to broader strategies that focus on building resilience and improving coping skills (Weisz et al., 2017; Merry et al., 2023). Among these approaches, cognitive behavioral therapy (CBT) is widely recognized and scientifically supported method to address different mental health challenges in school-aged children (Neil and Christensen 2019). Based on restructuring and behavioral changes, CBT equips children with practical tools to recognize negative thoughts, and adopt healthy coping mechanisms (Flessner et al., 2021). Studies show that implementing CBT in school environments leads to enhancements in anxiety, depression symptoms, enhancing children's mental well-being (Neil and Christensen, 2019; Tully et al., 2022).

Mindfulness-based programs are implemented in schools to support and enhance children's mental health. These programs emphasize practices that encourage individuals to become more aware of the present moment and accept their thoughts and feelings without judgment. These programs usually include organized mindfulness activities like meditation and mindful breathing, aiming to boost self-control, stress management, and emotional strength in children. Studies indicate that implementing interventions in school environments can reduce anxiety and depression symptoms while enhancing attention control and overall mental well-being.

Additionally, peer support interventions contribute to school-based mental health efforts by utilizing peer relationships to strengthen social connections, empathy, and emotional support among children. These initiatives often consist of peer mentoring schemes, peer support groups, or buddy systems where peers offer each other encouragement, validation, and help in dealing with various challenges. Studies have shown that peer support programs can have an effect on children's emotional well-being, self-confidence, and overall mental health. This suggests that incorporating interventions into school mental health frameworks could be beneficial (Rose et al., 2021; Neil and Christensen, 2019). In essence, evidence-based mental health interventions in schools encompass a variety of approaches, ranging from individualized therapies to broad prevention interventions. By implementing these interventions in schools, teachers and mental health professionals can better address the varied needs of school-aged children, fostering resilience, enhancing well-being, and reducing the negative impact of mental health challenges on academic and social performance.

Case Studies of Successful School-Based Interventions

Multiple case studies highlight how interventions implemented in schools can positively impact the well-being of school-age children. For example, a study by Johnson et al., in 2021 at a school showed the positive effects of implementing a mindfulness program for school-age children. In this study, by integrating mindfulness techniques into the school curriculum, school-age children developed skills to stay present and manage effectively (Johnson et al., 2021). The study showed decreases in anxiety levels and improvements in overall psychological health among the participants, highlighting the potential of mindfulness-based approaches to address mental health concerns in school-age children.

In this vein, Bradshaw et al., (2018) conducted research on school-wide intervention promoting positive behavior support, which showed promising results in terms of behavior outcomes and academic performance. By creating a supportive school environment that promoted positive behaviors and used proactive strategies to address challenges, the intervention resulted in a significant reduction in disciplinary incidents and increased student engagement in learning activities. These findings underscore the significance of creating a school atmosphere conducive to enhancing both social-emotional well-being and academic achievements, for school-age children.

Furthermore, a study by Smith and Jones (2023) supports the idea that mindfulness programs in schools can help reduce anxiety and improve children's mental well-being (Smith and Jones, 2023). Their research, conducted in primary schools, showed that students who participated in mindfulness sessions had lower anxiety levels and better emotional control than those who did not participate. These results highlight the importance of incorporating mindfulness techniques into school environments to support students' mental health needs.

In conclusion, these case studies stress the significance of using evidence-based strategies in schools to promote children's health and well-being. By implementing interventions like mindfulness programs and positive behavior support, educators and mental health professionals can create environments that foster the optimal growth and success of all school-age children.

Challenges and Limitations of School-Based Interventions

While school health interventions show promise in aiding students' well-being, they face various challenges that affect their effectiveness and sustainability. One major hurdle is the limited resources available, which often hinder the implementation of comprehensive intervention programs within school settings (Langley et al., 2010).

Insufficient funding allocated to health services in schools, including resources, personnel, and training, hinders the ability of schools to effectively meet the diverse needs of school-age children. Additionally, the lack of training for school staff poses a significant obstacle to successfully implementing mental health interventions (Langley et al., 2010). Educators and support staff may need training in evidence-based practices to deliver interventions with accuracy and skill. Without training and continuing professional development opportunities, school personnel may find it challenging to effectively assist school-age children with their mental health needs and execute intervention strategies correctly.

Another issue lies in reaching marginalized populations within school communities (Langley et al., 2010). Students from marginalized backgrounds, such as those from low-income families, ethnic minority groups, and non-native English speakers, may encounter obstacles in accessing mental health support services. Addressing the needs and cultural considerations of these populations requires specific outreach efforts and culturally sensitive approaches to intervention delivery.

Furthermore, maintaining the impact of interventions over time remains a challenge for schools and practitioners (Forman Hoffman et al., 2019). While initial progress may be made after implementing interventions sustaining long-term improvements, mental health outcomes necessitate monitoring, support, and reinforcement.

Without dedication and investment, the positive effects of interventions may fade over time, diminishing their long-term impact on students' well-being. Ensuring that program guidelines are consistently followed presents a significant challenge when implementing mental health interventions in schools (Forman-Hoffman et al., 2019). Variations in how practitioners and different settings adhere to these guidelines can undermine the reliability, as well as the uniformity of intervention delivery. Maintaining fidelity requires providing supervision, feedback, and quality control measures to uphold the integrity of intervention programs and to enhance their impact on student outcomes.

In conclusion, while school-based interventions hold promise for improving students' mental health, they encounter obstacles and constraints that require attention. Overcoming these challenges—such as securing sufficient resources, meeting training requirements for marginalized groups, addressing sustainability concerns, and ensuring adherence to program guidelines—is essential for enhancing the effectiveness and longevity of mental health interventions in educational settings.

Collaborative Approaches to School Mental Health

Effective mental health support in schools requires collaboration among school staff, mental health professionals, and other stakeholders (Atkins et al., 2019). This collaboration promotes a comprehensive approach that integrates resources, knowledge, expertise, and diverse perspectives to effectively address mental health needs (Levitt et al., 2007). Studies indicate that collaboration between schools and mental health professionals' benefits school-age children by enhancing their well-being and academic success. For example, partnerships facilitate the incorporation of mental health services into school settings, making it easier for students to access support, especially those facing barriers to care (Piscopo et al., 2021). By having health professionals present in schools, students can receive prompt evaluations, interventions, and continuous support tailored to their specific needs, leading to improved well-being and outcomes. Furthermore, collaboration empowers schools to benefit from the expertise of mental health professionals, such as psychologists, counselors, and social workers, to effectively address complex mental health issues. These professionals provide guidance, education, and direct services to students while also supporting teachers and staff in establishing a supportive and inclusive school environment (Atkins et al., 2019). Moreover, collaboration between school staff and health organizations ensures that school-age children receive coordinated care as they transition between school-based and community based services. This coordinated approach provides consistent support for school-age children and facilitates the implementation of evidence-based interventions across different settings (Levitt et al., 2007). School nurses are essential in this effort by providing hands-on care, educating on health topics, and promoting well-being within the school environment (National Association of School Nurses, 2017). School nurses collaborate with mental health professionals to identify students in need of support, and connect school-age children with appropriate community resources (Brennan et al., 2019). In summary, collaboration between school staff, mental health professionals, and school nurses is crucial in addressing the mental health needs of school-age children in educational settings.

Models of Collaboration for Promoting Mental Health in Schools

Collaboration strategies have been developed to support mental health interventions in schools, each with unique strengths and considerations. Key approaches include structured school health programs, multi-tiered support systems, and integrated care models. These approaches emphasize the importance of a coordinated strategy to address students' mental health needs (Adelman and Taylor 2019).

Organized school health models provide a structure for integrating various health promotion interventions within school, including those focused on mental health well-being. These models typically cover elements such as health education, physical activities, healthcare services, nutrition programs, counseling services, social environment, staff well-being, and involvement of families and communities (Centers for Disease Control and Prevention 2021). Additionally, these models enhance students' mental well-being by promoting collaboration between teachers, mental health professionals, and families.

Multi-tiered systems of support (MTSS) stand out established model for addressing students' mental health needs within educational settings. The MTSS is a system of supports and interventions aimed at identifying students with mental health issues and providing help to those at risk (Sugai and Horner 2009). MTSS helps schools identify and address students' mental health needs, through evidence-based practices.

Another model is integrated care models. Integrated care models, such as the collaborative care model, stress the importance of integrating health services into the broader healthcare system, including schools (Butler et al., 2008). These models promote cooperation among primary care providers, mental health professionals, educators, and other stakeholders to provide thorough and coordinated care to school-age children with mental health issues. Integrated care models improve communication and coordination across settings, ensuring early detection, timely support, and continuous care for school-age children facing mental health challenges.

In summary, collaborative models that promote well-being in schools emphasize the significance of a unified and systematic approach to addressing students' mental health needs. School nurses and mental health professionals can improve provide students' well-being by creating supportive environments through approaches such as MTSS, and integrated care models.

Examples of Successful Collaborative Interventions

Numerous successful collaborations underscore the positive impact of teamwork on the mental health of schools. A notable example is the collaboration between a school district and a local mental health center, as documented by Lyon et al., This collaboration increased students' access to counseling services leading to improved attendance and academic performance. Lyon et al., (2021a) discovered that students who received mental health counseling showed improvements in behavior and attendance, resulting in more involvement in school activities and better academic results. This collaboration demonstrates the effectiveness of integrating health services into schools to meet students' diverse needs and enhance their overall well-being (Lyon et al., 2021a).

Similarly, collaborations between schools, law enforcement, and community groups have produced results in addressing mental health issues among school-age children. For example, Bradshaw et al., (2021) demonstrated the effectiveness of collaborative efforts in addressing issues such as bullying and substance abuse in school communities. The study noticed improvements in students' sense of belonging to the school and their overall well-being (Bradshaw et al., 2021a). By involving different stakeholders, such as school staff, law enforcement, mental health professionals, parents, and community leaders, these interventions implemented comprehensive prevention strategies to create a safe and supportive school environment. These instances demonstrate the significance of collaboration among various groups in promoting mental health in schools. By building partnerships between schools, mental health facilities, law enforcement, community organizations, educators and health professionals can combine their knowledge and resources to comprehensively address students' health needs.

Recommendations for Policy, Practice, and Research

To progress health interventions in schools and improve emotional well-being support for school-age children, it is crucial for policymakers, practitioners, and researchers to collaborate and implement evidence-based policies and practices (Fazel et al., 2018). This collaborative effort should focus on key areas to effectively address students' mental health needs within the school setting. Firstly, policymakers should allocate funding for health services in schools to ensure adequate resources are available for the establishment and sustainability of comprehensive mental health programs (Domitrovich et al., 2021). This includes budgeting for hiring mental health professionals, providing training for school staff, and implementing evidence-based interventions that support students.' Secondly, enhancing training programs for educators and mental health professionals is vital in equipping them with the knowledge and skills to effectively assist students with their mental wellness (Fazel et al., 2018).

Additionally, there is a need for research to assess the impact of school-based interventions and guide evidence-backed practices (Domitrovich et al., 2021). Conducting studies can provide valuable insights into the impact of interventions on students' mental well-being. Moreover, addressing disparities in access to mental health resources is essential to ensure that all students can thrive at school. This involves tackling obstacles like stigma, cultural variations, and structural inequalities while implementing strategies for fairness and inclusivity within educational institutions (Forman Hoffman et al., 2020). By prioritizing these recommendations in policymaking, practical applications, and research efforts, stakeholders can collaborate to establish diverse school environments that focus on the well-being of every student.

Conclusion

In summary, supporting the well-being of school-age children is a multifaceted task that requires collaboration, creativity, and a strong dedication. Schools not only educate students but also play a crucial role in supporting their emotional and mental development. By focusing on health interventions for school staff, educators and stakeholders can establish environments that promote positive mental health outcomes for all school-age children. Research indicates that using evidence-based interventions can significantly impact students' mental health and success. Promoting health in schools involves creating a caring, inclusive school environment that values well-being and resilience.

School nurses are valuable members of the interdisciplinary team dedicated to enhancing the mental well-being of school-age children. School nurses employ a range of strategies to promote well-being and prevent mental health issues in school-age children. By integrating well-being lessons, offering mental health resources, and encouraging a sense of community, schools can create supportive environments where all students thrive. Essentially, prioritizing school-age children's mental health in schools is not only the right to do but also an investment in the future well-being of community. By addressing students' emotional needs alongside academic growth, schools can significantly impact the development of resilient, happy, and successful individuals.

Disclaimer

None.

References

Adelman, H. S., Taylor, L., Dwyer, K. P., & Mayer, M. J. (2019). Intersection of School Safety, Mental Health and Wellness, and Family and Community Issues. *Keeping Students Safe and Helping Them Thrive [2 volumes]: A Collaborative Handbook on School Safety, Mental Health, and Wellness* [2 volumes], 3.

Atkins, M. S., Frazier, S. L., Leathers, S. J., Graczyk, P. A., Talbott, E., Jakobsons, L., ... & Bell, C. C. (2019). Teacher key opinion leaders and mental health consultation in low-income urban schools. *Journal of Consulting and Clinical Psychology*, 87(2), 183-198.

Bradshaw, C. P., Waasdorp, T. E., Leaf, P. J., & Jenson, J. M. (2018). Effects of School-Wide Positive Behavioral Interventions and Supports on child behavior problems. *Pediatrics*, 140(2), e20163021.

Bradshaw, C. P., Johnson, S. L., Leaf, P. J., et al., (2021a). School partnerships with law enforcement: Lessons from a school-based bullying prevention program. *Journal of School Violence*, 20(1), 1-17.

Bradshaw, C. P., Waasdorp, T. E., Leaf, P. J., & Jenson, J. M. (2021b). Collaborative approaches to address bullying and substance abuse in schools: A systematic review. *School Psychology Review*, 50(1), 25-41.

Brennan, E. M., Bradley, K., Allen, D., & Perry, D. F. (2019). The role of the school nurse in addressing mental health in adolescents. *Journal of School Nursing*, 35(4), 253-260.

Butler, M., Kane, R. L., McAlpine, D., Kathol, R. G., Fu, S. S., Hagedorn, H., & Wilt, T. J. (2008). Integration of mental health/substance abuse and primary care (No. 173). *Agency for Healthcare Research and Quality.*

Centers for Disease Control and Prevention. (2021). *Coordinated school health.* Retrieved from https://www.cdc.gov/healthyschools/csh/index.htm.

Chang, L., & Lengua, L. J. (2018). Developmental cascades linking externalizing symptoms, internalizing symptoms, and academic competence in childhood. *Development and Psychopathology*, 30(2), 569-583.

Domitrovich, C. E., Bradshaw, C. P., Berg, J. K., Pas, E. T., Becker, K. D., Musci, R., ... & Frazier, S. L. (2021). How do school-based prevention programs impact teachers' mental health literacy? Results from a randomized controlled trial of the Good Behavior Game. *School Mental Health*, 13(3), 662-676.

Durlak, J. A., Weissberg, R. P., Dymnicki, A. B., Taylor, R. D., & Schellinger, K. B. (2011). The impact of enhancing students' social and emotional learning: A meta-analysis of school-based universal interventions. *Child Development*, 82(1), 405-432.

Fazel, M., Hoagwood, K., Stephan, S., & Ford, T. (2018). Mental health interventions in schools in high-income countries. *The Lancet Psychiatry*, 5(8), 738-748.

Fergusson, D. M., Boden, J. M., & Horwood, L. J. (2021). Childhood self-regulation and adult outcomes: Results from a 30-year longitudinal study. *Journal of the American Academy of Child & Adolescent Psychiatry*, 60(6), 746-754.

Flessner, C. A., Piacentini, J., Franklin, M. E., Keuthen, N. J., Moore, P. S., & Stein, D. J. (2021). Cognitive-behavioral therapy for pediatric obsessive-compulsive disorder: A meta-analysis. *Journal of Anxiety Disorders*, 86, 102483.

Forman-Hoffman, V. L., Kuklinski, M. R., Silverstein, M., et al., (2019). The role of schools in supporting mental health in children and adolescents. *Pediatrics*, 144(4), e20192758.

Gloppen, K. M., McDaniel, H. L., & Baruch, A. K. (2019). School-based mental health services: A review of clinical effectiveness. *School Mental Health*, 11(4), 707-727.

Greenberg, M. T., Brown, J. L., & Abenavoli, R. M. (2019). Teacher stress and health effects on teachers, students, and schools. *Applied Psychology: Health and Well-Being*, 11(1), 129-169.

Johnson, S. L., Burke, T. A., Taylor, S. K., et al., (2021). Mindfulness in schools: A randomized controlled trial of an online mindfulness intervention. *Mindfulness*, 12(1), 156-169.

Klapp, T., Klapp, A., & Gustafsson, J. E. (2024). Relations between students' well-being and academic achievement: evidence from Swedish compulsory school. *European Journal of Psychology of Education, 39*(1), 275-296.

Langley, A. K., Nadeem, E., Kataoka, S. H., Stein, B. D., & Jaycox, L. H. (2010). Evidence-based mental health programs in schools: Barriers and facilitators of successful implementation. *School mental health,* 2, 105-113.

Levitt, J. M., Saka, N., Romanelli, L. H., & Hoagwood, K. (2007). Early identification of mental health problems in schools: The status of instrumentation. *Journal of School Psychology*, 45(2), 163-191.

Lyon, A. R., Bruns, E. J., & Weathers, E. S. (2019). Can collaborative care be integrated into community-based services for youth? *Journal of Clinical Child & Adolescent Psychology*, 48(3), 366-378.

Lyon, A. R., Cook, C. R., Brown, E. C., et al., (2021a). Assessing the impact of a school district-university partnership in enhancing access to child and adolescent mental health services. *Journal of Clinical Child & Adolescent Psychology*, 50(1), 14-25.

Lyon, A. R., Whitaker, K., Ludwig, K., Hernandez, M., Stadnick, N., & McCauley, E. (2021b). The impact of school-based mental health services on academic outcomes: A systematic review. *School Mental Health,* 13(3), 509-524.

Merry, S. N., Hetrick, S. E., Cox, G. R., Brudevold-Iversen, T., Bir, J. J., & McDowell, H. (2023). Psychological and educational interventions for preventing depression in children and adolescents. *Cochrane Database of Systematic Reviews*, 2023(3), CD003380.

National Association of School Nurses (NASN). (2017). *Role of the school nurse in providing school health services.* Retrieved from https://www.nasn.org/advocacy/professional-practice-documents/position-statements/ps-role.

National Institute of Mental Health. (2020). *Child and adolescent mental health.* Retrieved from https://www.nimh.nih.gov/health/topics/child-and-adolescent-mental-health/index.shtml.

Neil, A. L., & Christensen, H. (2019). Efficacy and effectiveness of school-based prevention and early intervention programs for anxiety. *Clinical Psychology Review*, 70, 104-125.

Patel, V., Flisher, A. J., Hetrick, S., & McGorry, P. (2018). Mental health of young people: A global public-health challenge. *The Lancet,* 369(9569), 1302-1313.

Piscopo, K., Lipari, R., Cooney, J., et al., (2021). School-based mental health services: A comprehensive approach to serving students in need. *Children & Schools*, 43(1), 1-9.

Rones, M., & Hoagwood, K. (2018). School-based mental health services: A research review. *Clinical Child and Family Psychology Review*, 21(2), 233-250.

Schwartz, D., Kelly, B. M., Kim, B. K. E., Black, B. M., Goodrich, S., Gallion, K., & Godfrey, C. (2016). Effects of peer network interventions on adolescents' peer networks and mental health outcomes: A systematic review and meta-analysis. *Journal of Primary Prevention*, 37(3), 213-237.

Shoshani, A., & Steinmetz, S. (2021). Positive psychology at school: A systematic review. *Journal of Positive Psychology*, 16(1), 77-96.

Sink, H. E., Stroh, H. R., Wagner, L. M., Ligon, M., & Kemerer, F. R. (2015). The effectiveness of school-based mental health services for elementary-aged children: A meta-analysis. *Journal of School Psychology*, 53(5), 423-437.

Smith, A. B., & Jones, D. E. (2023). The impact of mindfulness programs on anxiety levels in primary school children: A randomized controlled trial. *Child Development*, 94(1), 102-117.

Sugai, G., & Horner, R. H. (2009). Responsiveness-to-intervention and school-wide positive behavior supports: Integration of multi-tiered system approaches. *Exceptionality*, 17(4), 223-237.

Tully, L. A., Piotrowska, P. J., Collins, D. A., Mairet, K. S., Hawes, D. J., & Kimonis, E. R. (2022). Effectiveness of school-based programs for the prevention of depression and anxiety in childhood and adolescence: A meta-analysis. Prevent*ion Science*, 23(1), 54-65.

Weare, K., & Nind, M. (2018). Mental health promotion and problem prevention in schools: What does the evidence say? *Health Promotion International*, 33(6), 986-1000.

Weisz, J. R., Kuppens, S., Ng, M. Y., Eckshtain, D., Ugueto, A. M., Vaughn-Coaxum, R. A., ... & Weersing, V. R. (2017). What five decades of research tells us about the effects of youth psychological therapy: A multilevel meta-analysis and implications for science and practice. *American Psychologist*, 72(2), 79-117.

Wyman, P. A., Brown, C. H., Inman, J., et al., (2018). *Randomized trial of a gatekeeper program for suicide prevention: 1-year impact on secondary school staff.*

Chapter 6

Anger Management in School-Age Children

Özden Erdem*, PhD

Department of Public Health Nursing, Health Science Faculty, Çanakkale Onsekiz Mart University, Çanakkale, Türkiye

Abstract

Anger is a universal emotion that is accompanied by physiological and biological changes that encourage aggression, which exist in every human being but whose expression and control vary from person to person. The onset of disruptive behavior in childhood is one of the most frequent parental challenges in clinics worldwide. Children with anger problems need to be dealt with at an early stage, as their sense of curiosity and learning are inhibited, and unhealthy and risky behaviors are observed, leading to personality disorders, violence, and crime. Many changes and developments at school age, such as hormonal changes, uncertainties in future life, internal conflicts, role confusion, mood confusion, and adjustment problems, make it difficult for the child to cope with anger. When the child cannot cope with anger, their relationships with others deteriorate, and life becomes increasingly difficult, leading to a cascade problems for both the child and their parents. Uncontrolled anger can result in the child harming themselves, their environment, or others in various ways. Without proper intervention, these issues can escalate, affecting the child's emotional well-being and overall development. Early support and teaching healthy anger management techniques are essential to prevent such negative outcomes. Thus, the child establishes strong and healthy relationships, and the child's violent and criminal behaviors are prevented. For this purpose, health professionals should learn about the situations that reveal anger in school-age children, the factors affecting it, anger expressions and behaviors, and the methods used in coping with anger. Thus, health professionals can help manage and reduce anger in school-age children. This proactive approach not only supports the emotional well-being of the child but also contributes to the overall mental health of society, especially during the school-age period when children first engage with social environments and begin to form long-lasting emotional patterns.

Keywords: adolescents and children, anger, behavior, community mental health, nurse

---

* Corresponding Author's Email: ozden85@gmail.com

In: Health Promotion and Prevention
Editor: Eda Kılınç İşleyen
ISBN: 979-8-89530-758-8

Introduction

Anger is a fundamental emotion that triggers physiological, psychological, and social changes in response to perceived violations, unmet needs, or obstacles, manifests through both constructive and destructive behaviors (Adana et al., 2023; Bierman, 2023; Dewi and Kyranides, 2022; Erdem et al., 2023). Anger is one of the earliest emotions experienced and triggers physiological responses such as numbness, muscle tension, dry mouth, sweating, and facial expression changes.

Over time, unmanaged anger leads to health problems such as pain, stomach, respiratory, circulatory, nervous system, and dermatological disorders. Anger problems in school-age children strain relationships with friends and family, lead to antisocial behavior, delinquency, aggressive, substance abuse, suicide attempts, and psychosocial problems (Adachi et al., 2022; Adana et al., 2023; Ahbab, 2019; Anjanappa et al., 2020; Cenkseven Önder and Bölükbaşı, 2019; Puff and Seghers, 2014; Rieffe et al., 2012; Serafini, Shipley and Stewart, 2016).

Generally, factors such as ridicule, deceit, disappointment, mistreatment, interference, inhibition, injustice, authoritative behavior, unmet expectations, arrogance, harassment, physical harm, jealousy, curiosity, loneliness, anxiety, and sadness can trigger anger in individuals. School-age children may become angry when they struggle to express themselves effectively (Adana et al., 2023; Ahbab, 2019; Akbaş and Yiğitoğlu, 2022; Dewi and Kyranides, 2022; Hashim and Alexiou, 2022; Puff and Seghers, 2014). School-age children who cannot control their anger may respond physically, hit objects, swear or cry, redirect their attention to other activities, sulk, avoid being in the same environment, withdraw, exhibit avoidance behavior, hide, worry, act timid, or fear the angry individual (Nasir & Ghani, 2014). If children recognize anger, identify anger-related behaviors, understand its symptoms, and use appropriate coping strategies, they control their emotions, express themselves correctly, plan their behavior, and relax. As a result, school-age children lead a healthy emotional life, which helps develop their emotional intelligence and prevents peer bullying (Hashim and Alexiou, 2022; Marín-Cortés et al., 2021; Puff and Seghers, 2014; Tryastuti, 2022; Zainel et al., 2023).

Adolescence is a period in which students experience emotional and physical changes. During this period, students feel strong emotions such as anger more intensely. Anger affects the way adolescents express their feelings and thoughts, and sometimes these emotions turn into aggressive behavior. When adolescents have difficulty coping with anger, this leads to aggressive attitudes and conflicts with their social environment. Adolescents, especially those who have difficulty controlling their anger, may overreact and exhibit violent behavior. Therefore, the development of adolescents' anger management interventions and emotional intelligence skills should be supported by families, teachers, school nurses and therapists (Elsayed et al., 2019). Early intervention in anger management is crucial to safeguarding the well-being of school-age children (World Health Organization, 2023).

Studies on anger have shown that school-age children who witness violent arguments between their parents, have more siblings, and do not want to attend university tend to be angrier (Kadan and Bilmez, 2018; Karslı, 2012; Loka et al., 2017). Studies show that factors anxiety, gender, family structure, age, grade level, and sports participation influence anger expression and anger styles (Erdem et al., 2023; Gümüş et al., 2018; Lafuente et al., 2021; Özmen et al., 2016; Puff and Seghers, 2014; Üstün et al., 2021; Uzunoğlu and Aktan, 2019; Uzunoglu and Arabaci, 2017).

Anger management is a critical aspect of adolescents' emotional development. Studies on adolescents show that they are moderately successful in expressing and controlling anger. Studies show that angry adolescents are more prone to substance use and destructive behaviors, while those who struggle to control their anger tend to act more aggressively (Adana et al., 2023; Bengisoy et al., 2019; Bierman, 2023; Puff and Seghers, 2014; Serin, 2019). However, male adolescents have lower anger control and higher levels of anger expression compared to females (Erdem et al., 2023; Özmen et al., 2016). Especially male adolescents tend to hit objects, engage in verbal and physical aggression when angry, whereas girls are more likely to cry and withdraw (Erdem et al., 2023)..

Anger can manifest in various ways among children and adolescents, particularly in the context of health challenges and environmental stressors. Studies show that children and adolescents aged 7-12 with stuttering have high levels of anger (Rocha et al., 2019). In street-dwelling youth, inward anger increases with prolonged exposure to street life and stress (Kaplan and Çuhadar, 2020). Children diagnosed with various illnesses (like cancer and multiple sclerosis) and disorders (like attention-deficit/hyperactivity disorder) are reported to exhibit heightened anger (Boufkhed vd., 2023; Yüksel Yılmaz, 2023; Mphahlele vd., 2023). Increases in anger behaviors have also been observed in children receiving inpatient treatment, particularly when the hospitalization period is prolonged (Suluhan et al., 2022; Selbes et al., 2021).

Effective anger regulation plays a significant role in shaping adolescents' behavioral and emotional outcomes. Adolescents can use inappropriate methods to cope with anger, including substance use (Adana et al., 2023; Serafini et al., 2016; Uzun and Kelleci, 2018). However, adolescents who are able to manage anger are less likely to attempt suicide and are more likely to be tolerant, kind, and versatile individuals (Cenkseven Önder & Bölükbaşı, 2019).

School nurses play a crucial role in supporting the emotional well-being of students. School nurses evaluate the anger levels of school-age children, provide counseling on anger management techniques, and implement effective interventions to prevent violence by addressing anger through various approaches (Adana et al., 2023; Akbaş and Yiğitoğlu, 2022; Elsayed and Hassan, 2023; Hafid Belhadj-Tahar and Aderrahim Mekhfi, 2023; Özmen et al., 2016; Saba et al., 2023; Temel et al., 2016; The Centre for Addiction and Mental Health, 2024). For this purpose, school nurses should be aware of situations that trigger anger in school-age children, the various ways anger is expressed, and how to effectively address anger issues. They should also be familiar with methods for anger control. The information in this section will serve as a guide for professionals working with anger-related issues and will provide insight for future studies.

Methods Used to Cope with Anger in School-Age Children

The ability to control the experience or expression of anger is known as anger control. Effectively managing and appropriately expressing anger is essential for personal development, and emotional well-being (Hashim and Alexiou, 2022; Puff and Seghers, 2014). By learning how to regulate anger, individuals can avoid destructive behaviors, improve relationships, and foster a positive mindset. Developing anger control skills contributes to emotional intelligence, helps maintain self-respect, and promotes a healthier, more balanced life.

Anger, when used appropriately, can be protective, stimulating, and mobilizing. It provides strength, shields against harm, and serves as a means to express anxiety. Additionally, it can drive motivation and contribute to the achievement of goals, acting as a powerful tool for self-assertion and personal growth. When managed properly, anger can help individuals address challenges, assert their needs, and navigate difficult situations more effectively (Elsayed et al., 2019; Tatlıoğlu and Karaca, 2013).

Many methods are used to control anger (Ahbab, Özdogan, and Sayar, 2022; Anjanappa et al., 2020; Puff & Seghers, 2014; Saba et al., 2023). When selecting a method for anger management, factors such as the child's age, personality, lifestyle, and individual differences should be considered. It is crucial to ensure that the chosen method is applied in a way that does not cause distress or negatively impact the child's daily life. The most effective method can vary from person to person. In many cases, several methods can be combined or integrated to tailor the intervention to the child's specific needs, providing a comprehensive approach to managing anger (Elsayed and Hassan, 2023; Jancy et al., 2023; Moorthi and Chandran, 2023; Saba et al., 2023; Shilpa Jayan et al., 2023).

Various therapeutic approaches have been found to be effective in addressing emotional and behavioral challenges in children. Among these, play therapy has proven particularly effective for children between the ages of three and thirteen (Ahbab, 2019; Ahbab et al., 2022; Şensoy and İpek, 2023). Play therapies can be categorized into structured forms (such as cognitive-behavioral play therapy, release play therapy, and sand play therapy/sand tray therapy), unstructured forms (such as child-centered play therapy), and family play therapies. While play therapy is specifically designed for children, psychotherapy is typically used for adults. In play therapy, the initial five-six sessions are focused on establish trust. Generally, problems addressed through play therapy are resolved in about 10-15 sessions (Şensoy and İpek, 2023; Türe and Barut, 2020). In children, aged five to ten years, with anger problems, child-centered play therapy was found to be effective in reducing anger when implemented for 45 minutes a week over a period of 12 weeks (Şensoy and İpek, 2023). In 12-year-old children, anger expression problems improved after attending sessions twice a week for three weeks (Ahbab et al., 2022). However, for some children, the solution to problems may take longer than one year (Türe and Barut, 2020).

Psychodrama provides an opportunity for children to enact and express their emotional experiences in a safe environment. Through role-playing and dramatization within the group, children can better understand and process their feelings of anger. These interventions allow the child to observe angry reactions. The child gains insight into the origin, triggers, and effects of anger, while exploring and practicing alternative behaviors to apply in daily life. Throughout this process, the counselor provides empathetic support, helping the child feel understood and guided in managing their emotions. As the child feels that their emotions and experiences are understood and accepted, anger-related behaviors tend to decrease. Psychodrama-based intervention programs have been shown to be effective in promoting positive emotional and behaviors changes across all age groups, according to systematic review (Şarlak and Öztürk, 2021). Creative drama has been found effective in reducing anger levels among adolescents aged 14 to 15 (Çapacıoğlu and Demirtaş, 2017).

Family therapy improves the relationships, communication, and functions of family members by addressing internal dynamics. It provides positive behaviors to replace learned patterns of anger and supports healthier parenting attitudes (Abdullah, 2019; Bhave et al., 2023). A study found that children raised with authoritarian and indifferent parental attitudes showed higher tendencies toward aggression, whereas those raised with democratic parenting styles exhibited lower levels of aggression (Yıldız & Erci, 2011). In this context, it is recommended that parents should have appropriate attitudes and positive approaches to their children and demonstrate a safe, and supportive attitude through family therapy (Bhave et al., 2023; Yıldız and Erci, 2011).

Acceptance and Commitment Therapy (ACT) helps individuals accept uncontrollable events or situations that negatively affect them, while promoting behaviors that support a meaningful and productive life. ACT is mostly used to reduce anger and aggression among adults (Berkout et al., 2019). ACT has been shown to reduce anger and aggression among children, adolescents, and young adults (Byrne and Cullen, 2024; Knight and Samuel, 2022). The use of ACT in combination with the model was found to be effective and in this direction, it was recommended to be used together with the Psychological Flexibility Model. This integrated approach enhances the individual's ability to cope with difficult emotions and adapt to challenging life circumstances (Berkout et al., 2019).

Mood regulation enables children to identify, express, and manage their anger in a healthy way. The emotions that accompany anger are recognized and controlled with a valid and reliable tool (Tatlı Harmancı and Güngör Aytar, 2023). Generally, visual and auditory messages are used to regulate the mood of children. The psychological flexibility model in coping with anger improves the emotional well-being of children aged five to six years (Arthur et al., 2023). Watching animated films combined with anger control-oriented cognitive behavioral therapy positively impacts the anger behaviors of children aged seven to nine years (Saba et al., 2023). In mood regulation, children can engage in activities such as reading books, painting, singing, diaries, watching animated films, and writing. The coping strategies used by the characters in these activities, when faced with negative emotions such as anger and sadness, become exemplary behavior models for children. A study showed that reading nine different stories to children aged five to eight years, three times per week for 14 weeks, helped improve their anger expressions (Kılıç and Büyüktaşkapu Soydan, 2022). In illustrated children's books, stories about anger are the most common negative emotions (Topçam and Yorulmaz, 2023). Tertiary emotions such as anguish, distress, depression, helplessness, grief, gloom, anguish, alienation, indifference, defeat, humiliation, insult, and pity are not very common in children's books. In addition, strategies to cope with the anger of the characters in the stories are not given enough space. In the books, cognitive development is prioritized, and emotional development may remain in the background. In this context, it is thought that there is a need for more use of auditory and visual tools in emotion regulation studies for anger control (Ceylan and Kılınç, 2022).

Cognitive Behavioral Therapy (CBT) aims to control anger through changes in thought, emotion, and behavior (Anjanappa et al., 2020; Bengisoy et al., 2019; Özdemir, 2015; Shilpa Jayan et al., 2023; Yalçın et al., 2023). It helps individuals recognize triggers for anger, challenge negative thoughts, and develop healthier coping strategies. CBT has been found effective in reducing anger in various groups, including adolescents aged 14-18 who were in prison (Yalçın et al., 2023), children with cancer (Melesse et al., 2022), and children aged 9-12 with Asperger's Syndrome (Sofronoff et al., 2007). Furthermore, a case report showed that CBT combined with Ayurveda was effective in reducing anger and behaviors such as running away from home and school in school-age children (Shilpa Jayan et al., 2023).

Forgiveness plays a significant role in emotional and psychological well-being, particularly in addressing negative emotional responses such as anger. Forgiveness interventions improve self-esteem, interpersonal relationships, trait anger, angry temperament, angry reaction, and anger management. It positively changes attitudes toward schools, teachers, and parents. In a meta-analysis study, it was proved that forgiveness interventions reduced the anger of children and adolescents who were harmed by injustice It was observed that forgiveness interventions with Enright's Forgiveness Model (2001) provided anger management in adolescents, and a six-week forgiveness program using the model in the 9-12 age range increased anger control and forgiveness (Brouzos et al., 2019; Burgess, 2010; Enright, 2001).

In addition to these techniques, relaxation methods and alternative medicine methods can be used to support anger control in school-age children. In a study, the Ayurveda method was applied to a 13-year-old girl diagnosed with Alternative Disruptive Mood Dysregulation, resulting in positive outcomes related to anger management (Jancy et al., 2023). In a study, a 17-year-old male diagnosed with adolescent Disruptive mood dysregulation was improved by individualized homeopathy (Jancy et al., 2023; Moorthi and Chandran, 2023). The feelings of anger of children and adolescents aged 7-17 years who were sexually abused with the support of domestic animals (dogs) were reduced (Dietz et al., 2012). It has been proven that rhythm training with music improves negative anger behaviors in adolescents with hearing impairment (Hafid Belhadj-Tahar and Aderrahim Mekhfi, 2023), and non-contact sports reduce aggression (Yang et al., 2023). Anger control has been achieved in children and adolescents through practices such as storytelling, reading books, listening to relaxing music, praying, and worshiping (Dağcı, 2021; Puff and Seghers, 2014; Tatlıoğlu and Karaca, 2013).

Anger problems in children and adolescents with disabilities during the school-age period are addressed through special training. In one study, it was proved that special training did not prevent tantrums in adolescents using hearing aids/cochlear implants but only reduced the feeling of tension and irritability experienced by adolescents (Çakıcı et al., 2022). Anger intensity was reduced in mentally retarded children and adolescents of primary school-age with a recreational behavior program of three (one session 30-minute) sessions per week for 6 weeks. In the program, both group and individual counseling and various behavioral techniques and leisure time activities such as reinforcement, modeling, role-playing, and response costs were used (Elsayed and Hassan, 2023). In another study, it was proven that an active rehabilitation program reduced anger and anxiety in children and adolescents aged 9-18 years with concussion symptoms in six weeks (Hunt et al., 2020).

Anger control should be ensured by providing children and adolescents with social skills, such as effective communication, empathy, and problem-solving through specialized social skills training programs (Abdullah, 2019; Bhave et al., 2023). School-age children should be supported to tell their teachers and friends how they feel (Hafid Belhadj-Tahar and Aderrahim Mekhfi, 2023; Puff and Seghers, 2014; Tatlıoğlu and Karaca, 2013). In a qualitative study, it was reported that excluding students from the classroom by sending them to isolation rooms and giving punishments led to feel injustice, hopelessness, frustration, and anger and that this practice negatively affected adolescents (Sealy et al., 2023). Consequently, it is believed that isolation is not an appropriate approach in schools, and its use in response to tantrums is not recommended.

It is recommended to stay calm, show empathy, provide a safe environment, listen attentively, suggest alternative behaviors, and apply calming techniques when approaching individuals experiencing an anger outburst. Especially those who made threats in the past should be treated with caution. If a school-age child expresses intentions to harm themselves, or others, they should be immediately referred for professional help (The Centre for Addiction and Mental Health, 2024). Involving both the family and school staff in anger management interventions enhances their effectiveness. It is recommended to include the school team in the process to ensure a collaborative and supportive approach for the child's emotional well-being (Puff and Seghers, 2014; Tekbaş and Koçtürk, 2023; Bhave et al., 2023).

Conclusion

Anger is the most important emotion for children to express negative emotions. Since it can lead to problems and escalate into aggression, it is crucial to address it early. Children should recognize and be aware of their feelings of anger, know when anger arises, in which situations it is triggered, and their behaviors during anger. They should also learn how to express themselves at that moment. Health professionals should support children and adolescents in this regard.

There are many interventions applied to anger management. The goal of these interventions is not for the child not to get angry at all or to suppress anger but to learn to express this emotion in a healthy way. Even when a child recognizes, accepts, and wants to control anger, the feeling of anger decreases. Releasing anger, allowing the emotion to emerge without controlling anger, is an increase in violence and loss of control. For this reason, children should be taught appropriate and alternative methods that they can use for anger control during the school period. When children manage their anger using effective methods, their self-esteem, cognitive flexibility, social competence, and personality are preserved. This positive change extends to their physical, mental, and social health, ultimately contributing to the well-being of society as a whole by promoting better mental health.

School nurses play a crucial role in guiding school-age children on anger control, offering support without leaving them isolated, and suggesting alternative behaviors to replace angry reactions. They also assist in the emotional development of angry children and adolescents by counseling parents on how to respond appropriately to their children's behavior. In addition, school nurses should prioritize male adolescents in anger control because they are at risk for aggressive behaviors, protect them from crimes, and protect them from environments where they are teased and peer bullying.

Parents, teachers, and health professionals should show empathy to children and adolescents, try to understand their feelings, and make appropriate approaches. The school team should create a safe environment where children and adolescents feel respected and valued, avoiding criticism. They should serve as role models by using calm and appropriate methods to address emotional events, fostering open dialogues instead of resorting to shouting.

Disclaimer

None.

References

Abdullah, S. M. (2019). Social Cognitive theory : A Bandura thought review. *Psikodimensia, 18*(1), 85. https://doi.org/10.24167/psifadanadim.v18i1.1708.

Adachi, T., Yamada, K., Fujino, H., Enomoto, K., & Shibata, M. (2022). Associations between anger and chronic primary pain: A systematic review and meta-analysis. *Scandinavian Journal of Pain, 22*(1), 1–13. https://doi.org/10.1515/sjpain-2021-0154.

Adana, F., Yeşilfidan, D., Mert, E., Öztaban, Ş., Türkal Gün, Z., & Demirkıran, F. (2023). The relationship between anger and substance use in adolescents: A systematic review. *Journal of Public Health Nursing, 5*(2), 190–203. https://doi.org/10.54061/jphn.1170791.

Ahbab. (2019). *Effect of Child-Centered Play Theraphy on Children with Anger Management*. Üsküdar University.

Ahbab, A., Özdogan, B., & Sayar, G. H. (2022). The effect of child-centered play therapy on children with anger control problems is true. *The Journal of Neurobehavioral Sciences, 9*(1), 31–35. https://doi.org/10.4103/jnbs.jnbs_35_21.

Akbaş, E., & Yiğitoğlu, G. (2022). Anger and adolescence. *Ordu University Journal of Nursing Studies, 5*(1), 139–147. https://doi.org/10.38108/ouhcd.972919.

Anjanappa, S., Govindan, R., & Munivenkatappa, M. (2020). Anger management in adolescents: A systematic review. *Indian Journal of Psychiatric Nursing, 17*(1), 51. https://doi.org/10.4103/IOPN.IOPN_37_19.

Arthur, A., McDevitt, M., Rooney, R. M., MacLeod, A., Kane, R. T., Tonta, K., … Baughman, N. (2023). Short-term effects of the "I Spy Feelings" program on emotion regulation in 5- to 6-year-old children. *Frontiers in Psychology, 14*. https://doi.org/10.3389/fpsyg.2023.1016521.

Bengisoy, A., Burak Özdemir, M., Erkıvanç Sacide Şahin, F., & Çelik İskifoğlu Geliş, T. (2019). The content analysis of the research articles about Cognitive Behavioural Therapy between 1997-2018. *Turkish Psychological Counseling and Guidance Journal, 9*(54).

Berkout, O. V., Tinsley, D., & Flynn, M. K. (2019, January 1). A review of anger, hostility, and aggression from an ACT perspective. *Journal of Contextual Behavioral Science*. Elsevier Inc. https://doi.org/10.1016/j.jcbs.2018.12.001.

Bhave, D. S., P, M., Patil, D. R., Kotwal, D. N., Jain, D. T., & Joshi, D. S. (2023). An analysis of anger expression in participants of a life skill education workshop from a school in Nagpur. *Journal of Pediatrics & Neonatal Care, 13*(2), 123–127. https://doi.org/10.15406/jpnc.2023.13.00503.

Bierman, K. L. (2023). Anger and aggression: A developmental perspective. In *Anger, Aggression, and Interventionsfor Interpersonal Violence* (pp. 215–238). https://doi.org/10.4324/9781003417989-12.

Boufkhed, S., Yurduşen, S., Alarjeh, G., Ahmed, F., Alrjoub, W., Guo, P., … Harding, R. (2023). Concerns and priority outcomes for children with advanced cancer and their families in the Middle East: A cross-national qualitative study. *Frontiers in Oncology, 13*. https://doi.org/10.3389/fonc.2023.1120990.

Brouzos, A., Vassilopoulos, S., Sourtzinou, A., & Baourda, V. (2019). Psychoeducational program for the enhancement of forgiveness in 9 to 12 year-old children. *Psychology, 24*(1), 32–50. https://doi.org/10.12681/psy_hps.22385.

Burgess, O. (2010). Forgiveness is a choice: A step-by-step process for resolving anger and restoring hope. *South Central Review, 27*(3), 170–174. https://doi.org/10.1353/scr.2010.a402545.

Byrne, G., & Cullen, C. (2024). Acceptance and Commitment Therapy for anger, irritability, and aggression in children, adolescents, and young adults: A systematic review of intervention studies. Trauma, violence, and abuse. *Trauma, Violence, and Abuse*. https://doi.org/10.1177/15248380231167393.

Çakıcı, S., Zeren, S., & Gümüş, N. M. (2022). Experiences of children with hearing aids or cochlear implants before and during special education. *Istanbul Gelisim University Journal of Health Sciences*, (18), 829–841. https://doi.org/10.38079/igusabder.992223.

Çapacıoğlu, G. K., & Demirtaş, V. Y. (2017). The effects of Creative Drama over the anger management skills of 9th grade secondary school students. *Elementary Education Online, 16*(3), 960–977. https://doi.org/10.17051/ilkonline.2017.330235.

Cenkseven Önder, F., & Bölükbaşı, A. (2019). Suicide probability in adolescents: relationship to self-esteem, and anger. *OPUS International Journal of Social Studies, 10*(17), 1–22. https://doi.org/10.26466/opus.528723.

Ceylan, Ş., & Kılınç, N. (2022). A review of children's picture books: Feelings of anger and sadness. *Yıldız Journal of Educational Research*, *6*(2), 106–121.

Dağcı, A. (2021). Perceptions regarding prayer: A metaphorical study. *Darulfunun Ilahiyat*, *32*(1), 179–198. https://doi.org/10.26650/di.2021.32.1.819178.

Dewi, I. D. A. D. P., & Kyranides, M. N. (2022). Physical, verbal, and relational aggression: The role of anger management strategies. *Journal of Aggression, Maltreatment and Trauma*, *31*(1). https://doi.org/10.1080/10926771.2021.1994495.

Dietz, T. J., Davis, D., & Pennings, J. (2012). Evaluating animal-assisted therapy in group treatment for child sexual abuse. *Journal of Child Sexual Abuse*, *21*(6), 665–683. https://doi.org/10.1080/10538712.2012.726700.

Elsayed, A. R., & Hassan, A. K. (2023). The effectiveness of a recreational behavioural programme in reducing anger among children with intellectual disabilities at the primary stage. *European Journal of Investigation in Health, Psychology and Education*, *13*(6), 948–963. https://doi.org/10.3390/ejihpe13060072.

Elsayed, D., Song, J. H., Myatt, E., Colasante, T., & Malti, T. (2019). Anger and sadness regulation in refugee children: The roles of pre- and post-migratory factors. *Child Psychiatry and Human Development*, *50*(5), 846–855. https://doi.org/10.1007/s10578-019-00887-4.

Enright, R. D. (2001). *Forgiveness is a choice: A step-by-step process for resolving anger and restoring hope.* APA LifeTools.

Erdem, Ö., Erol, S., Ergüven, N., & Kısaboyun, B. (2023). *Behavioral and psychological expression of anger and anger management in adolescents*.

Ergin, B., Ergin, E., & Hamarat, H. (2022). Hidden Gem in Christopher Robin's Jungle The Birth Of Winnie The Pooh: A content analysis. *Folklor Akademy Journal*, *5*(3), 817–832. https://doi.org/10.55666/folklor.1143587.

Gambaro, M. E., Enright, R. D., Baskin, T. W., & Klatt, J. (2008). School-based forgiveness education for the management of trait anger in early adolescence. *Journal of Research in Education*, *18*.

Gümüş, H., Yenen, İ., & Özyürek, A. (2018). The investigation the relationship between social skills and anger levels of adolescents. *Karaelmas Journal of Educational Sciences*, *6*, 51–61.

Hafid Belhadj-Tahar, & Aderrahim Mekhfi. (2023). Therapeutic impact of music in young deaf patients with aggressive behavior disorder. *World Journal of Advanced Research and Reviews*, *20*(2), 509–513. https://doi.org/10.30574/wjarr.2023.20.2.2277.

Hashim, H. T., & Alexiou, A. (2022). *The Psychology of anger*. (H. T. Hashim & A. Alexiou, Eds.) (1st ed.). Cham: Springer International Publishing. https://doi.org/10.1007/978-3-031-16605-1.

Hunt, A. W., Agnihotri, S., Sack, L., Tint, A., Greenspoon, D., Gauvin-Lepage, J., … Scratch, S. (2020). Mood-related changes in children and adolescents with persistent concussion symptoms following a six-week active rehabilitation program. *Brain Injury*, *34*(8), 1068–1073. https://doi.org/10.1080/02699052.2020.1776396.

Jancy K S, Jithesh M, & Aparna P M. (2023). Disruptive mood dysregulation disorder and its Ayurvedic management - A case report. *Ayushdhara*, 87–91. https://doi.org/10.47070/ayushdhara.v10i3.1247.

Kadan, G., & Bilmez, B. (2018). Examination of the levels of adolescent of child like and the expression of the anger according to some variables. *Journal of Child and Development*, *1*(1), 1–14. https://doi.org/10.36731/cg.414861.

Kaplan, V., & Çuhadar, D. (2020). The levels of anger and aggression in street children with substance dependence. *Journal of Child and Adolescent Psychiatric Nursing*, *33*(4). https://doi.org/10.1111/jcap.12275.

Karslı, N. (2012). An experımental study on relation between religiosity and anger management. *Ekev Akademy Journal*, *16*(50), 57–70.

Kılıç, S., & Büyüktaşkapu Soydan, S. (2022). The effect of the therapy program with stories on the emotional management skills of children with speech and language disorders. *Theory and Practice in Child Development*, *2*(2), 1–24. https://doi.org/10.46303/tpicd.2022.14.

Knight, L., & Samuel, V. (2022). Acceptance and commitment therapy interventions in secondary schools and their impact on students' mental health and well-being: A systematic review. *Journal of Contextual Behavioral Science*. https://doi.org/10.1016/j.jcbs.2022.06.006.

Lafuente, J. C., Zubiaur, M., & Gutiérrez-García, C. (2021). Effects of martial arts and combat sports training on anger and aggression: A systematic review. *Aggression and Violent Behavior*. https://doi.org/10.1016/j.avb.2021.101611.

Lee, E. J. (2015). The effect of positive group psychotherapy on self-esteem and state anger among adolescents at korean immigrant churches. *Archives of Psychiatric Nursing*, *29*(2). https://doi.org/10.1016/j.apnu.2014.10.005.

Liu, Z. (2023). The effect of emotion regulation on pupils' peer relationships. *BCP Education & Psychology*, *9*, 323–329. https://doi.org/10.54691/bcpep.v9i.4701.

Loka, W. P., Sumadja, W. A., & Resmi. (2017). The effects of interparental conflict on preadolescent behaviour: the case of primary schools in dar es salaam and coast region. *Journal of Chemical Information and Modeling*, *21*(2), 1689–1699. Retrieved from https://www.oecd.org/dac/accountable-effective-institutions/Governance Notebook 2.6 Smoke.pdf.

Marín-Cortés, A., Herrera-Pérez, V., & Aguirre-Mosquera, M. (2021). Anger and cyberbullying among adolescents: friendship, injustice and image in digital environments. *Psicologia Em Estudo*, *26*, 1–13. https://doi.org/10.4025/psicolestud.v26i0.51343.

Melesse, T. G., Chau, J. P. C., & Nan, M. A. (2022). Effects of cognitive-behavioural therapy on psychological, physical and social outcomes of children with cancer: A systematic review and meta-analysis. *Journal of Psychosomatic Research*. https://doi.org/10.1016/j.jpsychores.2022.110805.

Moorthi, S. K., & Chandran, K. C. M. (2023). Role of individualised homoeopathic medicine in the management of disruptive mood dysregulation disorder - A case report. *Journal of Integrated Standardized Homoeopathy*, *6*. https://doi.org/10.25259/jish_34_2022.

Mphahlele, R. M., Pillay, B. J., & Meyer, A. (2023). Symptoms of oppositional defiant disorder, conduct disorder and anger in children with ADHD. *South African Journal of Education*, *43*(1), 1–14. https://doi.org/10.15700/saje.v43n1a2136.

Nasir, R., & Ghani, N. A. (2014). Behavioral and emotional effects of anger expression and anger management among adolescents. *Procedia - Social and Behavioral Sciences*, *140*, 565–569. https://doi.org/10.1016/j.sbspro.2014.04.471.

Neukel, C., Bullenkamp, R., Moessner, M., Spiess, K., Schmahl, C., Bertsch, K., & Herpertz, S. C. (2022). Anger instability and aggression in Borderline Personality Disorder – an ecological momentary assessment study. *Borderline Personality Disorder and Emotion Dysregulation*, *9*(1). https://doi.org/10.1186/s40479-022-00199-5.

Özdemir, M. B. (2015). The impact of activity based group along with psychological consultation and intervention programme to reduce anger and aggression in children. *Education and Society in the 21st Century Journal of Educational Sciences and Social Research*, *4*(10), 221–238. Retrieved from http://turkegitimsen.dergipark.gov.tr/egitimvetoplum/issue/5134/69906%0Ahttp://dergipark.ulakbim.gov.tr/egitimvetoplum/article/view/5000119700/0.

Özmen, D., Özmen, E., Çetinkaya, A., & Akil, İ. (2016). Trait anger and anger expression styles in adolescents. *Anatolian Journal of Psychiatry*, *17*(1), 65–73. https://doi.org/10.5455/apd.176085.

Puff, R., & Seghers, J. (2014). *The everything guide to anger management : proven techniques to understand and control anger* (1st ed.). Avon, Massachusetts: F W Media;Everything;Adams Media.

Rapp, H., Wang Xu, J., & Enright, R. D. (2022). A meta-analysis of forgiveness education interventions' effects on forgiveness and anger in children and adolescents. *Child Development*. https://doi.org/10.1111/cdev.13771.

Rieffe, C., Camodeca, M., Pouw, L. B. C., Lange, A. M. C., & Stockmann, L. (2012). Don't anger me! Bullying, victimization, and emotion dysregulation in young adolescents with ASD. *European Journal of Developmental Psychology*, *9*(3), 351–370. https://doi.org/10.1080/17405629.2012.680302.

Rocha, M. S., Yaruss, J. S., & Rato, J. R. (2019). Temperament, executive functioning, and anxiety in school-age children who stutter. *Frontiers in Psychology*, *10*. https://doi.org/10.3389/fpsyg.2019.02244.

Saba, P., Qi, H., Saleem, A., Chen, I. J., Kausar, F. N., & Iqbal, M. F. (2023). Effects of animated movies on the aggression and behavior performance of primary school students and their control using a Cognitive Behavioral Anger-Control Training (CBACT) program. *Behavioral Sciences*, *13*(8). https://doi.org/10.3390/bs13080659.

Şarlak, D., & Öztürk, E. (2021). Psychodrama-based intervention programs: A Systematic evaluation. *Karya Journal of Health Science*, *2*(1), 21–29.
Sealy, J., Abrams, E. J., & Cockburn, T. (2023). Students' experience of isolation room punishment in UK mainstream education. 'I can't put into words what you felt like, almost a dog in a cage.' *International Journal of Inclusive Education*, *27*(12), 1336–1350. https://doi.org/10.1080/13603116.2021.1889052.
Selbes, M., Manav, G., & Karayağız Muslu, G. (2021). Investigation of psychosoial symptoms of children in hospital in terms of children's variables. *Journal of Anatolia Nursing and Health Sciences*, *4*(4), 420–428. https://doi.org/10.17049/ataunihem.650615.
Şensoy, P., & İpek, M. (2023). The effect of preschool children's attachment styles on emotion regulation and interpersonal problem-solving skills. *Aydın Journal of Health*, *9*(3), 185–205.
Serafini, K., Shipley, L., & Stewart, D. G. (2016). Motivation and substance use outcomes among adolescents in a school-based intervention. *Addictive Behaviors*, *53*, 74–79. https://doi.org/10.1016/j.addbeh.2015.10.004.
Serin, N. B. (2019). The impact of anger management training on anger, aggression and problem-solving skills of primary school students. *International Online Journal of Education and Teaching*, *6*(3), 525–543.
Shilpa Jayan T, Satheesh K, & Aparna P.M. (2023). Ayurvedic management along with cognitive behavioural therapy in conduct disorder - A case report. *International Journal of Ayurveda and Pharma Research*, 120–124. https://doi.org/10.47070/ijapr.v11i5.2826.
Sofronoff, K., Attwood, T., Hinton, S., & Levin, I. (2007). A randomized controlled trial of a cognitive behavioural intervention for anger management in children diagnosed with Asperger syndrome. *Journal of Autism and Developmental Disorders*, *37*(7), 1203–1214. https://doi.org/10.1007/s10803-006-0262-3.
Suluhan, D., Nurdan, A., Yıldız, D., & İslamoğlu, A. (2022). A Social psychological evaluation about anger. *Izmir Democracy University Health Sciences Journal*, *5*(2), 467–479. https://doi.org/10.52538/iduhes.1166110.
Tatlı Harmancı, S., & Güngör Aytar, A. (2023). Study of Turkish Adaption of the Emotion Regulation Scale for Children Child Form (ÇDDÖ) and Adult Form (ÇDDÖ-YF). *Milli Eğitim Dergisi*, *52*(237), 71–106. https://doi.org/10.37669/milliegitim.1072215.
Tatlıoğlu, K., & Karaca, M. (2013). A social psychological evaluation about anger. *International Journal of Social Science*, *6*(6), 1101–1123.
Tekbaş, G., & Koçtürk, N. (2023). Parent participation in Cognitive Behavioral Therapy for children and adolescents: A Scoping review. *Psikiyatride Güncel Yaklaşımlar*, *15*(3), 418–429. https://doi.org/10.18863/pgy.1150920.
Temel, A. B., Bahar, Z., Ergün, A., Kadıoğlu, H., Erol, S., Öncel, S., … Şişman, F. N. (2016). *Improving the health of school children.* (S. Gözüm, Ed.) (1st ed.). Ankara: Vize.
The Centre for Addiction and Mental Health. (2024). *Aggressive behaviour in children and youth. The Centre for Addiction and Mental Health.* Retrieved from https://www.camh.ca/en/health-info/guides-and-publications/aggressive-behaviour-in-children-and-youth.
Topçam, A. B., & Yorulmaz, B. (2023). Best selling illustrated children's books: What values do they have? *Medya ve Din Araştırmaları Dergisi*, *6*(1), 47–72. https://doi.org/10.47951/mediad.1160959.
Tryastuti, D. (2022). The effectiveness of anger management training in reducing bullying behavior among school-age children. *International Journal of Nursing and Health Services (IJNHS)*, *5*(2), 203–209. https://doi.org/10.35654/ijnhs.v5i2.598.
Türe, E., & Barut, Y. (2020). Investigation of play therapy studies conducted in Turkey. *Life Skills Journal of Psychology*, *4*(8), 127–138. https://doi.org/10.31461/ybpd.837024.
Üstün, G., Akan, B., & Küçük, L. (2021). Examining the relationship between psychosocial symptoms in hospitalized children and the anxiety levels of their mothers. *E-Journal of Dokuz Eylul University Nursing Faculty*, *14*(3), 207–216. https://doi.org/10.46483/deuhfed.832698.
Uzun, S., & Kelleci, M. (2018). Substance abuse in high school students: Their self-efficacy to avoid substance abuse and related factors. *Dusunen Adam - The Journal of Psychiatry and Neurological Sciences*, *31*(4), 356–363. https://doi.org/10.5350/DAJPN2018310404.
Uzunoğlu, G., & Aktan, Z. D. (2019). The relationship between premenstrual syndrome and mental health variables in adolescents. *Current Approaches in Psychiatry*, *11*, 37–50. https://doi.org/10.18863/pgy.521549.

Uzunoglu, G., & Arabaci, L. B. (2017). The effect of psychoeducation on the anger management of adolescents diagnosed with conduct disorder. *Dusunen Adam - The Journal of Psychiatry and Neurological Sciences*, *30*(4). https://doi.org/10.5350/dajpn2017300409.

World Health Organization. (2023). *Youth violence*. Retrieved from https://www.who.int/news-room/fact-sheets/detail/youth-violence.

Yalçın, M., Arıtürk, S., Görgü Akçay, N. S., & Tekinsav Sütcü, S. (2023). Cognitive behavioral group therapy for anger management in juvenile delinquents: Effectiveness study in a Turkey child prison. *International Journal of Offender Therapy and Comparative Criminology*, 0306624X2311654. https://doi.org/10.1177/0306624X231165418.

Yang, Y., Zhu, H., Chu, K., Zheng, Y., & Zhu, F. (2023). Effects of sports intervention on aggression in children and adolescents: a systematic review and meta-analysis. *PeerJ*, *11*. https://doi.org/10.7717/peerj.15504.

Yıldız, E., & Erci, B. (2011). The investigation of relation between parental behavior and adolescence aggressiveness behavior. *Düzce Üniversitesi Sağlık Bilimleri Enstitüsü Dergisi*, *1*(3), 6–11.

Yüksel Yılmaz, D. (2023). Having Multiple Sclerosis from childhood to youth according to uncertainty theory: A case report. *Celal Bayar University Journal of Health Sciences Institute*, *10*(1), 67–70. https://doi.org/10.34087/cbusbed.1065743,

Zainel, A. A., Daher-Nashif, S., Al-Maadeed, A. N., Qotba, H. A., Al Mujalli, H., & Al-Kohji, S. M. (2023). Children and adolescents coping with home isolation and social distancing during Covid-19 in Qatar: A cross sectional study with qualitative items. *BMC Psychology*, *11*(1). https://doi.org/10.1186/s40359-023-01183-6,

Chapter 7

Preventing Violence, Bullying, Discrimination and Stigma in Schools

Betül Kaplan[1], PhD
and Metin Yıldız[2,*], PhD
[1]Gaziantep Islamic Science and Technology University, Faculty of Health Sciences, Department of Midwifery, Gaziantep, Türkiye
[2]Sakarya University, Faculty of Health Sciences, Department of Midwifery, Sakarya, Türkiye

Abstract

Preventing violence, bullying, discrimination, and stigmatization at school is an important issue aiming to make educational environments safer, inclusive, and supportive. These problems can negatively affect students' academic achievement, social development, and psychological health. Therefore, schools need to develop effective strategies to prevent such negative behaviors. A safe learning environment should be created in schools to prevent violence and bullying. This requires teachers and school administrators to be sensitive and respond quickly to cases of violence and bullying. In addition, teaching school-age children values such as empathy, respect, and tolerance are critical in preventing bullying and violence. Preventing discrimination and stigmatization is based on the acceptance and celebration of differences. Students should be consistently given the message that diversity is a strength that every individual holds equal value. This can help students from various cultural, ethnic, and social backgrounds to better understand and respect each other. It is important for schools to implement programs that support the development of healthy relationships between students. These programs should cover topics such as communication skills, conflict resolution techniques, and emotional intelligence. This encourages the resolution of conflicts between students in more positive ways. The prevention of violence, bullying, discrimination, and stigmatization at school requires the cooperation of the entire school community (teachers, students, parents, and school administration). A zero-tolerance policy towards such negative behavior should be adopted, and continuous training and awareness programs should be organized. These measures can transform schools from places of academic learning into safe and supportive environments where students can develop socially, emotionally, and ethically.

---

* Corresponding Author's Email: yildizzmetin@gmail.com

In: Health Promotion and Prevention
Editor: Eda Kılınç İşleyen
ISBN: 979-8-89530-758-8

Keywords: students, violence, bullying, discrimination, stigmatization, prevention

Introduction

Violence is a phenomenon that has existed since the existence throughout human history (Golan et al., 2018). Violence is defined as the use of force, rudeness, resorting to brute force, and engaging in damaging behavior. According to the Turkish Language Association (TLA), violence is defined as "hitting, damaging behavior and psychological pressure on people who do not think like oneself and who are different from oneself" (TLA, 2016). This definition emphasizes not only physical aggression but also the psychological dimension of violence, highlighting its impact on individuals who are perceived as different.

Violence at school refers to criminal behaviors and aggressive acts that disrupt the educational environment, hinder students' development and learning processes, and negatively affect the overall school climate (Hoşgörür and Orhan, 2017). At one end of violence, there are relatively innocent acts, such as humiliating and insulting a student, and at the other end, there are acts that may result in death. According to reports on school violence, the most common forms of violence in schools are bullying (physical bullying, sexual bullying, psychological bullying, and cyberbullying), physical fights, and physical assaults. Importantly, both girls and boys are affected by school violence and bullying, which significantly disrupts students' sense of safety and well-being (UNESCO, 2019). Studies in the literature have demonstrated that violence and bullying are common phenomena observed in school environments. In the study conducted by Davli-Temel (2018) with high school students, it was found that students who evaluated their relationship with their family as "very good" or "good" had lower levels of violent behavior compared to those who rated their relationship as "moderate," "poor," or "very poor." Furthermore, the tendency toward violence decreased as the level of perceived social support from the family increased (Davli Temel, 2018). In the study conducted by Emiroğlu (2018) with secondary school-age children aged 10-14, it was found that male students had a higher tendency toward violence than female students. As the educational level of parents decreases, the tendency toward violence increases among school-age children. Additionally, students who reported higher levels of family life satisfaction demonstrated lower levels of violent tendencies (Emiroğlu, 2018). In the study conducted by Omidi et al., (2014) with adolescents, it was found that violent behaviors decreased when there was more love and attention in the family, increased when there were violent behaviors within the family (Omidi et al., 2014). When the literature on coping with violence at school is examined, there is a lack of research on how to address violence directed at teachers. Most studies focus on conflict resolution and anger management for students, while research on parenting attitudes and enhancing parental skills are primarily aimed at families. For example, Kubar and Kıral (2019) found in their study that school violence could be prevented by raising awareness about violence among students, encouraging teachers and other school staff to take responsibility, and ensuring the active participation of all stakeholders in violence prevention programs. It is observed that studies primarily focus on violence against students. It is concluded that it is not possible to cope with violence at school by working alone with students who are at the center of the research (Kubar and Kıral, 2019).

The Non-violent Resistance Programme (NRP) is gaining recognition as an effective approach to managing conflict and fostering peaceful solutions in various environments. The program based on a systemic psychotherapy approach, is a new model developed by Haim Omer and colleagues with a different perspective on resisting violence. The program is an approach or intervention designed to help individuals or communities manage conflict and resolve issues without resorting to violence. NRP is typically used in a variety of contexts, such as in schools, communities, or for individuals experiencing difficulties in relationships or in situations involving aggression or violence. The NRP model has emerged to help and empower parents and educators (Van Holen et al., 2016). When the literature is examined, it is seen that research on this model for parents and educators has been conducted in countries such as Israel, (Lavi-Levavi et al., 2013) Germany (Ollefs et al., 2009), and Belgium (Van Holen et al., 2016). As the application of NRP expands, its impact on reducing violence and promoting peaceful conflict resolution continues to be explored in various cultural and societal contexts.

Violence and bullying are also seen in the form of discrimination and stigmatization. Prejudices and stereotypes based on race, ethnicity, gender, or socioeconomic background often lead to the exclusion or negative labeling of certain students. Discrimination and exclusion based on ethnic background can have profound effects on young people's well-being. Young people who experience discrimination or exclusion based on their ethnic origin are more likely to engage in risky behavior. These marginalized young people may be more prone to using cannabis as they may try to numb the social pain associated with discrimination (i.e., the self-medication hypothesis). They may also seek acceptance in alternative groups, such as substance-using peer groups (Bakhtiari et al., 2020). Addressing discrimination and providing supportive environments is crucial in mitigating the harmful effects on vulnerable youth and reducing risky behaviors.

Preventing violence in schools is important to maintain a safe and supportive learning environment for students. Research has shown that it is important to understand teachers' awareness of peer bullying, their intervention strategies, and their suggestions for prevention (Kutlu and Karaca, 2022). Understanding the perspectives of school administrators regarding the causes of conflicts and potential solutions can provide valuable insights for developing effective conflict resolution strategies (Bayar, 2015). Addressing student misbehavior in classrooms is vital, and studies have shown that there is a significant relationship between teachers' beliefs about self-efficacy and the methods they use to manage these behaviors (Aslan and Alpaslan, 2020). Difficulties in implementing inclusive education practices in schools, such as negative attitudes of educators and lack of experience, can also affect the effectiveness of violence prevention initiatives (Özbek and Taneri, 2023). A comprehensive approach to preventing violence in schools includes understanding teachers,' principals,' and students' perspectives on various forms of violence, implementing effective conflict resolution strategies, promoting inclusive educational practices, and tailoring interventions to address specific health and behavioral issues.

Prevention of Violence at School

Violence can include behaviors such as coercion, physical attacks, he use of brute force, inflicting serious physical or psychological harm, hitting, injuring, or forcing someone to do something against their will, either through physical means or the use of objects. These behaviors disrupt the learning environment and pose significant risks to students' safety and well-being. As can be understood from its definition and the behaviors it includes, violence is a phenomenon that goes beyond the use of brute force or physical harm. It also involves psychological harm and can manifest in various forms, including emotional, verbal, and social violence (Çakır and Özkan, 2021). While violence is more often the subject of research as domestic violence, violence is generally experienced more among adolescents in the school environment. Schools are the main institutions that aim to protect children and young people from physical and psychological violence (Körük, 2020). Although violence contradicts the fundamental purpose of education and the role of schools, unfortunately, individuals continue to face violence in their educational lives (İnandı and Yıldız, 2014). School violence is considered one of the factors that negatively affect learning within an educational environment, as it undermines students' motivation to learn. School violence is defined as all kinds of destructive and disruptive actions that prevent schools from performing their educational duties, target the lives and property of students and employees at school, and prevent the creation of a safe environment. According to the results of a report published by United Nations Educational, Scientific and Cultural Organization (UNESCO), exposure to violence and bullying at school occurs all over the world. It is estimated that approximately 246 million children and adolescents are exposed to violence and bullying at school every year (UNESCO, 2017). A study conducted in Türkiye revealed that adolescents are frequently exposed to violence and bullying. Among the environments where adolescents are exposed to violence, the school environment ranks first (Ünlü, 2019). As a result of this situation, there are security problems in schools, and the quality of education decreases (MOE, 2015). UNICEF's research in 2018 revealed that students are exposed to violence at school and out of school. It was observed that 35% of students worldwide were physically exposed to violence (UNICEF, 2018). It is not possible to attribute the cause of violence to a single event (MOE, 2015). When analyzing the causes of school violence, several factors come to light. These include class conflict, pressure and restrictions, an inappropriate environment, negative teacher attitudes, the wrong choice of friends, the lack of self-confidence, academic failure, family problems, broken families, adolescence-related challenges, and lack of family education (Ankaralı and Savaş, 2021). Studies have concluded that the primary causes of violence in schools are often rooted in family dynamics (Çubukçu and Dönmez, 2012). Violence in schools has a detrimental impact on students' health, increasing their stress and fear levels (Coşkun and Bebiş, 2014). Studies have revealed that 1-2% of students exposed to psychological violence by educators at school are diagnosed with Post Traumatic Stress Disorder (PTSD) and that students show behavioral disorders such as aggression, anti-social behavior, fighting, and have serious emotional problems as long as they live (Bulut and Aktaş, 2022). For some children, violence, bullying, sexual assault, or fear at school has resulted in death (UNICEF, 2018). A safe school environment is needed for learning to take place (Çoban, 2021). In many studies, it has been concluded that violence at school can be prevented by raising awareness about violence among students, ensuring that teachers and other personnel at school take responsibility, and ensuring that stakeholders within the school participate in violence prevention programs (Çubukçu and Dönmez, 2012; Kubar and Kıral, 2019; Milner, 2020; Uzbaş, 2009).

Prevention of Bullying at School

Bullying is a top concern among parents of school-age children. The answer to the question of whether the increase in the prevalence of violence increases bullying or whether the experience of bullying at a young age fuels violence has still not been answered to this day (Aslan and Polat, 2023).

Today, the most widely used definition of bullying is made by Dan Olweus (Qiu, 2021). Bullying is defined as repeated aggressive negative behavior by a group or individual with the intention of causing discomfort. It is characterized by intentionality, repetition, and power imbalance (Borgen et al., 2021). Peer bullying, which often begins in preschool age, remains prevalent among school-age children (Tanrıkulu et al., 2021). Bullying is a situation that students face almost every day and is seen as a vital and important social problem in many countries when its effects and consequences on students and schools are considered (Garmy et al., 2018; Salmivalli, 2010). The impact of bullying on students' mental health, academic performance, and overall well-being makes it a priority for intervention and prevention in educational systems.

Bullying affects approximately one-third of children worldwide (UNESCO, 2022). Data from 96 countries and territories show that in the past six months, about one in five students (19.4%) were bullied one or two days, one in 20 (5.6%) three to five days, and one in 13 (7.3%) every day (UNESCO, 2019). In the study conducted by Karakuş Şahbaz (2019) with 5th, 6th, 7th, and 8th-grade students, it was determined that 36.7% of the students were bullies, 57.5% were victims, and 32.7% were bully victims. In terms of gender, 61% of male students and 54.5% of female students were found to be bullies. The rates of physical and verbal bullying tend to increase as students progress through higher grade levels (Karakuş Şahbaz, 2019). According to a study conducted by Polat and Sohbet (2020) with 1,743 students, 40.4% of the participants reported that bullying was a common occurrence at their school. In the study, 47.9% of the bullying incidents were verbal, while 26.7% were physical. Additionally, 41.9% of the participants stated that bullying was seen as a way to deal with the bully (Polat and Sohbet, 2020).

With the recent technological developments all over the world, phones and the internet have become the easiest tools to access in daily life, and in addition to physical and verbal bullying, another type of bullying has emerged. Cyberbullying is defined as disturbing a person in an unwanted and continuous manner through phone, e-mail, and social media. While classifying peer bullying, cyberbullying should also be included in this classification (Akça et al., 2014). Furthermore, Sipahi (2019) found a relationship between students' tendencies toward peer bullying and their tendencies toward cyberbullying in his study with 383 secondary school students (Sipahi, 2019).

In peer bullying, school-age children may assume the roles of bully, victim, bully-victim, or bystander. Children who engage in bullying often have difficulty adapting to social norms and integrating into society. Bullying behaviors in children often show up as signs of emotional or behavior problems they are dealing with inside. They tend to exhibit health problems and aggressive personality traits (Mercan and Sarı, 2018). Conflicts are seen within the families of children who bully. Typically, the father of a child, who engages in bullying, is uninvolved, emotionally distant from both the home and the child, and may exhibit violent behavior, while the mother is often not respected by her husband and tends to be angry. Children who engage in bullying are often neglected at home and are lacking sufficient attention and love; they may grow into individuals angry toward their environment(Gürhan, 2017).

Bullying negatively affects the health and academic performance of school-age children. Studies have found that victims of bullying show somatic symptoms such as sleep disturbances, bedwetting, headaches, stomachaches, fatigue, and school-related problems. They may also experience psychological issues, including low self-esteem, anxiety, depression, and suicidal ideation and may feel socially rejected or isolated (Brown et al., 2005). Although, peer bullying can not be completely prevented despite various interventions, it can be significantly reduced through effective measures (Basım and Şeşen, 2005).

In the World Health Organization's (2019) report on the prevention of bullying in schools, three basic strategies are emphasized: developing children's life skills, teaching safe behaviors, and fighting to change social and cultural norms that encourage bullying. These strategies target various groups, including bullies, victims, parents, and teachers (WHO, 2019).

Prevention of Discrimination and Stigmatization in Schools

Discrimination refers to actions that hinder individuals or social groups from receiving equal treatment. The grounds for discrimination can vary widely. In Western contexts, researchers commonly categorize discrimination into two main types: discrimination based on personal characteristics and discrimination based on group membership. Discrimination based on personal characteristics occurs when an individual faces prejudice due to traits such as age, appearance or other personal characteristics. On the other hand, discrimination based on group membership arises when an individual is subjected to bias or unfair treatment due to their affiliation with a particular social group, such as an ethnic group (Zhao and Ngai, 2022).

Stigma refers to the social devaluation, discrimination, or possession of a profoundly discrediting trait rooted in negative stereotypes directed at a specific population. The notion of stigma is categorized into three distinct but interconnected realms: perceived, enacted, and internalized stigma. Perceived stigma relates to an individual's awareness or fear of being unfavorably treated due to a specific condition or trait. Enacted stigma involves the actual discriminatory actions faced by an individual because of a certain characteristic. Internalized stigma, which is often considered the most harmful, occurs when individuals accept and internalize the negative stereotypes and prejudices held against them by society due to their particular condition or characteristic (Feingold and Drossman, 2021). Moreover, internalized stigma can lead to manifestations of self-hatred, self-isolation, shame, and a fear of experiencing further stigmatization (Li et al., 2020).

Broadly, there are significant reports of frequent encounters with discrimination in schools. Specifically, among young adolescents in Australia, data indicate that 22.1% experience racism daily, while 47.3% witness it occurring around them. These results underscore the urgent need for interventions aimed at preventing discrimination in schools (Priest et al., 2014). Simultaneously, a recent report by the Department for Children, Equality, Disability, Integration, and Youth reveals that nearly half (47%) of young individuals under the age of 18 in Ireland encounter discrimination specifically related to their age. This significant percentage underscores the prevalence of age-based discrimination among youth, highlighting a widespread issue that affects a substantial portion of young people in Ireland and pointing to the need for targeted interventions and policy adjustments to address and mitigate ageism in various societal sectors (Költő et al., 2023).

School stigmatization can negatively affect school-age children's health and behavior, primarily due to diminished school quality and increased exposure to racial discrimination. This environment not only hinders their academic success but also significantly harms their psychological well-being and social development (Wang et al., 2022). The learning process for a stigmatized individual occurs in stages: first, learning the societal norms of self-perception and realizing one's inadequacy according to these norms; then, learning how to navigate belonging to a particular group and coping with the way others treat individuals from that group; and finally, learning to adopt a deceptive appearance. School-age children usually discover their stigma when they start school, sometimes directly on the first day of school, with teasing, exclusion, and conflict (Goffman and Ağırnaslı, 2014). Consequently, early interventions and a supportive school environment are crucial in addressing these challenges and promoting the well-being of stigmatized children.

Emotional reactions due to the decrease in the quality of life and self-confidence of the victim as a result of stigmatization sometimes manifest themselves in the form of fear and anger. The fear of stigmatization is a sufficiently frightening threat perception for school-age children. While the social life of the stigmatized individual is disrupted, it can sometimes results in complete exclusion from their social group (Bayramlık and Feyzi, 2019). For school-age children, the emotional impact of stigmatization can be particularly severe, leading to heightened feelings of loneliness and insecurity, which may interfere with their ability to build healthy social connections. The process of discrimination has been observed to impact mental and physical health during childhood and adolescence in several ways, serving as a predictor for antisocial behavior and substance use. A study found a significant negative correlation between experiences of discrimination and the value students place on their school environment. Additionally, perceived discrimination negatively affects collective self-esteem, indicating that its consequences extend beyond immediate emotional distress, influencing broader aspects of well-being, social behavior, and academic engagement. These findings highlight the critical need for interventions and support systems within educational settings to address and mitigate the effects of discrimination, fostering a more inclusive and supportive environment for all students (Flores et al., 2021). In addition to the profound effects on self-esteem, perceived discrimination has other harmful effects on a wide range of undesirable and negative impacts on health, well-being, and development. Perceived discrimination is linked to behavioral risk factors such as depression, anxiety and distress, and substance use. All forms of discrimination are inhumane because they devalue individuals and diminish people's sense of dignity and pride (Assari and Caldwell, 2018).

The mere observation of discrimination has been proven to compromise an individual's sense of belonging and commitment. This evidence demonstrates that students do not have to directly experience discrimination to be adversely affected by it; rather, the discrimination they observe within the school environment can have significant negative impacts. Specifically, students from minority groups who witness discrimination report higher levels of fatigue. The phenomenon indicates that the more students are exposed to instances of discrimination against their peers, the less they identify with school. Furthermore, their levels of anxiety and depression are notably higher. This underscores the pervasive effects of discrimination, affecting not just those who are directly targeted but also those who are bystanders (Baysu et al., 2023). Therefore, creating an inclusive and supportive school environment is essential to mitigate the harmful effects of discrimination, not only on those directly targeted but also on the wider student body.

The substantial body of evidence highlighting the adverse effects of perceived discrimination on health and well-being, particularly among school-age children, underscores the urgency of implementing anti-discrimination policies and interventions. These measures are essential to curtail social exclusion and bullying, thereby fostering a more inclusive environment. Enhancing cultural awareness, tolerance, and empathy plays a significant role in the integration and acceptance of minority students. It is imperative that teachers, school nurses, and school staff providers receive comprehensive education tailored to meet the diverse needs of all minority students. This education should address not only prejudicial perceptions and stigmatization but also equip these professionals with the necessary skills to intervene effectively when discrimination occurs. This approach not only supports the immediate needs of minority youth but also contributes to the creation of a more inclusive and supportive community for future generations (Költő et al., 2023).

Conclusion

School violence, bullying, discrimination, and stigmatization are serious problems that negatively affect students' physical, emotional, and academic development. These behaviors undermine the safety and supportiveness of the learning environment and prevent equal educational opportunities for all students. Studies show that victimized students' academic achievement declines, school attendance rates decrease, and they face mental health problems. In particular, it is known that psychological problems such as depression, anxiety, and low self-esteem are more common among victims of bullying and discrimination. Schools should take proactive measures to create a safe and supportive environment among students. These measures should include developing policies to prevent bullying and discrimination, training teachers and administrators on these issues, implementing awareness and education programs for students, and providing support services to victims. In addition, schools need to work on fostering positive relationships between students and creating a culture that respects differences. In conclusion, combating violence, bullying, discrimination, and stigmatization at school requires a comprehensive approach that not only changes individual behavior but also extends to the whole education system. This struggle can be achieved through the joint efforts of educators, administrators, school nurses, students, parents, and all members of society. Such an approach will not only reduce these problems but also strengthen society at large by ensuring that every student receives education in a safe, supportive, and equitable learning environment.

Disclaimer

None.

References

Akca, E. B., Sayimer, İ., Sali, J. B., & Başak, B. E. (2014). Okulda siber zorbalığın nedenleri, türleri ve medya okuryazarlığı eğitiminin önleyici çalışmalardaki yeri [Causes and types of cyberbullying in schools and the role of media literacy education in preventive efforts]. *Electronic Journal of Professional Development and Research*, 2(2), 17-30.

Ankarali, F., & Savaş, G. (2021). Okul öncesi çocuklarda öğretmen açısından helikopter ebeveyn tutumlarının şiddet bağlamında değerlendirilmesi [Evaluation of helicopter parenting attitudes in terms of violence by preschool teachers]. *Journal of Sociology*, (41-42), 117-143.

Aslan, H., & Alpaslan, S. (2020). The correlation between classroom teachers' using methods in coping with unwanted student behaviors and self-efficacy: Sınıf öğretmenlerinin istenmeyen öğrenci davranışlarına karşı kullandıkları baş etme yöntemleri ile öz yeterlilikleri arasındaki ilişki [The correlation between classroom teachers' coping methods with unwanted student behaviors and self-efficacy]. *Journal of Human Sciences*, 17(4), 1177-1203.

Aslan, M., & Polat, M. O. (2023). Tüm boyutlarıyla akranlar arası zorbalık [Peer bullying in all aspects]. *Hacettepe University Journal of Social Sciences*, 5(1), 43-82.

Assari, S., & Caldwell, C. H. (2018). Teacher discrimination reduces school performance of African American youth: Role of gender. *Brain Sciences*, 8(10), 183.

Bakhtiari, F., Boyle, A. E., & Benner, A. D. (2020). Pathways linking school-based ethnic discrimination to Latino/a adolescents' marijuana approval and use. *Journal of Immigrant and Minority Health*, 22(6), 1273-1280.

Basım, H. N., & Şeşen, H. (2005). Çalışma yaşamında tükenmişlik: Sosyal hizmet uzmanları ile hemşireler üzerine karşılaştırmalı bir çalışma [Burnout in working life: A comparative study on social workers and nurses]. *Community and Social Service*, 16(2), 57-70.

Bayar, A. (2015). Bir örgüt olarak okulda meydana gelen çatışma nedenleri ve çözüm yollarına yönelik okul müdürlerinin görüşleri [School conflict causes and solutions according to school administrators]. *Sakarya University Journal of Education*, 5(3), 130-141.

Bayramlık, H. A., & Feyzi, U. (2019). Öğretmenlerin kişilik özellikleri ile damgalama davranışları arasındaki ilişkinin incelenmesi [Examination of the relationship between teachers' personality traits and stigmatizing behaviors]. *Journal of Contemporary Management Sciences*, 6(1), 4-17.

Baysu, G., Agirdag, O., & De Leersnyder, J. (2023). The association between perceived discriminatory climate in school and student performance in math and reading: A cross-national analysis using PISA 2018. *Journal of Youth and Adolescence*, 52(3), 619-636.

Borgen, N. T., Olweus, D., Kirkebøen, L. J., Breivik, K., Solberg, M. E., Frønes, I., ... Raaum, O. (2021). The potential of anti-bullying efforts to prevent academic failure and youth crime: A case using the Olweus Bullying Prevention Program (OBPP). *Prevention Science*, 22, 1147-1158.

Brown, S. L., Birch, D. A., & Kancherla, V. (2005). Bullying perspectives: Experiences, attitudes, and recommendations of 9-to-13-year-olds attending health education centers in the United States. *Journal of School Health*, 75(10), 384-392.

Bulut, S., & Aktaş, A. (2022). Öğretmenlerin gösterdikleri psikolojik, sosyal ve fiziksel şiddet davranışları ve sonuçları [Teachers' psychological, social, and physical violence behaviors and their consequences]. *Humanistic Perspective*, 4(2), 448-465.

Coşkun, S., & Bebiş, H. (2014). Şiddetin okul sağlığına etkisi ve hemşirelik [The impact of violence on school health and nursing]. *Cumhuriyet Hemşirelik Dergisi*, 3(1), 15-23.

Çakır, Ç., & Özkan, M. (2021). Okulda şiddet ve yansımaları: Eğitim ortamlarındaki şiddete yönelik uluslararası raporların incelenmesi [School violence and its reflections: An analysis of international reports on violence in educational environments]. *International Innovative Education Researcher (IEdRes)*, 1(2).

Çoban, G. S. (2021). Maslow'un ihtiyaçlar hiyerarşisi kendini gerçekleştirme basamağında gizil yetenekler [Latent talents at the self-actualization stage of Maslow's hierarchy of needs]. *European Journal of Educational and Social Sciences*, 6(1), 111-118.

Çubukçu, Z., & Dönmez, A. (2012). İlköğretim okullarında görev yapan öğretmenlerin okuldaki şiddet üzerine görüşleri [Teachers' views on violence in elementary schools]. *Electronic Journal of Social Sciences*, 11(40), 89-108.

Davli Temel, D. (2018). Ergenlerde algılanan sosyal destek ve şiddet eğilimi [Perceived social support and violence tendency in adolescents] [Unpublished master's thesis]. Sağlık Bilimleri Enstitüsü.

Emiroğlu, Z. (2018). Examining the effects of basic psychological needs and life satisfaction levels on tendencies to violence of 10-14 aged middle school students [Unpublished master's thesis]. Eğitim Bilimleri Enstitüsü.

Feingold, J. H., & Drossman, D. A. (2021). Deconstructing stigma as a barrier to treating DGBI: Lessons for clinicians. *Neurogastroenterology & Motility*, 33(2), e14080.

Flores, J., Caqueo-Urízar, A., Quintana, L., Urzúa, A., & Irarrázaval, M. (2021). Perceived discrimination and contextual problems among children and adolescents in northern Chile. *PloS One*, 16(2), e0246998.

Garmy, P., Vilhjálmsson, R., & Kristjánsdóttir, G. (2018). Bullying in school-aged children in Iceland: A cross-sectional study. *Journal of Pediatric Nursing*, 38, e30-e34.

Goffman, E., & Ağırnaslı, S. (2014). *Damga: Örselenmiş kimliğin idare edilişi üzerine notlar* [Stigma: Notes on the management of spoiled identity]. Heretik Yayıncılık.

Golan, O., Shilo, H., & Omer, H. (2018). Non-violent resistance parent training for the parents of young adults with high functioning autism spectrum disorder. *Journal of Family Therapy*, 40(1), 4-24.

Gürhan, N. (2017). Her yönü ile akran zorbalığı [Peer bullying in all aspects]. *Turkiye Klinikleri J Psychiatr Nurs-Special Topics*, 3(2), 175-181.

Hoşgörür, V., & Orhan, A. (2017). Okulda zorbalık ve şiddetin nedenleri ve önlenmesinin yönetimi (Muğla merkez ilçe örneği) [The causes of bullying and violence in schools and management of prevention (The case of Muğla city center)]. Bayburt Faculty of Education Journal, 12(24), 859-880.

İnandi, Y., & Yildiz, S. (2014). Lise okul yöneticilerinin okullarda şiddeti önleme yeterlikleri: Mersin ili örneği [The competencies of high school administrators in preventing violence in schools: The case of Mersin]. *Trakya Üniversitesi Eğitim Fakültesi Dergisi*, 4(2), 137-147.

Karakuş Şahbaz, Y. (2019). Ortaokul öğrencilerinde akran zorbalığı: Adana ili Yüreğir ilçesi pilot çalışma [Peer bullying among secondary school students: The pilot study in Yüreğir, Adana] [Unpublished master's thesis]. Çağ University.

Költő, A., Gavin, A., Vaughan, E., Molcho, M., Kelly, C., & Nic Gabhainn, S. (2023). Perceived discrimination among adolescents in Ireland. *Health Education & Behavior*, 50(2), 193-198.

Körük, S. (2020). Saldırganlık ve şiddeti açıklayan yaklaşımlar [Approaches explaining aggression and violence]. In N. Ş. Özabacı (Ed.), *Çağımızın çözüm arayan sorunu şiddet* [The issue of violence seeking a solution in our age] (pp. 93-104).

Kubar, Y., & Kıral, G. (2019). Lise öğrencilerinin şiddet algısı üzerine bir araştırma: Elazığ merkez ilçe örneği [A study on high school students' perception of violence: The case of Elazığ central district]. *Journal of Çukurova University Social Sciences Institute*, 28(2), 354-374.

Kutlu, M., & Karaca, N. H. (2022). 3. ve 4. sınıf öğretmenlerinin akran zorbalığına yönelik görüşlerinin incelenmesi [An examination of 3rd and 4th grade teachers' views on peer bullying]. *e-Kafkas Journal of Educational Research*, 9(2), 621-641.

Lavi-Levavi, I., Shachar, I., & Omer, H. (2013). Training in nonviolent resistance for parents of violent children: Differences between fathers and mothers. *Journal of Systemic Therapies*, 32(4), 79-93.

Li, H., Zheng, L., Le, H., Zhuo, L., Wu, Q., Ma, G., & Tao, H. (2020). The mediating role of internalized stigma and shame on the relationship between COVID-19 related discrimination and mental health outcomes among back-to-school students in Wuhan. *International Journal of Environmental Research and Public Health*, 17(24), 9237.

Mercan, H., & Sarı, H. Y. (2018). Lise öğrencilerinde akran zorbalığı ve sosyodemografik değişkenlerle ilişkisi [Peer bullying among high school students and its relationship with sociodemographic variables]. *Florence Nightingale Journal of Nursing*, 26(1), 21-29.

Ministry of Education (MOE). (2015). *Çocuğa yönelik şiddetin önlenmesi teknik destek projesi: Revize erken uyarı uygulamaları* [Technical assistance project for preventing violence against children: Revised early warning practices]. Ministry of National Education Project Office. https://siddetinonlenmesi.meb.gov.tr/meb_iys_dosyalar/2015_09/17121034_1.2.4._erken_uyari_uygulamalari_programi.pdf.

Milner, H. R. (2020). Fifteenth annual AERA Brown lecture in education research: Disrupting punitive practices and policies: Rac (e) ing back to teaching, teacher preparation, and Brown *Educational Researcher*, 49(3), 147-160.

Ollefs, B., Schlippe, A., Omer, H., & Kriz, J. (2009). Youngsters with externalizing behavior problems: Effects of parent training. *Familiendynamik*, 34, 256-265.

Omidi, R., Heidari, K., Davari, H., Espanani, M., Poursalehi, M., Naeini, S. E., ... Zakizadeh, M. (2014). The relationships between environmental factors and violent behaviors in adolescent students of Isfahan, Iran. *International Journal of Preventive Medicine*, 5(Suppl 2), S97.

Özbek, Ö. Y., & Taneri, P. O. (2023). Okul yöneticilerinin kapsayıcı eğitime ilişkin farkındalıkları üzerine sanat-temelli bir çalışma [A study on school administrators' awareness of inclusive education through art-based methods]. *Çankırı Karatekin University Karatekin Faculty of Letters Journal*, 11(1), 75-96.

Polat, F., & Sohbet, R. (2020). Ortaöğretim öğrencilerinde akran zorbalığı [Peer bullying among secondary school students]. *Kahramanmaraş Sütçü İmam University Medical Faculty Journal,* 15(2), 41-51. https://doi.org/10.17517/ksutfd.608921.

Priest, N., Perry, R., Ferdinand, A., Paradies, Y., & Kelaher, M. (2014). Experiences of racism, racial/ethnic attitudes, motivated fairness and mental health outcomes among primary and secondary school students. *Journal of Youth and Adolescence*, 43, 1672-1687.

Qiu, H. (2021). Explore the factors of school bullying from the ecosystem theory. *Open Access Library Journal*, 8(12), 1-10.

Salmivalli, C. (2010). Bullying and the peer group: A review. *Aggression and Violent Behavior*, 15(2), 112-120.

Sipahi, E. (2019). Ortaokul öğrencilerinin siber zorbalık ve akran zorbalığı eğilimlerinin örgütsel yabancılaşma ve örgütsel güven algılarına etkilerinin incelenmesi [The impact of secondary school students' tendencies towards cyberbullying and peer bullying on their perceptions of organizational alienation and trust] [Unpublished master's thesis]. Ankara University.

Tanrıkulu, İ., Özdinç, N. K., & Besnili, Z. N. (2021). Okul öncesi dönemde akran zorbalığı ve okul yapısı ile ilgili değişkenlerin incelenmesi [Peer bullying in preschool and analysis of school structure-related variables]. *Erzincan University Faculty of Education Journal,* 23(3), 857-873.

TLA (Turkish Language Association). (2016). *Türkçe sözlük* [Turkish dictionary]. Turkish Language Association Publications.

UNESCO. (2017). *School violence and bullying: Global status report.* United Nations Educational, Scientific and Cultural Organization.

UNESCO. (2019). *Behind the numbers: Ending school violence and bullying.* UNESCO Publishing.

UNESCO. (2022). *International day against violence and bullying at school including cyberbullying.* https://www.unesco.org/en/articles/international-day-against-violence-and-bullying-school-including-cyberbullyin.

UNICEF. (2018). *An everyday lesson: End violence in schools.* New York: USA. https://www.unicef.org/publications/files/An_Everyday_Lesson_END_violence_in_Schools.pdf.

Uzbaş, A. (2009). Okul psikolojik danışmanlarının okulda saldırganlık ve şiddete yönelik görüşlerinin değerlendirilmesi [Evaluation of school counselors' views on aggression and violence in schools]. *Mehmet Akif Ersoy University Faculty of Education Journal*, (18), 90-110.

Ünlü, M. (2019). Öğretmen şiddeti ve akran zorbalığına maruz kalan lise öğrencilerinin saldırganlıklarının ve okula ilişkin tutumlarının incelenmesi [*Examination of aggression and school attitudes of high school students exposed to teacher violence and peer bullying*] [Unpublished master's thesis]. Institute of Educational Sciences.

Van Holen, F., Vanderfaeillie, J., & Omer, H. (2016). Adaptation and evaluation of a nonviolent resistance intervention for foster parents: A progress report. *Journal of Marital and Family Therapy*, 42(2), 256-271.

World Health Organization (WHO). (2019). *School-based violence prevention: A practical handbook.* World Health Organization. https://apps.who.int/iris/handle/10665/324930.

Wang, G., Schwartz, G. L., Kim, M. H., White, J. S., Glymour, M. M., Reardon, S., ... Hamad, R. (2022). School racial segregation and the health of Black children. *Pediatrics*, 149(5).

Zhao, L., & Ngai, S. S.-y. (2022). Perceived discrimination at school and developmental outcomes among Bai adolescents: The mediating roles of self-esteem and ethnic identity. *International Journal of Environmental Research and Public Health*, 19(2), 657.

Chapter 8

Infection Control in Schools

Zahide Aksoy*, **PhD**
Department of Nursing, İstanbul Kent University, İstanbul, Turkiye

Abstract

Schools are environments that provide ideal conditions for the spread of infectious diseases. School-age children are susceptible to many infections. Situations such as students being in close contact for a long time, sharing and using some objects, limited opportunities for hand hygiene, inadequate personal hygiene materials, and students or staff going to school despite having symptoms of contagious diseases accelerate the spread of infections. Infectious disease control in schools, vaccination, hand hygiene, respiratory etiquette, environmental cleaning and disinfection, food hygiene, ventilation, practices for infectious disease outbreaks, and management of emergencies in infectious diseases should be taken as a basis. These are effective methods to prevent the spread of most infectious diseases. Therefore, it should be implemented consistently in schools. In schools, students and school staff, as well as parents and other community members, can be educated about health behaviors to prevent infections. Healthy behaviors learned in schools can contribute to future health and well-being.

Keywords: school health, infection control, health promotion

Introduction

Schools, which cover a large part of the population, are environments where diseases can spread rapidly. Situations such as children being in close contact for a long time, sharing and using some objects, limited opportunities for hand hygiene, inadequate personal hygiene materials, and students or school staff going to school despite having symptoms of contagious diseases are factors that play an important role in the spread of infections (Centre for Health Protection, 2023). By effectively preventing infectious diseases in schools, the damage caused by diseases is minimized, and the health of children and staff is protected. Schools are ideal environments for children and staff to learn effective ways to prevent infections (Public Health England,

---

* Corresponding Author's Email: zahide.aksoy@kent.edu.tr

In: Health Promotion and Prevention
Editor: Eda Kılınç İşleyen
ISBN: 979-8-89530-758-8

2014). Infections are a major cause of school absenteeism for both children and school staff. Outbreaks can cause school closures and major disruptions for all members of the school. Therefore, it is important to comply with and maintain existing hygiene regulations and develop new strategies and action plans for infection prevention with the active participation of all school members (Centre for Health Protection, 2023).

Vaccination

Vaccines are important in protecting against the serious consequences of many infectious diseases. Students and school staff should be educated on all recommended vaccines for infectious diseases. Compliance with the mandatory immunization program should be ensured, and immunization status should be recorded. Unvaccinated children should be included in the immunization program again, and unvaccinated children should be followed up against vaccine-preventable diseases (Minnesota Department of Health, 2023).

Hand Hygiene

Hand hygiene is an essential infection control measure to prevent the spread of infectious diseases. Research shows that proper hand washing is the most effective way to prevent the spread of infectious diseases (Bolon, 2016). Common hand hygiene practices include hand washing and proper use of 70-80% alcohol-based hand sanitizer. Hand washing should be done if hands are visibly dirty. If the hands are not visibly dirty, the application of 70-80% alcohol-based hand sanitizer is equally effective (Centre for Health Protection, 2023).

To ensure infection control in schools, everyone must perform regular hand hygiene. All students and school staff should be taught to perform hand hygiene, especially before eating, after using the restroom, and after coughing or sneezing into a tissue (Minnesota Department Health, 2023). Children should be taught how to perform hand hygiene with a 70-80% alcohol-based hand sanitizer. To prevent unsupervised use, 70-80% alcohol-based hand sanitizer should be kept out of reach of children. Wearing gloves does not eliminate the indication of hand hygiene. The hands should always be washed after the gloves are removed. Improper hand drying may also cause cross-infection with others through contaminated hands. Disposable paper towels and a hand dryer are suitable tools for hand drying (WHO, 2021). Adequate hand hygiene facilities should be provided in schools/centers (Centre for Health Protection, 2023).

School health personnel are also required to perform hand hygiene. If school health personnel neglect hand washing, they become carriers of different infective agents and cause cross-infection. Therefore, both hands should be washed with liquid soap before and after caring for each child (Public Health England, 2014).

Respiratory Etiquette

To prevent respiratory transmission, students should be taught to cover their noses and mouths with tissues when coughing or sneezing. Hands should also be washed immediately after contact with respiratory secretions or after touching objects contaminated with respiratory secretions (Public Health Ontario, 2023).

Students and school staff with respiratory symptoms should avoid attending class or working at school. Students with respiratory symptoms detected at school should be physically separated from others as soon as possible, and a mask should be worn on these students (Centre for Health Protection, 2023).

Lid waste bins should be used to dispose of used masks and tissues. Visual warnings can be posted in prominent places to remind students to practice coughing patterns. Maintaining ventilation in classrooms is part of comprehensive measures to prevent and reduce the transmission of respiratory infections, especially in schools (Minnesota Department of Health, 2023).

Environmental Cleaning and Disinfection

Surfaces in the school should be cleaned at least once a day to reduce the risk of spreading germs. Cleaning with products containing soap or detergent reduces germs on surfaces by removing contaminants and reducing the risk of infection from surfaces. School nurses should develop protocols with care staff for the correct use of cleaning and disinfection products (Public Health England, 2014). The infirmary should be cleaned and disinfected daily. The number of people who can use the infirmary should be determined, the person coming to the infirmary should take precautions for the use of personal protective equipment, and case tracking records of people applying to the infirmary should be kept. The waste generated in the infirmary should be disposed of in accordance with waste management (Centre for Health Protection, 2023). The number of users of the elevator capacity should be stated at the elevator entrance. Alcohol-based hand antiseptics should be kept at elevator entrances. Posters/voice announcements should be provided to ensure that cough/sneeze etiquette is observed in the elevator and, if possible, to avoid talking. The places where each person should stand should be determined on the elevator floor (Public Health England, 2014).

The lids of the garbage cans should be kept closed. Garbage should be properly wrapped before being disposed of in lidded bins. Litter bins should be emptied at least once a day. Hands should be washed after handling garbage. The clean and hygienic conditions of toilets, changing rooms, and bathrooms must be maintained. Liquid soap and disposable paper towels or hand dryers should be provided for hand washing. It should be ensured that the toilet's flush system is working properly Centre for Health Protection, 2023). The type and frequency of cleaning of the school zones are shown in Table 1.

Food Hygiene

Hygiene rules must be observed during food purchasing, storage, preparation, cooking, and service processes. Foodborne infections are common, especially in places where public meals are eaten, such as schools. The school nurse should effectively inspect the school cafeteria and canteen for health compliance and provide training to the relevant personnel. If food services are to be purchased in schools, catering companies must be licensed and inspected (Centre for Food Safety, 2023; Centre for Health Protection, 2023).

Table 1. Cleaning according to school environments

Area	Cleaning	Frequency
Tables, windowsills, door, and cabinet handles	Cleaning with neutral detergent, warm water, and clean cloth	It should be cleaned daily, but if it becomes dirty, it should be cleaned immediately. Additionally, sterilization is required. If contaminated with blood and body fluids, cleaning, disinfection, rinsing, and drying procedures must be carried out.
Chair, dining table	Drying with neutral detergent, warm water, clean cloth, and disposable paper towels	It should be cleaned before and after use. Additionally, sterilization is required. If contaminated with blood and body fluids, cleaning, disinfection, rinsing, and drying procedures must be carried out.
Washable floor	Detergent, the material should be washed with warm water, and clean.	It should be cleaned daily. However, if there is pollution due to spillage, it should be cleaned immediately with a vacuum cleaner.
Carpets	Washing Sweeping	It should be cleaned at least once a month in areas where adults are present, and once every three months in other areas, and if it gets dirty, it should be cleaned immediately. It should be vacuumed daily with a vacuum cleaner.
Rugs	Laundry	It should be washed weekly.
Walls, interior coverings	It should be cleaned with general-purpose detergent and warm water. If it is contaminated with blood and body fluids, it must be cleaned and disinfected.	There is no need for routine cleaning in areas where hand contact is not frequent.
Trash can	Unloading Should be cleaned with neutral detergent, warm water	Daily It should be cleaned weekly, but if it becomes dirty, it should be cleaned immediately.
Mop	The mop head is washed with detergent and warm water, rinsed, and air-dried. After being tumble dried, it should be washed daily in the machine at least 60°C.	It should be cleaned and sterilized after daily use. After daily use
Sink, Soap dispenser, Faucet, Toilet seat, handle, door handles	The detergent should be cleaned with warm water.	It should be cleaned daily, but if it becomes dirty, it should be cleaned immediately. Additionally, sterilization is required. If contaminated with blood and body fluids, cleaning, disinfection, rinsing, and drying procedures must be carried out.
Closet	The toilet should be cleaned with cleaning products. The manufacturer's instructions must be followed.	It should be cleaned daily, but if it becomes dirty, it should be cleaned immediately. Additionally, sterilization is required.

From: Public Health England. (2014).

Infectious Disease Outbreak

The fact that schools are crowded environments, exposure to risk factors, and the difficulty of applying effective infection control measures in such environments increase the risk of transmission of infectious diseases. Early detection of infectious diseases is important to prevent the spread of the disease (Donaldson, 2023). If similar symptoms develop in students or school personnel and the incidence is higher than normal, an epidemic is suspected. For this, information on daily infectious disease cases should be followed (Centre for Health Protection,

2023). To this end, the school nurse is responsible for closely monitoring the emergence and outbreaks of infectious diseases, including legally notified diseases. Contact between children and staff on different floors should be minimized. At the same time, the same team of staff should be provided to care for a fixed group of children whenever possible (Minnesota Department of Health, 2023). All parents should be informed about a suspected or confirmed infectious disease outbreak and reminded that sick children should stay at home. Close communication should be maintained with parents about the children's condition. Students, staff, visitors, and relevant people should be encouraged to practice hand hygiene, respiratory hygiene, and cough etiquette for potential measures to minimize the transmission of epidemic diseases (Alaska Department of Health, 2013).

Recommendations for Managing Some Infectious Disease Outbreaks

Acute Gastroenteritis or Food Poisoning Outbreak

Items or places contaminated with feces or vomit should be disinfected. Toilets should be cleaned with household bleach diluted 1/49. Personal, food and environmental hygiene should be maintained in schools. A hygienic environment should be maintained in the kitchen, and it should be ensured that the refrigerator is working properly. The person who spreads the disease, especially the food processing personnel, should be provided with sick leave to prevent the spread of the disease. Affected children and staff should be out of school for at least 2 days or as long as the doctor recommends (Donaldson, 2023).

Respiratory Infection Outbreak

Medical records of suspected patients should be prepared. Students and staff should be informed to wear a well-fitting surgical mask and seek medical attention immediately if they experience flu symptoms such as fever, sore throat, or cough. They should be reminded that they must notify the school in case of hospitalization. Those who are sick should rest until their symptoms improve. Other children should be followed up on, such as body temperature measurements. Indoor ventilation should be performed frequently. Group activities should be avoided during the pandemic. Appropriate protective equipment should be provided when necessary (Alaska Department of Health, 2013).

Sexually Transmitted Diseases

Students need to receive proper education about sexuality. Many infections can be transmitted through sexual contact. Syphilis, gonorrhea, chlamydia, and chancroid bacterial viral infections include herpes, HIV, hepatitis B, and human papillomavirus (HPV). Sexually transmitted diseases (STDs) may not cause any symptoms. The most common symptoms are vaginal or penile discharge, pain during urination, skin ulcers, or warts. HPV causes warts and cervical cancer. Untreated genital infections can lead to infertility and other medical complications

(Kılınç İşleyen et al., 2024). Accurate diagnosis is important for appropriate treatment and counseling, and partner assessment is essential to limit the spread of infections (Amu and Adegun, 2015). Hepatitis B is an STD that can be prevented by vaccination. In preventing other STDs, abstinence, barrier methods such as condoms, and limiting the number of sexual partners are important (Centre for Health Protection, 2023).

Skin Infections

Herpes simplex is a common viral infection that causes recurrent fever blisters. All students should be advised to avoid contact with other students' oral secretions and not to share cups or bottles. There is no need to exclude children with herpes symptoms from routine school activities. However, in contact sports, students with open mouths or skin lesions may be excluded. Impetigo is a local skin infection caused by bacteria. It may show redness and pus discharge in one or more areas of the skin. Antibiotics may need to be used in such skin infections (Hartman-Adams et al., 2014).

Ringworm (tinea corporis), a fungal infection involving the face, trunk, or limbs, is usually red, circular, and scaly. Itching is common. Local medication applied to the affected areas is usually successful in treatment. Ringworm (tinea capitis) on the scalp requires more aggressive treatment. Fungi are acquired through contact with the skin scales of an affected person or through contact with fungi in moist areas such as swimming pools, locker rooms, and shower rooms (Ba et al., 2021).

The risk of ringworm in schools can be reduced by not sharing towels, washing towels properly, and disinfecting shower areas. Students with tinea pedis should avoid swimming pools and walking barefoot on the locker room and shower floors until treatment is initiated. Scabies is a red rash caused by mites found in the upper layers of the skin. Severe itching, especially at night, is an important feature. Inside the home, scabies are transmitted on clothing and bedding. In schools, direct skin contact is the main route of transmission. Several medications are available to treat scabies. Lice usually occur in the head, but they can also occur in the body or genital area. The most common symptom of head lice is itching; however, many children are asymptomatic. Lice or nits can be found in the hair, behind the ears, or around the neck. Transmission occurs through direct contact with the affected person's hair or through contact with objects such as combs, hairbrushes, and hats. Children with scabies or head lice should be excluded from school until treatment is initiated (Centre for Health Protection, 2023).

Emergencies in Infections in School-Age Children

In students with compromised immune systems, a febrile illness requires immediate medical evaluation. Especially children with sickle cell anemia, children with an abnormal immune system, children receiving chemotherapy, children receiving post-transplant immunosuppressive therapy, or children receiving immunosuppressive therapy for diseases such as rheumatoid arthritis or inflammatory bowel disease require close monitoring. Any child experiencing a cough and significant difficulty breathing should receive an immediate medical evaluation. Signs of brain infection, such as headache, neck stiffness, seizures, or change in mental status, should be evaluated immediately. Signs of bone/joint infection, such as difficulty and pain in limb movement, should also be evaluated (Centre for Health Protection, 2023).

Conclusion

There are many conditions in schools that are prone to the transmission of infections. Infections in school environments can be controlled with some precautions. These measures are vital to ensuring a healthy and safe learning environment. In schools, students, school staff, parents, and other community members can be educated about health behaviors to prevent infections. Healthy behaviors learned in schools can contribute to future health and well-being. Infection control protects student and staff health and ensures the continuation of education. It also reduces community spread and lowers healthcare costs.

Disclaimer

None.

References

Alaska Department of Health & Social Services. (2013). *Infectious disease management.* https://health.alaska.gov/dph/wcfh/Documents/school/assets/InfectiousDiseaseManagementGuidelinesForAlaskaSchools.pdf.

Amu, E. O., & Adegun, P. T. (2015). Awareness and knowledge of sexually transmitted infections among secondary school adolescents in Ado Ekiti, South Western Nigeria. *Journal of Sexually Transmitted Diseases*.

Ba, O., Kébé, M., Groun, S. A., Sy, O., Sidiya, M. A., Eibih, A. B. A., & Bollahi, M. A. (2021). Epidemiology of scalp ringworms and superficial fungal infections in schools in Mauritania. *La Tunisie Medicale*, 99(12), 1126-1133.

Bolon, M. K. (2016). Hand hygiene: an update. *Infectious Disease Clinics*, 30(3), 591-607.

Centre for Food Safety. (2023). *Safe food at school.* Retrieved from https://www.cfs.gov.hk/english/index.html.

Centre for Health Protection. (2023). *Guidelines on prevention of communicable diseases in schools-kindergartens-cum-child care centres-child care centres*. Hong Kong Department of Health. Retrieved from https://www.chp.gov.hk/files/pdf/guidelines_on_prevention_of_communicable_diseases_in_schools_kindergartens_kindergartens_cum_child_care-centres_child_are_centres.pdf.

Donaldson, A. L. (2023). *Infectious intestinal disease (IID) in schools and school-aged children* (Doctoral dissertation, The University of Liverpool, United Kingdom).

Hartman-Adams, H., Banvard, C., & Juckett, G. (2014). Impetigo: diagnosis and treatment. *American Family Physician*, 90(4), 229-235.

Kılınç İşleyen, E., Korkmaz Aslan, G., & Kartal, A. (2024). Knowledge and perceptions about cervical cancer and human papillomavirus, and relationship with e-health literacy, and affecting factors among female university students. *Journal of Adolescent and Young Adult Oncology*.

Minnesota Department of Health. (2023). *School health services.* Retrieved from https://www.health.state.mn.us/people/childrenyouth/schoolhealth/infection.html#:~:text=Infection%20Control%20Measures&text=Standard%20precautions%20include%20the%20following,of%20needles%20and%20other%20sharps.

Public Health England. (2014). *Guidance on infection control in schools and other childcare settings*. Retrieved from https://www.gov.uk/government/uploads/system/uploads/attachment_data/file/353953/Guidance_on_infection_control_in_schools_11_Sept.pdf.

Public Health Ontario. (2023). *Respiratory etiquette*. Retrieved from https://www.publichealthontario.ca/en/About/News/2023/01/Respiratory-Etiquette#:~:text=Respiratory%20etiquette%20is%20a%20simple,or%20elbow%2C%20not%20your%20hands.

World Health Organization (WHO). (2021). *Guideline on school health services*. Retrieved from https://www.who.int/publications/i/item/9789240029392.

Chapter 9

A Safe and Healthy School Environment

Sultan Kayan*, **MSc**
Bilecik Seyh Edebali University, Health Science Faculty, Department of Nursing, Bilecik, Türkiye

Abstract

Creating a safe and healthy school environment is crucial for promoting the success of school-age children. Achieving this requires a holistic approach that addresses school-age children's physical well-being, emotional development, and academic needs. In addition to addressing issues such as physical security, fire safety, hygiene standards, and emergency plans, schools must also consider school-age children's psychosocial needs. A safe school environment provides that school-age children are protected from aggression, bullying, and other forms of harmful behaviors. Such an environment is characterized by the establishment of positive relationship between school staff and students, as well as the fair and consistent implementation of disciplinary policies. In parallel, a healthy school environment supports the physical and emotional well-being of students through the integration of health-promoting policies and practices. These may include comprehensive nutrition programs, access to physical activity and sports facilities, and the provision of psychosocial support services. This helps students develop healthy lifestyle habits and meet their emotional needs. In conclusion, a safe and healthy school environment is a fundamental factor in ensuring student success. Creating such an environment requires collaboration among school management, educators, school nurses, students, and parents. Through this collaboration, a school environment can be created where every student can maximize their developmental potential.

Keywords: school-age children, safe school, healthy school

Introduction

Schools serve as important environments where school-age children grow, develop, and acquire lifelong habits that influence their physical, mental, and social well-being (WHO, 2018a). A safe and healthy school environment encompasses a broad spectrum of factors, including

* Corresponding Author's Email: sultan.kayan@bilecik.edu.tr

In: Health Promotion and Prevention
Editor: Eda Kılınç İşleyen
ISBN: 979-8-89530-758-8

physical infrastructure, hygiene standards, mental health support, nutrition, and protection from violence, abuse, and neglect. These elements contribute to school-age children's ability to learn effectively, interact positively with peers and teachers, and develop a strong foundation for healthy living (Castanheira et al., 2024).

Global organizations such as the World Health Organization (WHO) and UNICEF emphasize the importance of school settings in promoting child health and resilience (WHO, 2018a; Godfrey et al., 2012). Extensive research consistently associates supportive and protective school environments with reduced absenteeism, improved academic performance, and lower rates of behavioral and emotional problems (Geller et al., 2007). The presence of clean water, proper sanitation, secure infrastructure, inclusive policies, and a culture of respect and equity strengthens students' capacity to thrive both academically and personally (Eppler-Wolff and Martin, 2021).

Safe and healthy schools operate through a multidisciplinary framework, where educators, health professionals, school nurses, families, and communities collaborate to address the diverse needs of school-age children. In this context, school health programs, and access to on-site or community-based health services play a vital role. The school climate, including social relationships and institutional norms, also holds significant influence over students' well-being (Bonell et al., 2013).

This comprehensive subject encompasses various elements, including the physical surroundings of the school, hygiene standards, nutrition, opportunities for physical activity, and the preservation of the natural environment.

A safe and healthy school environment aims to protect students' well-being considering both indoor building conditions and external environmental factors. The concept of the school environment includes aspects such as the location, building, grounds, social atmosphere, infrastructure, play areas, water sources, waste management, restrooms, heating, ventilation, lighting, desks, and classrooms. The school environment should incorporate necessary measures to safeguard students from discrimination, harassment, abuse, accidents, violence, and entrapments related to tobacco, alcohol, drugs, and stimulants (Jones et al., 2007). Schools should strategically implement interventions that not only enhance learning but also promote behavioral norms that support students' health. Research indicates that schools implementing such initiatives witness students more inclined to adopt healthy lifestyle behaviors, whereas schools without or with insufficiently implemented interventions tend to have students joining risky peer groups and engaging in risky health behaviors (Bonell et al., 2013). Moreover, preserving natural habitats within the school environment and fostering environmental awareness among students contributes to shaping future generations of environmentally conscious individuals. These students will be better prepared to assume responsibility for environmental stewardship in the future.

In this regard, it is crucial for schools to take the necessary measures and conduct awareness campaigns to support students' health. This chapter highlights the essential components and determinants of a safe and healthy school environment, supported by current evidence and best practices from international guidelines and public health frameworks.

Physical School Environment

The physical school environment is a crucial and multifaceted aspect that profoundly impacts students' health, well-being, and overall learning potential. It includes a wide array of elements, ranging from the physical structure of the school itself to the safety measures in place to protect students, as well as opportunities for physical activity, recreation, and nutrition (Terrón-Pérez et al., 2021). The design and condition of school buildings, including classrooms, hallways, restrooms, and common areas, play a fundamental role in ensuring that students are both comfortable and able to focus on their studies. Well-maintained, clean, and organized physical spaces not only foster a positive learning atmosphere but also contribute to the mental and emotional well-being of students (WHO, 2018a).

In addition to the structural elements, student safety is of paramount importance in any school environment. Ensuring that the school is free from hazards, whether related to physical accidents, security threats, or exposure to harmful substances, is a key responsibility. Schools must implement effective safety measures, including surveillance systems, well-trained staff, and clear emergency protocols, to create a secure environment for all students. This sense of safety enhances students' ability to focus on their education without unnecessary distractions or concerns about personal safety (WHO, 2018a).

Furthermore, the availability of sports and recreational opportunities is a vital component of the physical school environment. Access to well-equipped playgrounds, gymnasiums, and sports facilities encourages students to engage in physical activity, which is crucial for their physical health and cognitive development. Physical activity not only improves students' physical fitness but also has significant positive effects on their mental health, reducing stress and boosting concentration and mood. Encouraging active play and structured physical education programs helps students develop important social skills, teamwork, and discipline (Mason et al., 2022).

Another important issue for school conditions is hygiene standards. Maintaining high hygiene standards within the school environment (ensuring clean restrooms, safe food preparation areas, and promoting proper handwashing practices) help prevent the spread of illness and ensure the health of students and staff (Teo et al., 2019). By creating a safe, clean, and supportive physical space, schools can positively influence students' health, enhance their learning experiences, and help foster their holistic development.

Indoor and Outdoor Environments

It is widely recognized that school buildings have significant implications not only for the educational process but also for economic, social, and environmental sustainability. Within this context, school infrastructure projects should be guided by key principles such as ensuring a healthy indoor environment, implementing energy-efficient systems, utilizing environmentally sustainable building materials, adopting intelligent architectural designs, and embracing environmentally conscious forms. These components are essential for fostering a healthy and safe school environment. For instance, a study by Çelik and Ünver (2019) revealed that approximately 50% of educational facilities are over 25 years old and were constructed based on architectural paradigms prevalent three decades ago (Çelik and Ünver, 2019). This statistic highlights a critical concern regarding the adequacy of existing school infrastructures and signals the potential emergence of significant challenges in the future due to outdated physical conditions.

Şahin (2018) concluded that there is a significant positive relationship between the physical conditions of school building and students' life satisfaction. Supporting this, a study by Cradock et al., (2017), conducted with students aged 12 to 14, found that increases in the school campus area, playground area, and school building area per student were associated with higher levels of physical activity during school hours. These findings underscore the direct and measurable impact of the physical school environment on various dimensions of school health, including students' well-being and physical activity levels. The quality and design of school facilities, therefore, play a crucial role in promoting healthy behaviors and enhancing the overall educational experience.

One of the conditions that school buildings must fulfill is the provision of full participation and equal opportunity for all students. Ensuring equal access to educational environments is fundamental to upholding the right to education for every individual, regardless of physical ability, socio-economic background, or other potential barriers (Sandoval, 2018). Accessibility in school infrastructure includes, but is not limited to, the presence of ramps, elevators, accessible restrooms, appropriate classroom layouts, and clear signage. The accessibility needs of disabled students vary depending on the type, severity, and duration of the disability. In summary, disability encompasses diversity within itself, and inclusivity is expected in accessibility. It is stated that the graduation rate of disabled students from schools with inclusive school policies is 60%, while the graduation rate of other schools is 38% (Sanford et al., 2021). Another study on this matter indicates that disabled students in schools lacking inclusive policies experience more bullying, school-related anxiety, loneliness, absenteeism, and low academic achievement issues (Adams et al., 2016). In conclusion, the removal of physical barriers encountered by disabled students during their education and the provision of an appropriate learning environment is of great importance for these students to lead healthy school life. Furthermore, making the physical conditions of schools suitable for disabled students will not only enhance their participation in the educational process but also enable them to engage more actively in society. Therefore, necessary steps should be taken to make schools accessible, and efforts should be made to create an appropriate learning environment. These features not only support students with disabilities but also promote an inclusive educational environment where diversity is respected and accommodated. Therefore, ensuring accessibility is a critical step toward achieving equity in education and fostering a school culture that values participation and inclusivity.

Physical activity is important for students to adopt a healthy lifestyle and maintain their physical health. Therefore, the sports facilities available in schools provide students with the opportunity to engage in regular physical activity. These activities contribute to the prevention of health problems such as obesity, heart disease, and diabetes, both in this age group and in the future (Sales et al., 2023). Engaging in sports not only benefits physical health but also has positive effects on mental health. Regularly engaging in physical activities and sports has been shown to significantly reduce students' stress levels while enhancing their concentration and attention span (Sampasa-Kanyinga et al., 2020). A systematic review reveals that the presence of sports facilities within schools exerts positive effects on various parameters such as students' health-related quality of life, self-esteem, mental resilience, mental health, and sleep quality. However, it also shows negative impacts on factors such as anxiety, depression, aggressive behaviors, and screen time (Andermo et al., 2020). These research findings underscore the multifaceted and substantial correlation between school health and the availability of sports facilities. The contribution of sports facilities to students' physical, mental, and social development underscores their pivotal role in establishing a healthy school environment. As such, efforts should be directed toward not only establishing sports facilities but also promoting their utilization and encouraging participation in sports activities to foster the adoption of healthy lifestyle behaviors among students.

A crucial element indispensable for ensuring a safe and healthy school environment is the presence of green spaces and natural surroundings. Green spaces represent a vital aspect that embodies the revitalizing effects of nature and offers numerous benefits for overall well-being. Particularly, green spaces within or adjacent to schools play a significant role in aiding students' healthy growth and development. They achieve this through their stress-reducing effects, provision of opportunities for physical activity, exposure to natural light and clean air, reinforcement of the connection with nature, and enhancement of social interactions. Therefore, the existence of green spaces within and around schools, coupled with regular maintenance, substantially contributes to the health and well-being of students.

School Accidents

Accidents are defined as preventable and unintentional incidents that can cause physical or emotional harm. Approximately 30% of child deaths in the 5-14 age group occur due to accidents (WHO, 2018b). Furthermore, 10-25% of these injuries occur within schools (Akçay et al., 2018). For an incident to be considered a school accident, it must occur during school hours or while the student is being transported to a location outside the school premises for school-related activities or instruction, using a vehicle provided by the school administration (Kılınç and Gür, 2018). The period when a child starts school is believed to contribute to the child acquiring autonomous behaviors, leading to increased exposure to risks due to greater independence. A study examining the factors contributing to injuries among school-age children revealed that 53.6% of the risks were associated with the children's own actions, including aggressive behavior, locomotor skills, physical activity. In contrast, only 3.6% of injury risks were attributed to environmental conditions within the school setting, such as ecological characteristics, hazardous school activities, sports participation, and playgrounds infrastructure (Akçay et al., 2018; Gür, 2016). However, it is estimated that acquiring safe and protective behaviors that prevent the onset of illnesses or deaths resulting from accidents would prevent the occurrence of most accidents (Malta et al., 2016; Margeson and Gray, 2017).

It is believed that schools are an ideal setting for approaching accident prevention and first aid from childhood onward. Educational activities in this area within schools are essential initiatives to increase school-age children's awareness of risks related to accidents and preventive measures. Moreover, implementing simple yet effective safety measures -such as removing sharp objects and cleaning agents from accessible areas, restricting access to hazardous materials, providing handrails on stairs and steps, and ensuring that exits and passageways are free of furniture, or other obstructions- can significantly reduce the risk of accidents among school-age children (Kılınç and Gür, 2023). Increasing school-age children's awareness of risk factors and encouraging their participation in activities and games suitable for their competence levels are crucial steps. In this context, schools provide the most appropriate environment for school-age children to acquire healthy lifestyle behaviors that they can benefit from throughout their lives.

Lighting

The main function of light is not only vision but also to regulate the human circadian system. The timing of every biological function is guided by this system regulated by light, impacting both physical and mental health. Considering the school commuting hours, it can be argued that school-age children do not benefit from daylight adequately throughout the year, leading to adverse effects on their health. The positive impact of daylight on academic performance, the preservation of the natural environment, the support of healthier conditions, and also the achievement of energy savings are particularly important for schools (Michael and Heracleous, 2017). On the contrary, insufficient daylight has been associated with a range of symptoms, including sleep disturbances, increased stress levels, obesity, fatigue, and seasonal affective disorder (Tureková et al., 2017). A study conducted in the European region found a positive relationship between the ratio of window/floor area and the percentage of windows facing south with students' achievement scores (Nguyen and Korkina, 2021). This result proves that benefiting from daylight also affects academic success. However, due to factors such as local time practices and physical conditions of buildings, students spend time in classrooms with lighting that does not resemble natural light. Studies have demonstrated that lighting conditions can significantly influence students' behaviors. Shapiro, Roth, and Marcus (2010) reported an increase maladaptive behaviors among school-age children exposed to fluorescent lighting. Additionally, artificial lighting accounts for a total of 14% of electricity consumption in the European region (Shapiro et al., 2010), therefore, the use of natural lighting is an important factor in energy conservation. In this context, the integration of natural lighting in school environments not only supports students' health and academic performance but also contributes to sustainability by reducing energy consumption.

Noise

Background noise refers to auditory disturbances that hinder an individual's ability to hear desire or necessary information. In classroom settings, such noise can stem from various possible reasons, including external noise, generally categorized as external noise (e.g., traffic, construction), internal noise (e.g., hallway chatter, adjacent classrooms), and room noise (e.g., heating and ventilation systems, reverberation). Research shows that noise has direct negative effects on students' learning processes, particularly impairing cognitive functions such as attention, memory, and motivation (Shield and Dockrell, 2018; Woolner and Hall, 2020).

To compensate for the noise level in classrooms, teachers often find themselves speaking loudly during lessons; this habit of speaking loudly is known to be a risk factor for voice disorders among teachers (Araújo-Alves et al., 2019). A study by Knecht et al., (2012) reported that classroom noise levels often fail to meet recommended standards, with measurements reaching up to 65 dB(A) even in empty classrooms—significantly exceeding the suggested maximum of 40 dB(A). While noise levels are naturally higher when students are present, prolonged exposure to such elevated levels has been associated with an increased risk of hearing disorders among teachers, highlighting the occupational health risks posed by inadequate acoustic conditions in educational settings (Knecht et al., 2012). Walinder et al., (2007) investigated the physiological and psychological stress responses of school-age children to classroom noise and found that noise levels ranging from 59 to 87 dB(A) were associated with increased symptoms such as fatigue and headaches. Similarly, Evans et al., (2010) reported that children attending schools in noisier environments exhibited higher resting systolic blood pressure and elevated nighttime urinary cortisol levels, indicating heightened physiological stress. In line with these findings, Forns et al., (2016) observed that exposure to road traffic noise in school environments was significantly associated with hyperactivity and inattention among children aged 7 to 11 years. These studies collectively underscore the detrimental impact of environmental noise on teachers' and school-age children's physical health, cognitive functioning, and behavioral regulation.

Although noise has become an indispensable part of modern life, it emerges as a factor that negatively affects teachers' and school-age children's health and learning performance in school environments. Therefore, measures should be taken to control noise in schools and necessary steps should be taken for students to learn in a healthy environment. Continuous awareness and efforts are crucial to maintaining both physical and mental health in this regard.

Temperature, Humidity, and Ventilation

In school environments, a significant part of learning takes place indoors; this means that the thermal environment indoors has a significant impact on learning efficiency. Unlike general indoor activities, learning requires high concentration and attention, so it is essential to create a suitable indoor environment considering temperature and relative humidity. Richardson and colleagues (2018) found that increasing the temperature from 20°C to 25.8°C significantly improved learning efficiency. Abbasi et al., (2019), on the other hand, noted that excessively high or low temperatures not only affect learning performance but also significantly influence heart rate and brain activities. It is known that thermal discomfort caused by high temperatures in classrooms reduces students' ability to perform typical school tasks and lowers their academic achievement (Porras-Salazar et al., 2018; Wargocki and Wyon, 2017). Additionally, it has been shown that heat stress induced by high outdoor temperatures reduces students' pass rates in exams (Park et al., 2020).

Studies on relative humidity have reported that low relative humidity easily leads to an increase in common mucosal-associated symptoms, such as dry and tired eyes, which hinder performance (Razjouyan et al., 2020). It is stated that individuals exposed to relative humidity between 30% and 60% are more likely to reduce eye dryness and fatigue caused by respiratory mucosa compared to those exposed to a drier environment for a long time (Shan et al., 2016). In addition to these findings, it is indicated that being in a moist environment throughout the day triggers feelings of fatigue and that indoor relative humidity should be around 50-70% (Tsutsumi et al., 2017).

In addition to temperature and humidity values, ventilation is also an important factor affecting school-age children's health. A study conducted in California showed that increasing ventilation by 1 l/s per person reduced illness-related absenteeism by 1.6% (Mendell et al., 2013). Similarly, another study suggests that proper ventilation methods can lead to a 9% increase in student performance in mathematics and a 7% increase in reading (Haverinen-Shaughnessy et al., 2011). Low ventilation rates are also a concern because they can lead to increased exposure to indoor air pollutants, which need to be controlled.

Indoor Air Quality

Particle air pollution is a major environmental factor contributing to the global disease burden and has become one of the most important causes of preventable diseases over time. It is known that air pollution has negative effects not only on the respiratory and cardiovascular systems but also on brain development (Rivas et al., 2018). School-age children are particularly vulnerable to environmental effects as they are still in their developmental stages. Additionally, due to physiological factors such as high respiratory rate and behavioral differences such as increased physical activity, school-age children may be exposed to higher doses of air pollutants compared to adults (Cohen et al., 2017). Therefore, it is especially important for air quality to be good in environments where school-age children spend long periods of time, such as schools.

A study conducted in Barcelona detected high levels of fine particulate matter ($PM_{2.5}$), nitrogen dioxide (NO_2), equivalent black carbon, and ultrafine particle concentrations in schools (Rivas et al., 2018). Another study in Italy found that indoor particle concentrations during school hours were influenced by outdoor particle concentrations (Fuoco et al., 2015). It is also essential to consider the presence of heavy metals indoor dust, given their persistence in the environment, high toxicity, and harmful effects on human health. Since school-age children spend most of their time at school, classroom dust, considered indoor dust, poses a significant risk by exposing school-age children to heavy metals. The main routes of exposure include ingestion, dermal contact, and respiratory pathways (Tan et al., 2018). Indoor air quality in schools has a significant impact on students' health and learning performance. Conscious and preventive steps should be taken regarding indoor air quality to protect the health of both students and staff. A clean and healthy indoor environment fosters improved concentration, promotes physical well-being, and contributes to a more successful educational experience for school-age children. Therefore, measures should be taken to improve indoor air quality in schools, and it should be constantly monitored.

Hygiene Practices

School hygiene is essential components inseparable from students' ability to receive education in a healthy manner. Measures taken regarding cleanliness, healthy nutrition, and hygiene support students in growing and developing healthily. Considering that the behavioral patterns of future adult populations are shaped during their school years, the acquisition of behaviors such as toilet and hand hygiene plays a crucial role in determining a child's future health (Horner and Sugai, 2015). Improving children's health and protecting them from infectious diseases and infections are significantly influenced by proper hygiene education. Factors such as inadequate genital hygiene and post-toilet handwashing habits, as well as the lack of toilet paper usage, play a significant role in exposing school-age children to infectious diseases. Additionally, school-age children are more vulnerable to infectious diseases compared to adults due to their immature immune systems (Glynn and Moss, 2020). This makes the school an important environment for the prevention and control of disease transmission.

In schools, the most common diseases, such as diarrhea and respiratory tract infections, account for 80% of childhood illnesses (Abdulhussein and Abdul Hussein, 2023). Therefore, regardless of past and current school curricula, hygiene education programs are implemented, especially targeting school-age children. The outcomes of these hygiene education initiatives have shown effectiveness in reducing the infectious diseases experienced by students and the resulting school absenteeism (Mbakaya et al., 2019; Azor-Martinez et al., 2016). This situation highlights the need for cleanliness and hygiene-related education programs in schools to address knowledge and skill gaps, increase awareness, and improve attitudes toward hygiene practices.

Nutrition and Physical Activity Environment

An adequate, safe, and nutritious diet is crucial for human growth and development and for reducing the risk of chronic diseases later in life. Therefore, establishing healthy eating behaviors early on is important, as evidence suggests that eating habits and patterns persist in adulthood (Dudley et al., 2015). WHO (2004) emphasized the importance of developing and implementing school policies that encourage physical activity and healthy eating habits. This enables interventions aimed at healthy and active lifestyle behaviors to be integrated into existing systems, such as schools, ensuring sustainability and success.

The school nutrition environment plays a vital role in shaping students' dietary habits by offering them the chance to learn and practice healthy eating behaviors. This environment encompasses the types of food and beverages available on campus, the quality and content of nutrition education integrated into the curriculum, and the choices presented in the school canteen. All members of the school community play a crucial role in fostering a healthy school nutrition environment. This includes promoting and marketing healthier food and beverage options, encouraging student participation in school meal programs, modeling healthy eating behaviors, and ensuring access to free drinking water throughout the school day (Lewallen et al., 2015). Despite these recognized best practices, many schools continue to offer sugar-sweetened beverages and snack foods high in fat and sodium (Black et al., 2015).

It is extremely important to follow hygiene rules in school canteens, as these settings directly influence students' health and well-being. Improper handling, storage or preparation of food in canteens can lead to the proliferation and spread of foodborne pathogens, posing serious health risks to school-age children (Grace et al., 2020). Despite their negative outcomes, intervention can be achieved by ensuring food safety. Food safety refers to minimizing the risk of harmful microorganisms, chemicals, or other contaminants being present in food that could pose a threat to health. Giving importance to food safety in schools involves taking the necessary precautions in storing, preparing, and handling food to ensure that students consume healthy and safe food. Ensuring that food handlers are adequately trained in food safety, maintaining clean kitchen environments, implementing proper temperature control, and adhering to sanitation standards are essential components of a safe food service system. Regular inspections and strict enforcement of hygiene protocols help minimize the risk of contamination and ensure that the food served is both nutritious and safe for consumption.

In addition to food safety, water quality is also critical for students to have a healthy learning environment. Water sources can become contaminated due to chemical and microbiological pollutants, inadequate treatment and disposal of waste from humans and animals, industrial discharges, and overuse of limited water resources. Heavy metal pollution, such as arsenic, in drinking water poses a serious threat to human health due to its high toxicity and potential carcinogenicity. Identified organisms and chemicals can cause water-related illnesses, which can have serious health effects, especially for school-age children. A clean and hygienic school environment, along with access to safe drinking water that meets health standards, are fundamental factors in preserving students' physical and mental health. Therefore, water quality should be regularly monitored in schools, and necessary measures should be taken accordingly.

Waste Management

Waste management in schools is an important step towards creating an environmentally friendly learning environment. Proper collection, segregation, and recycling of waste contribute to reducing environmental pollution and conserving natural resources. Waste management involves the effective collection, segregation, recycling, or safe disposal of waste. Implementation of waste management practices in schools not only fosters environmental awareness among students and staff but also ensures a healthy school environment. A study conducted on waste management in elementary schools found that paper recycling increased by 4.3%, while recycling rates for glass, metal cans, and textile products increased by 8.7% (Lee et al., 2022).

It is noted that waste generated in educational institutions has a high potential for recycling, with 55-90% of the waste stream in schools being recyclable (Sağlam and Aydın, 2024). Especially schools are expected to be leaders in environmental protection actions and are obligated for ethical and moral reasons to behave responsibly toward the environment. Therefore, the most effective implementation of waste reduction strategies is necessary in schools.

Disaster Management

Disasters are events that profoundly affect life and the environment. Children become vulnerable in disaster situations due to their physiology, developing organ systems, behaviors, emotional and developmental understanding, and responses to events (Kousky, 2016). Therefore, schools should take necessary precautions for the safety and health of students and act in a planned and effective manner in disaster situations. In this way, damage can be minimized during disasters, and society can become more resilient.

Schools are responsible for providing adequate disaster management education, developing awareness of disaster management in society, and strengthening the disaster management capabilities of communities. Every school should have an effective and region-specific school safety plan that includes preparation, response, and recovery procedures. A study conducted in Indonesia shows that disaster management training is effective in dealing with post-disaster injuries and infectious diseases (Pascapurnama et al., 2018). Schools should implement a management approach covering all hazards by creating a concrete, continuous, and controllable disaster management framework.

Psychological and Social School Environment

The psychological and social environment of a school plays a vital role in shaping students' academic performance, emotional development, mental health, and overall well-being. While physical infrastructure and health services are essential components of a healthy school, the psychological climate and social dynamics within the school have an equally profound impact on students' success and their ability to thrive (Podiya et al., 2025). The psychological school environment aims to provide a safe and supportive environment that meets students' emotional needs. In this environment, healthy communication should be established among students, teachers, and other staff members, sensitivity to emotional needs should be shown, and support services should be provided when necessary (Hawkins et al., 2023).

The social school environment refers to the quality of interpersonal relationships and the sense of community within the school setting. Peer interactions, group belonging, opportunities for collaboration, and a climate of social justice and equity are critical for student development.

Bullying, social exclusion, discrimination, or unequal treatment undermine this environment and can lead to significant long-term consequences, such as decreased self-esteem, academic disengagement, and mental health problems (Morin, 2022). A positive school climate has the potential to help students feel socially, emotionally, and physically safe at school. School climate is described as a combination of physical safety, emotional security, order, and discipline (conflict resolution, fairness, and consistency of rules) (Fossum et al., 2023). It is anticipated that aggressive behaviors in school are intertwined with the school climate, and an increase in aggressive behaviors is associated with a decline in the school climate. A positive teacher-student relationship can function as a protective factor in addressing behavioral and emotional difficulties, preventing school dropout, and improving school performance. In summary, when implementing safe school initiatives, the school climate should also be taken into consideration.

Educators, school administrators, families, and health professionals share responsibility in shaping and sustaining a psychologically and socially healthy school environment. This involves creating policies that protect students from violence, harassment, and discrimination, as well as offering access to mental health services, counseling, and psychoeducation. In conclusion, the psychological and social dimensions of the school environment are fundamental to the holistic development of students. A healthy school is not only free of physical hazards but also rich in emotional support and positive social interactions. Investing in the psychological and social well-being of students contributes to safer, more inclusive, and more effective learning environments (Podiya et al., 2025; Hawkins et al., 2023; Morin, 2022).

Conclusion

A safe and healthy school environment is indispensable for students to be successful, as it directly influences their academic performance, emotional well-being, and overall development. The development of such an environment is not only a fundamental objective of the education system but also an investment in the future of society, as it lays the foundation for the holistic growth of the next generation. Creating and maintaining this environment requires the collective commitment and active involvement of all stakeholders, including school management, educators, staff, school nurses, students, and parents. Through this collaboration, a school environment can be created where every student can maximize their potential.

Disclaimer

None.

References

Abbasi, A. M., Motamedzade, M., Aliabadi, M., Golmohammadi, R., & Tapak, L. (2019). The impact of indoor air temperature on the executive functions of human brain and the physiological responses of body. *Health Promotion Perspectives*, 9(1), 55.

Adams, R., Taylor, J., Duncan, A., & Bishop, S. (2016). Peer victimization and educational outcomes in mainstreamed adolescents with autism spectrum disorder. *Journal of Autism and Developmental Disorders*, 46, 3557-3566.

Akcay, D., & Yıldırımlar, A. (2018). Investigation of children's school accidents and behavior of their parents' safety measures. *DEUHFED*, 11(1), 48-55.

Andermo, S., Hallgren, M., & Nguyen. (2020). School-related physical activity interventions and mental health among children: A systematic review and meta-analysis. *Sports Med Open*, 6, 25.

Araújo-Alves, J., Neto-Paiva, F., Torres-Silva, L., & Remoaldo, P. (2020). Low-frequency noise and its main effects on human health—A review of the literature between 2016 and 2019. *Applied Sciences*, 10(15), 5205.

Azor-Martinez, E., Carrascosa, E., Seijas-Vazquez, M. L., & Torres-Alegre, P. (2016). Hand hygiene program decreases school absenteeism due to upper respiratory infections. *Journal of School Health*, 86(12), 873-881.

Black, J. L., Velazquez, C. E., & Ahmadi, N. (2015). Sustainability and public health nutrition at school: Assessing the integration of healthy and environmentally sustainable food initiatives in Vancouver schools. *Public Health Nutrition*, 18(13), 2379-2391.

Bonell, C., Parry, W., Wells, H., Jamal, F., Fletcher, A., Harden, A., & Moore, L. (2013). The effects of the school environment on student health: A systematic review of multi-level studies. *Health Place*, 21, 180-191.

Celik, K., & Unver, F. R. (2019). Eğitim yapılarında sürdürülebilir aydınlatma tasarımı yaklaşımı [Sustainable lighting design approach in educational buildings]. *Çukurova Üniversitesi Mühendislik-Mimarlık Fakültesi Dergisi*, 34(3), 49-64.

Cohen, A. J., Brauer, M., Burnett, R., Anderson, H. R., Frostad, J., Estep, K., & Forouzanfar, M. H. (2017). Estimates and 25-year trends of the global burden of disease attributable to ambient air pollution: An analysis of data from the Global Burden of Diseases Study. *The Lancet*, 389, 1907-1918.

Cradock, A. L., Melly, S. J., Allen, J. G., Morris, J. S., & Gortmaker, S. L. (2017). Characteristics of school campuses and physical activity among youth. *American Journal of Preventive Medicine*, 33(2), 106-113.

Dudley, D. A., Cotton, W., & Peralta, L. R. (2015). Teaching approaches and strategies that promote healthy eating in primary school children: A systematic review and meta-analysis. *International Journal of Behavioral Nutrition and Physical Activity*, 12, 28.

Forns, J., Dadvand, P., Foraster, M., Alvarez-Pedrerol, M., Rivas, I., & López-Vicente, M. (2016). Traffic-related air pollution, noise at school, and behavioral problems in Barcelona schoolchildren: A cross-sectional study. *Environmental Health Perspectives*, 124, 529-535.

Fossum, S., Skokauskas, N., Handegård, B. H., Hansen, K. L., & Kyrrestad, H. (2023). The significance of traditional bullying, cyberbullying, and mental health problems for middle school students feeling unsafe in the school environment. *Scandinavian Journal of Educational Research*, 67(2), 281-293.

Grace, D., Alonso, S., Bett, B. K., Lindahl, J. F., Patel, E., Nguyen-Viet, H., & Dominguez-Salas, P. (2020). The impact of the International Livestock Research Institute (eds J. McIntire and D. Grace). In *Food safety and nutrition*. Bell and Bain Ltd, Glasgow.

Gür, K. (2016). Special problems in school health; school accidents. In S. Gözüm (Ed.), *Developing the health of children in school period* (pp. 854-865). Istanbul: Vize, Turkey.

Haverinen-Shaughnessy, U., Moschandreas, D. J., & Shaughnessy, R. J. (2011). Association between substandard classroom ventilation rates and students' academic achievement. *Indoor Air*, 21(2), 121-131.

Hung, D. T., Thi, V., & Thi Bich Phuong, V. (2020). Evaluation of drinking water quality in schools in a district area in Hanoi, Vietnam. *Environmental Health Insights*, 14.

Kılınç, E., & Gür, K. (2018). The effect of health belief model-based initiatives in preventing school injuries. *HSP*, 5(3), 467-475.

Kılınç, E., & Gür, K. (2023). Health protection and promotion: Risk groups, living environments and disease protection. In A. Bayık Temel (Ed.), *Childhood involuntary injuries and prevention* (pp. 859-886). Ema Tıp Kitabevi.

Knecht, H. A., Nelson, P. B., Whitelaw, G. M., & Feth, L. L. (2012). Background noise levels and reverberation times in unoccupied classrooms: Predictions and measurements. *American Journal of Audiology*, 11, 65-71.

Lee, S. A., Mork, J., Voća, N., Voronova, V., Virsta, A., Daraban, A. E., & Banks, C. E. (2022). A comparison of waste education in schools and colleges across five European cities. *International Journal of Sustainable Development & World Ecology*, 29(4), 338-348.

Lewallen, T. C., Hunt, H., Potts-Datema, W., Zaza, S., & Giles, W. (2015). The whole school, whole community, whole child model: A new approach for improving educational attainment and healthy development for students. *Journal of School Health*, 85(11), 729-739.

Malta, D. C., Mascarenhas, M. D. M., Silva, M. M. A., Carvalho, M. G. O., Barufaldi, L. A., Avanci, J. Q., & Bernal, R. T. I. (2016). The occurrence of external causes in childhood in emergency care: Epidemiological aspects. *Cien Saude Colet*, 21(12), 3729-3744.

Mbakaya, B. C., Lee, P. H., & Lee, R. L. T. (2019). Effect of a school-based hand hygiene program for Malawian children: A cluster randomized controlled trial. *American Journal of Infection Control*, 47(12), 1460-1464.

Margeson, A., & Gray, S. (2017). Interventions aimed at the prevention of childhood injuries in the indigenous populations in Canada, Australia, and New Zealand in the last 20 years: A systematic review. *International Journal of Environmental Research and Public Health*, 14, 589.

Michael, A., & Heracleous, C. (2017). Assessment of natural lighting performance and visual comfort of educational architecture in Southern Europe: The case of typical educational school premises in Cyprus. *Energy and Buildings*, 140, 443-457.

Moyano, D. B., & Lezcano, R. (2021). The importance of light in our lives: Towards new lighting in schools. In *Advancements in Sustainable Architecture and Energy Efficiency* (pp. 239-256).

Nguyen, T. P., & Korkina, E. V. (2021). Connectivity of the window to floor area ratio and the daylighting assessment criteria. *Iranian Journal of Science and Technology, Transactions of Civil Engineering*, 45(3), 2035-2045.

Park, R. J., Goodman, J., Hurwitz, M., & Smith, J. (2020). Heat and learning. *American Economic Journal: Economic Policy*, 12(2), 306-339.

Pascapurnama, D. N., Murakami, A., Chagan-Yasutan, H., Hattori, T., Sasaki, H., & Egawa, S. (2018). Integrated health education in disaster risk reduction: Lessons learned from disease outbreak following natural disasters in Indonesia. *International Journal of Disaster Risk Reduction*, 29, 94-102.

Porras-Salazar, J. A., Wyon, D. P., Piderit-Moreno, B., Contreras-Espinoza, S., & Wargocki, P. (2018). Reducing classroom temperature in a tropical climate improved the thermal comfort and the performance of elementary school pupils. *Indoor Air*, 28(6), 892-904.

Razjouyan, J., Lee, H., Gilligan, B., Lindberg, C., Nguyen, H., Canada, K., & Najafi, B. (2020). Wellbuilt for wellbeing: Controlling relative humidity in the workplace matters for our health. *Indoor Air*, 30(1), 167-179.

Richardson, M. B., Li, P., Gohlke, J. M., & Allison, D. B. (2018). Effects of indoor thermal environment on human food intake, productivity, and comfort: Pilot, randomized, crossover trial. *Obesity*, 26(12), 1826-1833.

Rivas, I., Querol, X., Wright, J., & Sunyer, J. (2018). How to protect school children from the neurodevelopmental harms of air pollution by interventions in the school environment in the urban context. *Environment International*, 121, 199-206.

Sağlam, B. S., & Aydın, N. (2024). Investigation of waste characteristics and recycling behavior at educational institutes. *Waste Management*, 180, 115-124.

Sahin, S. (2018). The relationship between school building and school life satisfaction. *Journal of Human Sciences*, 15(4), 2113-2126.

Sales, D., Silva Junior, J. P., & Bergamo, R. R. (2023). Association between school environment with sedentary behavior and physical activity intensity in children. *Scientific Reports*, 13, 6995.

Sanford, C., Newman, L., Wagner, M., Cameto, R., Knokey, A. M., & Shaver, D. (2021). The post-high school outcomes of young adults with disabilities up to 6 years after high school: Key findings from the National Longitudinal Transition Study-2 (NLTS2). *National Center for Special Education Research*.

Sandoval, J. M. J. (2018). Accessibility, heritage, and project: Re-architectures for everyone. *Millenium*, 2(7), 103-111.

Shan, X., Zhou, J., Chang, V. W. C., & Yang, E. H. (2016). Comparing mixing and displacement ventilation in tutorial rooms: Students' thermal comfort, sick building syndromes, and short-term performance. *Building and Environment*, 102, 128-137.

Shapiro, M., Roth, D., & Marcus, A. (2010). The effect of lighting on the behavior of children who are developmentally disabled. *Journal of International Special Needs Education*, 4, 19-23.

Shield, B. M., & Dockrell, J. E. (2018). The effects of environmental and classroom noise on the academic attainments of primary school children. *Journal of the Acoustical Society of America*, 123, 133-144.

Tan, S. Y., Praveena, S. M., & Abidin, E. Z. (2018). Heavy metal quantification of classroom dust in school environment and its impacts on children's health from Rawang (Malaysia). *Environmental Science and Pollution Research*, 25, 34623-34635.

Tobler, A. L., Komro, K. A., Dabroski, A., Aveyard, P., & Markham, W. A. (2021). Preventing the link between SES and high-risk behaviors: "Value-added" education, drug use, and delinquency in high-risk, urban schools. *Prevention Science*, 12, 211-221.

Tsutsumi, H., Tanabe, S. I., Harigaya, J., Iguchi, Y., & Nakamura, G. (2017). Effect of humidity on human comfort and productivity after step changes from warm and humid environment. *Building and Environment*, 42(12), 4034-4042.

Tureková, I., Lukáčová, D., & Gabriel, B. (2017). Monitoring of lighting in a school classroom. In *Prevention of Accidents at Work* (pp. 339-344).

Wargocki, P., & Wyon, D. P. (2017). Ten questions concerning thermal and indoor air quality effects on the performance of office work and schoolwork. *Building and Environment*, 112, 359-366.

Woolner, P., & Hall, E. (2020). Noise in schools: A holistic approach to the issue. *International Journal of Environmental Research and Public Health*, 7, 3255-3269.

World Health Organization (WHO). (2018). *Road traffic injuries*. https://www.who.int/news-room/fact-sheets/detail/road-traffic-injuries.

Chapter 10

Immunizations in School-Age Children and Adolescents

Gülbahar Korkmaz Aslan[1,*], PhD
and Ebru Öztürk Çopur[2], PhD
[1]Pamukkale University, Faculty of Health Sciences, Department of Public Health Nursing, Denizli, Turkiye
[2]Kilis 7 Aralık University, Yusuf Şerefoğlu Faculty of Health Sciences/Department of Public Health Nursing, Kilis, Turkiye

Abstract

Immunization is the process of protecting a person against a disease by vaccination. It is one of the most reliable and effective ways to prevent mortality and morbidity. To maintain this success, it is necessary to continue vaccination practices by adhering to the principle of vaccination from birth to death. Recognition of the importance of booster doses to extend the protection of infant and early childhood vaccines and the development of new vaccines for children and adolescents, such as human papillomavirus vaccines, have led to increased interest in immunization strategies for school-aged children and adolescents. Low vaccination coverage in this age group may pose a risk not only for this age group but also for public health. Therefore, immunization services for school-aged children and adolescents are important. Countries' immunization strategies for school-aged children and adolescents vary. Although they vary according to national immunization policies, recommended vaccines for school-aged children and adolescents include tetanus, diphtheria, pertussis, HPV (human papillomavirus), and influenza. Hepatitis B, inactivated polio, MMR (measles, rubella, mumps), and hepatitis A are recommended for those who have missed their vaccinations. Hib, conjugated pneumococcal, meningococcal, and varicella are recommended for those at risk.

Keywords: adolescent, school-age children, immunization

Introduction

Immunization is the process of protecting a person against a disease by vaccination. It is one of the most reliable and effective ways to prevent mortality and morbidity. Developed vaccines

---

* Corresponding Author's Email: gkorkmazaslan@gmail.com

In: Health Promotion and Prevention
Editor: Eda Kılınç İşleyen
ISBN: 979-8-89530-758-8

prevent 25 life-threatening infectious diseases (WHO, 2024b; Eskiocak and Marangoz, 2019). The World Health Organization (WHO) reports that immunization prevents 3.5-5 million deaths each year from life-threatening diseases such as diphtheria, tetanus, pertussis, influenza, and measles. Vaccination is also essential for preventing and controlling outbreaks of infectious diseases. Immunization is a cost-effective public health intervention, demonstrating high returns in terms of reduced healthcare costs and improved quality of life (WHO, 2024b). However, infectious diseases remain the leading cause of morbidity and mortality. Widespread immunization programs have significantly decreased the incidence of vaccine-preventable diseases, leading to the eradication of smallpox and near-elimination of polio in many regions (WHO, 2024a; Ministry of Health, 2024). To maintain this success of vaccination, it is necessary to continue vaccination programs by adhering to the principle of vaccination from birth to death (Karakuş, 2021).

Immunization in School-Age Children and Adolescents

Vaccination is a tool to protect health not only in infancy and childhood but also throughout life (WHO, 2024a). Recognition of the importance of booster doses to extend the protection of infant and early childhood vaccines and the development of new vaccines for children and adolescents, such as human papillomavirus (HPV) vaccines, have led to increased interest in immunization strategies for school-aged children and adolescents (Mackroth et al., 2010). The Global Immunization Vision and Strategy (GIVS) 2006-2015, developed jointly by WHO and UNICEF, promotes the expansion of immunization beyond the traditional target groups of infants and young children (Wolfson et al., 2008). Immunization of school-age children and adolescents is important to make up for missed doses, boost waning immunity, and provide primary immunization with new vaccines (Abdullahi et al., 2020).

School-age children and adolescents usually go to health institutions only when they are ill. They may not benefit from preventive and curative health services sufficiently due to the lack of information and negligence of their families (Durmaz et al., 2018). This can lead to a decrease in vaccination coverage, increasing the risk of outbreaks of vaccine-preventable diseases. Low vaccination coverage in this age group may pose a risk not only for this age group but also for public health. Therefore, immunization services provided to school-aged children and adolescents are important (Abdullahi et al., 2020; Durmaz et al., 2018). Public health nurses should assess the vaccination history of this age group when encountering them at school or in primary health care facilities. Those with missing vaccines and those in at-risk groups should be vaccinated as soon as possible (Abdullahi et al., 2020; Göl ve Açıkgöz, 2021).

Countries' immunization strategies for school-age children and adolescents vary (Vandelaer and Olaniran, 2015). Schools can be an appropriate setting for vaccinating school-age children (Abdullahi et al., 2020; Göl and Açıkgöz). Several strategies can be used to increase vaccination coverage among school-aged children and adolescents, including health education programs, financial incentives, and compulsory vaccination (Cadeddu et al., 2021 al., 2021).

Recommended Vaccinations for School-Aged Children and Adolescents

Vaccination policy varies from country to country, influenced by factors such as national health priorities, disease prevalence, healthcare infrastructure, cultural beliefs, and socioeconomic conditions. Vaccines to be included in the national immunization program are determined as a result of long-term and broad-based scientific research (Ministry of Health, 2024; Eskiocak and Marangoz, 2021). WHO reports that there are currently 25 vaccines in use worldwide to protect against infectious diseases (WHO, 2024). In Turkey, the Ministry of Health implements an immunization program for all school-age children against 13 diseases (hepatitis A and B, diphtheria, pertussis, tetanus, pneumococcal diseases, Haemophilus influenzae b, polio, measles, rubella, mumps, varicella, and tuberculosis) through the Expanded Vaccination Programme (Ministry of Health, 2024). However, the rotavirus, HPV, inactivated influenza, and meningococcal vaccines recommended by the Centers for Disease Control and Prevention (CDC) and WHO are not included in the national immunization schedule. These vaccines, approved for use by the Ministry of Health, are administered for a fee at the request of families (Ministry of Health, 2024; WHO, 2024a; CDC, 2024). Although they vary according to national vaccination policies, recommended vaccines for school-aged children and adolescents include DTP (diphtheria, tetanus, and pertussis), HPV (human papillomavirus), and influenza (Table 1). Hepatitis B, inactivated polio, MMR, and hepatitis A are recommended for those who have missed their vaccinations. Hib, conjugated pneumococcal, meningococcal, and varicella are recommended for those at risk (Chiara et al., 2021; CDC, 2024). According to the Expanded Immunisation Programme (EIP) implemented in Turkey, the Td (diphtheria, tetanus) vaccine is enhanced at school age. Rubella and hepatitis B vaccines are required for children who have not been vaccinated on time (until the unvaccinated age group is completed) (Ministry of Health, 2024) (Table 2).

Table 1. Recommended vaccinations for children aged 6-18 (CDC 2024)

Vaccinations	7-10 years	11-12 years	13-15 years	16 years	17-18 years
Hepatitis B					
[1]Hib					
Conjugate					
Influenza			1 dose per year		
[2]MMR					
Hepatitis A					
[3]DTP					
Human papillomavirüs					
Meningokok B					
Chickenpox					

[1]Haemophilus influenza type b (Hib) vaccination.
[2]Measles, mumps, and rubella vaccine.
[3]Diphtheria, Tetanus, and Pertussis.

It shows the recommended vaccinations for all children.

Vaccinations for people at risk.

Recommended vaccinations for children with missed vaccinations.

Table 2. Republic of Türkiye ministry of health childhood immunization schedule

Vaccinations	given at birth	1st month	2st month	4st month	6st month	9st month	12st month	18st month	24st month	48st month	13 years
Hepatitis B	I	II			III						
BCG		I									
[1]DTP-IPV-Hİb			I	II	III			R			
Conjugate P											
[2]MMR						AD*	I			II	
DTP-IPV										B	
OPA					I			II			
Td											B
Hepatitis A								I	II		
Chickenpox							I				

[1]Diphtheria, Tetanus, and Pertussis-inactivated polio vaccine (IPV).
[2]Measles, mumps, and rubella vaccine.
*Aditional dose.

Diphtheria-Pertussis and Tetanus Vaccines (DPT)

Diphtheria is caused by a micro-organism called Corynebacterium diphtheriae. It can lead to severe complications, including breathing difficulties, heart failure, paralysis, and even death if left untreated. Diphtheria is spread from person to person through airborne droplets. Symptoms of the disease include a sore throat and loss of appetite (WHO, 2015a). The diphtheria vaccine is administered as a 5-mixed vaccine (DPT-IPA-Hib) at 2,4,6 months and 18 months. A booster dose of quadrivalent mixed vaccine (DPT-IPA) is administered at 48 months. A separate booster dose of the adult diphtheria-tetanus (DT) vaccine is administered to the adolescent age group at the age of 13 (156th month). The diphtheria vaccine should not be administered to those with a history of a severe allergic reaction (anaphylaxis) to the vaccine or vaccine ingredients (Ministry of Health, 2024; Demiroğlu, 2021). No serious adverse reactions have been reported with the diphtheria vaccine alone. Common side effects are generally mild and may include redness, swelling, or tenderness at the injection site, as well as a low-grade fever (WHO, 2015a).

Pertussis is a respiratory disease caused by the bacterium Bordetella pertussis. Although pertussis is more severe in infants and young children, it can affect people of all ages. Pertussis is mostly spread from person to person through droplets from coughing or sneezing (WHO, 2015a). The only reliable way to prevent pertussis is through vaccination. The pertussis vaccine is a highly effective vaccine, administered as a 5-mixed vaccine (DPT-IPA-Hib) at 2,4,6 months and 18 months. The vaccination schedule includes a booster dose in the form of a quadrivalent mixed vaccine (DPT-IPA) at 48 months. The WHO recommends that countries decide on booster doses in adolescents and adults according to their own conditions (WHO, 2015a). Rarely, there may be redness, swelling, and pain at the injection site. School-aged children may have crying spells and mild fever (Demiroğlu, 2021).

Tetanus is an infection caused by a bacterium called Clostridium tetani, which is found in soil. A toxin released by the bacterium causes severe, painful muscle spasms that can lead to death. Bacteria can enter people of all ages through objects such as dirty fingernails, knives, nails, or deep penetrating wounds from animal bites (WHO, 2015a). The most effective way to prevent tetanus is to be fully vaccinated (Demiroğlu 2021, Ministry of Health, 2024). The tetanus vaccine is administered as a quadrivalent mixed vaccine (DPT-IPA-Hib) at 2,4,6 months and 18 months. The booster dose is administered as a quadrivalent mixed vaccine (DPT-IPA) at 48 months. The adult diphtheria-tetanus (Td) vaccine is administered as a separate booster dose at the age of 13 (156th month). Tetanus vaccination in adults with an unknown previous vaccination status is the Td (adult diphtheria-tetanus) vaccine (Ministry of Health, 2024).

Human Papillomavirus (HPV) Vaccine

HPV causes cancer of the cervix, vagina, and vulva in women, penile cancer in men, and anal and oropharyngeal cancer in women and men (Kutlu, 2021). There are more than 200 HPV types, which can be classified into different groups according to their oncogenic risk. However, two HPV types (16 and 18) are responsible for approximately 50% of high-grade cervical cancers (WHO, 2024). An effective and safe vaccine is available against the two cancer-causing types of HPV (HPV16 and 18), which are the main cause of cervical cancer. Vaccination against HPV types 16 and 18 significantly reduces the risk of developing cervical cancer. As part of the Global Strategy to Accelerate the Elimination of Cervical Cancer, WHO (2024) recommends that girls be vaccinated before the age of 15 years (WHO, 2024). HPV vaccination is routinely recommended by the Advisory Committee on Immunization Practices (ACIP) of the CDC for all adolescents aged 11-12 years (CDC, 2024). It is not yet included in the routine childhood immunization schedule in our country. The vaccine can be given from nine years of age. The vaccination schedule varies according to age. The HPV vaccine is given in two doses for those aged 9-14 years and in three doses for those aged 15 years and older (Kutlu, 2021). There should be at least 5 months between doses. It is important to be vaccinated before the sexual activity (CDC, 2024).

Influenza Vaccine

Influenza is a common infection in the community that can cause hospitalization and even death in certain risk groups. It is spread by respiratory particles expelled by coughing and sneezing from sick people (Azap, 2021). Annual vaccination is recommended to prevent seasonal influenza, especially for high-risk groups (WHO, 2015a; WHO, 2024). Today, there are three types of influenza vaccines produced by different methods: Live Attenuated Virus (LAIV), Inactivated Virus (IIV), and Recombinant Hemagglutinin (RIV). Influenza vaccines are prepared from four influenza viruses (two type A and two type B) that are expected to cause disease in humans that year. The only contraindication for the inactivated influenza vaccine is anaphylaxis to the vaccine or its components. As with all vaccines, local side effects (pain, redness, etc. at the injection site) are the most common. Rarely, complaints such as fever, headache, muscle aches, and weakness may also be observed (Azap, 2021; WHO, 2015a).

Hepatitis B Vaccine

Hepatitis B is a viral infection that affects the liver and can cause both acute and chronic diseases. The hepatitis B virus spreads through contact with infected blood and other body fluids (WHO, 2015a). The most effective way to protect against hepatitis B virus infection is vaccination. As HBV infection in childhood has a high rate of chronicity, the HBV vaccine has been included in the WHO Expanded Programme on Immunisation to protect newborns and young children (WHO, 2015a; Durmaz et al., 2018; Ministry of Health, 2024). The hepatitis B vaccine is administered free of charge to people in risk groups outside childhood as part of the Expanded Programme on Immunisation. It is administered as a single dose at 0, 1, and 6 months in unvaccinated adolescents. The most commonly reported side effects are pain at the injection site, mild fever, malaise, headache, and restlessness (Saltoğlu et al., 2021).

Hepatitis A Vaccine

Hepatitis A infection is a serious liver infection caused by the hepatitis A virus. It is mainly transmitted by the fecal-oral route, person-to-person contact, or consumption of contaminated food or drink (Mutlu, 2021). In our country, it is administered in 2 doses at 18 and 24 months. Children who have not been vaccinated before the age of two can be vaccinated at later visits (Ministry of Health, 2024). Those who live in the same house as a person with hepatitis A and those who have sexual intercourse are considered contacts. A single dose of vaccine should be administered to contacts aged 12-40 years within 2 weeks of contact. Adult vaccination consists of two doses at least 6 months apart, as in children. However, a blood test should be carried out before vaccination in adults to check whether the person has been previously vaccinated (Mutlu, 2021; Ministry of Health, 2024). Side effects are very rare. Pain, mild redness, swelling, headache, fever, chills, weakness, diarrhea, nausea, and loss of appetite may be observed at the injection site (Ministry of Health, 2024).

Measles, Mumps, Rubella Vaccine (MMR)

Measles is a highly contagious disease caused by the measles virus. It is spread through the respiratory tract, and symptoms include fever, rash, cough, runny nose, weakness, and redness of the eyes. Measles is spread by contact with the nasal and throat secretions of infected people or by droplets spread in the air (WHO, 2015a). It can cause serious complications in children under one year of age and adults. The only way to prevent the disease is through vaccination. The measles vaccine is administered free of charge in the form of MMR as two doses in the childhood vaccination schedule to all children aged 12 months and 48 months (Ministry of Health, 2024).

Rubella is an often mild infection in children caused by the rubella virus. Symptoms may include a rash, mild fever, a sore throat, swollen lymph nodes, and a runny nose. Rubella is spread by airborne droplets when infected people sneeze or cough (WHO, 2015a). Rubella, a mild viral infection of childhood, is important because it causes congenital rubella syndrome (CRS). The main purpose of rubella vaccination is to prevent CRS, which leads to hearing loss, blindness, and mental retardation (Durmaz et al., 2018). The only way to prevent the disease is vaccination (Ministry of Health). The WHO recommends that countries use the rubella vaccine in combination with the measles vaccine for the rubella elimination target (WHO, 2015a).

Mumps infection is common in children, and a third of cases are asymptomatic. The mumps virus is spread by airborne droplets when an infected person sneezes or coughs and by direct contact with an infected person (WHO 2015). Mumps infection can lead to complications such as hearing loss, orchitis, oophoritis, meningitis, and post-infectious encephalitis. As mumps infection is more severe in adolescents and adults, vaccination history should be sought in this age group (Durmaz et al., 2018; Ministry of Health, 2024). The World Health Organization recommends the mumps vaccine, which is a mixed vaccine containing measles, mumps, and rubella (WHO, 2015a).

Chickenpox Vaccine

Chickenpox, caused by the varicella-zoster virus (VZV), is characterized by widespread, itchy, fluid-filled rashes that usually appear in early childhood and are often accompanied by fever. It is a highly contagious disease. After primary infection, VZV remains in the body (sensory nerve ganglia) as a latent infection. Primary infection with VZV causes varicella. Reactivation of the latent infection causes herpes zoster (shingles). Based on the history of chickenpox infection and vaccination of all adolescents, it is recommended that adolescents aged 13 years and older who are incompletely vaccinated receive a single dose and those who have never been vaccinated receive two doses of vaccine at least 4 weeks apart (WHO, 2015a; CDC, 2024).

Common Side Effects of Vaccines and How to Deal with Them

Vaccines are very safe medical products administered to protect and maintain public health (Korkmaz, 2020; Song and Katial, 2004). Most developed countries understand the importance of vaccination and have reduced the prevalence of vaccine-preventable diseases by providing positive behavioral changes to parents through education about vaccines (Shukla and Shah, 2018). With immunization, the antigen that activates the body's immune system is injected into the body. Furthermore, after the vaccine is administered, side effects may occur, which are thought to be caused by the vaccine and are an undesirable but natural process (Sezen, 2022). While the side effects that occur after vaccination are mild and short-lived, in some cases, rare serious reactions may occur. These side effects that develop after vaccination cause parents to be hesitant about vaccines and refuse vaccination; parents cannot be sure about getting the next vaccine (Korkmaz, 2020). Today, undesirable side effects are still a source of concern for parents because vaccines contain harmful components (Song and Katial, 2004). Starting with the hepatitis B vaccine in the neonatal period, all children in our country are vaccinated with BCG (tuberculosis), DaBT-IPA-Hib (diphtheria, whooping cough, tetanus, polio, Haemophilus influenza), MMR (measles, rubella, mumps), chickenpox, hepatitis A and pneumococcal vaccines against infections. It is implemented free of charge to protect against (Akman and Yıldız, 2022).

Side effects that develop after vaccination may be regional, systemic, or allergic reactions (Sezen, 2022). Local reactions are an inflammatory response of the body to antigens, seen after many vaccine applications (Öneş and Palanduz, 1996). Symptoms such as pain, redness, burning, swelling, and limitation of movement in the injection area are the most common local/regional symptoms after vaccination (Sezen, 2022). Fever and accompanying weakness, fatigue, headache, and muscle aches may be seen as systemic symptoms (Öneş and Palanduz, 1996). The incidence of fever is higher in premature births and in babies with birth weight below normal, and the fever is usually above 39 °C (Korkmaz, 2020).

When we look at the side effects of the poliomyelitis vaccine, Paralytic Polio is one of the rare and scary complications of the polio vaccine (Shukla and Shah, 2018). DaTB: Fever, local pain, swelling, and erythema are some of the common side effects of DaTB, which is in the five-valent mixed vaccine group (Shukla and Shah, 2018). The most common side effects are mild local symptoms such as pain and hypersensitivity (50%), edema (40%), and rashes (33%) (Song and Katial, 2004). Rare but possible side effects such as hyperpyrexia - fever >40.5°C, seizures due to high fever, long-term uncontrollable crying attacks in the child, and decreased interest in environmental stimuli (hyporesponsiveness) may also be observed (Shukla and Shah, 2018). After the administration of the MMR vaccine, possible side effects such as skin rash, cough, rhinorrhea, redness in the eyes, high fever, and swelling in the parotid gland may occur, while some complications such as encephalitis may also occur (Kaçmaz et al., 2019). According to studies, thrombocytopenia, febrile seizures, anaphylaxis, and arthritis have also been associated with the MMR vaccine. While the thrombocytopenia level returned to normal after one month in 80.7% of individuals who received the MMR vaccine, 8.2% developed persistent thrombocytopenia lasting more than 3 months (Song and Katial, 2004).

Özer et al., reported the incidence of side effects observed within the first 14 days following varicella vaccination as follows: 29.5% experienced pain at the injection site, 6.6% redness, 3.2% swelling, and 6.6% fever (Özer et al., 2016). While there were only five serious cases related to the Varicella vaccine, it was determined that these individuals were not healthy enough and had insufficient immunity before vaccination (Song and Katial, 2004). The BCG vaccine is safer than other vaccines, and serious complications are very rare. The most common side effects are ulceration at the vaccination site, lymph node inflammation, and lupus vulgaris, with a rate of 1-10% (Turhan et al., 2017). Mild local pain and swelling and low-grade fever symptoms may be observed in individuals after pneumococcal vaccination (Shukla and Shah, 2018). Adverse negative events after Haemophilus influenza type b (Hib) vaccination have been found to occur approximately 18 times per 100,000 doses. While the most common symptoms after vaccination are redness, swelling, increased temperature, and fever at the injection site, local or systemic findings are less common (Song and Katial, 2004).

Despite the rare negative side effects of vaccines, side effects remain relatively unimportant because they prevent many diseases that cause disability and death (Song and Katial, 2004). When we consider the impact of the pandemic we have experienced in recent years on global health, we see again the importance of vaccination. Therefore, individuals/society should be educated about the importance of immunization. Healthy individuals form the foundation of healthy families, and in turn, healthy families are the building blocks of a healthy society (Akman and Yıldız, 2022).

Safety of Vaccines/Safe Vaccination

Throughout history, keeping food intact has been a very important issue for humanity. Nowadays, with the influence of developing technology, food can be stored for a long time without spoiling. Advances in the field of medicine have led to the need to preserve the produced drugs at appropriate temperatures, and cooling technologies have begun to be used in this field (Çevik, 2021). Cooling systems are needed to ensure the safety of vaccines, which have an important role in protecting and improving public health (Ağırtıcı and Güler, 2023). All equipment used to preserve vaccines in the appropriate environment and temperature, away from sunlight and ultraviolet rays, from the production stage to the application to individuals in the society, and all the healthcare professionals who monitor these storage conditions are a link to the cold chain system (Uzun, 2007). Cold chain rules should be given due importance during the storage and transfer of vaccines, which are highly sensitive and whose effectiveness decreases due to the slightest temperature changes (Bozkurt and Erdim, 2004). Since the area where the temperature change is greatest when opening and closing the refrigerator is the lid, vaccines should never be placed on the shelves in the lid but on the appropriate inner shelf of the refrigerator according to the type of vaccine (Çimşir Soran, 2022). For vaccines to effectively protect individuals against infectious diseases and create long-term immunity, they must be administered before the expiration date of the vial (Sezen, 2022). Frozen vaccines such as oral polio, measles, and mumps can be stored in the central warehouse for 6 months and can be stored in the refrigerator between -15 and -25 C°. Vaccines that should not be frozen, such as DBT, HepB, DT, Td, and BCG, can be stored in the central warehouse for 6 months and can be stored in the refrigerator. It should be stored between +2 and +8 C° temperature values (Küçüktürkmen and Bozkır, 2018).

To reliably preserve vaccines in the cold chain system, the cold chain range required is +2 to +8C°. Since conditions other than these temperature values damage the vaccine, temperature deviations are referred to as cold chain breaks (Çimşir Soran, 2022). It is the nurse's responsibility to store and administer heat-sensitive vaccines in a manner that preserves the integrity of their active ingredients and formulation. Failure to adhere to proper storage and administration protocols may compromise vaccine efficacy (Küçüktürkmen and Bozkır, 2018).

Vaccine Hesitancy

Distrust of vaccines, hesitancy, and anti-vaccine thoughts emerged with the discovery of the vaccine and began to become more effective in the world since 1990 and in our country since 2010 (Yüksel and Topuzoğlu, 2018). Nowadays, it is increasing, especially among families of children with chronic or congenital diseases. This situation, which seriously affects the success rate of immunization services, attracted the attention of the WHO and directed it to studies on the subject. For this purpose, a vaccine hesitancy working group was established by WHO. Vaccine hesitancy is defined by the WHO as "delaying or refusing to accept vaccines despite the availability of vaccination services" and is among the top ten situations that threaten health (WHO, 2015b). However, the concept of vaccine hesitancy includes not only vaccine rejection but also anxiety, anxiety, reluctance, and distrust experienced when getting vaccinated (Peretti Peretti Watel et al., 2015; Peretti Watel et al., 2019). Factors that cause vaccine hesitancy include religious beliefs, economic concerns (the idea that vaccines are paid, not affordable, or that companies produce vaccines for commercial reasons), the desire to gain natural immunity, the epidemic period, disbelief in the benefits of vaccines, low health literacy, lack of information, and the content of vaccines. The lack of understanding, preference for alternative or complementary medicine, speculative discourses and rumors about side effects, and the negative influence by social media contribute significantly to growing vaccine hesitancy (Yiğit et al., 2020; Etesamınıa and Bağcı Derinpınar, 2021; Saada et al., 2015). Although the degree of credibility and provability of these factors is debated, vaccine hesitancy is increasing day by day (Gesser Eldesburg et al., 2017).

Vaccine hesitancy is mostly experienced by parents in societies. The level of vaccine hesitancy is higher among parents, especially mothers who are primarily responsible for the care and health of children (Smith, 2017; Özceylan et al., 2020). Studies show that the rate of vaccine rejection and vaccine hesitancy is higher in parents of children with chronic or congenital diseases (Çıklar and Güner, 2020; Tezol et al., 2020; Tunç and Öztürk Çopur, 2022). Zerbo et al., it was found that children diagnosed with autism and their younger siblings were vaccinated at a lower rate than the general population (Zerbo et al., 2018). Similarly, in the study conducted by Keşli et al., with parents of children with autism, the rate of vaccine rejection was found to be 63.8%, and the rate of suspicion about the content of the vaccines was 73.1% (Keşli et al., 2021). It is likely that parents' thoughts and attitudes about a subject will direct their children's attitudes toward that subject. For this reason, families of adolescents and school-age children should be informed about the benefits of vaccines by providing education about them. Factors that cause vaccine hesitancy should be examined, and solutions should be offered (Tanrıkulu and Tanrıkulu, 2021). Protecting and improving public health depends on the success of immunization services. In order for immunization services to be successful, anti-vaccine sentiment and vaccine hesitancy must be prevented. To prevent vaccine hesitancy in adolescents and school-age children, who constitute the future of society, adding additions to the curriculum in the education program, eliminating vaccine-related information pollution and increasing health literacy levels, using mass media, creating content that will appeal to young people and sharing on social media networks. And parents and the school community need to be included in all these processes. Additionally, facilitating access to immunization services, explaining vaccine contents in an understandable language, and collaborating with leaders of society on this issue will also help reduce vaccine hesitancy (Özmen and Aksoy, 2022; Attwell et al., 2018). It should not be forgotten that although vaccine hesitancy is an individual decision, it is a problem that concerns the whole society.

Conclusion

In conclusion, immunization during school-age and adolescence plays a vital role in safeguarding individual and public health. Adhering to the recommended vaccination schedules ensures protection against various preventable diseases at a critical stage of growth and development. While common side effects of vaccines are generally mild and manageable, addressing concerns about vaccine safety through transparent communication is essential. Promoting safe vaccination practices and combating vaccine hesitancy through education and trust-building are key to maintaining high immunization coverage. Ultimately, protecting school-aged children and adolescents through timely and safe vaccinations contributes to healthier communities and a more resilient future.

Disclaimer

None.

References

Abdullahi, L. H., Kagina, B. M., Ndze, V. N., Hussey, G. D., & Wiysonge, C. S. (2020). Improving vaccination uptake among adolescents. *The Cochrane Database of Systematic Reviews*, 1(1).

Ağırtıcı, D. Y., & Güler, H. (2023). Determining the knowledge of health professionals working in a family health center about cold chains. *Cumhuriyet University Health Sciences Institute Journal*, 8(3), 457-465. https://doi.org/10.51754/cusbed.1364898.

Akman, N., & Yıldız, A. (2022). Evaluation of mothers' opinions regarding routine childhood vaccinations. *Journal of Pediatric Infection*, 16(4), 251-257. https://doi.org/10.5578/ced.20229621.

Attwell, K., Smith, D. T., & Ward, P. R. (2018). The unhealthy other: How vaccine-rejecting parents construct the vaccinating mainstream. *Vaccine*, 36(12), 1621–1626.

Azap, A. (2021). *Influenza Vaccination.* In Esin Şenol, Ali Acar, Selma Alp Çavuş, & Çiğdem Erol (Eds.), *Turkish Clinical Microbiology and Infectious Diseases Association Publications*, Konya. https://asi.klimik.org.tr/kutuphane. Accessed: 6.04.2024.

Bozkurt, G., & Erdim, L. (2010). Responsibilities of midwives and nurses in safe immunization. *Anatolian Journal of Nursing and Health Sciences*, 8(3), 119-126.

Cadeddu, C., Castagna, C., Sapienza, M., Lanza, T. E., Messina, R., Chiavarini, M., Ricciardi, W., & de Waure, C. (2021). Understanding the determinants of vaccine hesitancy and vaccine confidence among adolescents: A systematic review. *Human Vaccines & Immunotherapeutics*, 17(11), 4470-4486. https://doi.org/10.1080/21645515.2021.1961466.

Centers for Disease Control and Prevention. (2024). *Child and adolescent immunization schedule. Recommendations for ages 18 years or younger, United States, 2024.* https://www.cdc.gov/vaccines/schedules/hcp/imz/child-schedule-notes.html#note-hpv. Accessed: 6.04.2024.

Çevik, V. A. (2021). The most comprehensive cold chain application in history: Challenges encountered in the logistics of the coronavirus (Covid-19) vaccine. *Üsküdar University Journal of Social Sciences*, (12), 155-204. https://doi.org/10.32739/uskudarsbd.7.12.88.

Çıklar, S., & Güner, P. D. (2020). Annelerin çocukluk çağı aşıları hakkındaki bilgi, davranış ve tutumları ve aşı reddi nedenleri: Nitel ve nicel bir araştırma. *Ankara Medical Journal*, 20(1), 180-195. https://doi.org/10.5505/amj.2020.80148.

Çimşir Soran, T. (2022). *Evaluation of the knowledge, attitudes and behaviors of adults applying to the family medicine clinic about adult vaccines* (Thesis No. 751580) [Expert thesis, Zonguldak Bülent Ecevit University]. YÖK Thesis Center. https://tez.yok.gov.tr/UlusalTezMerkezi/tezSorguSonucYeni.jsp.

Çoklar, S., & Güner, P. D. (2020). Mothers' knowledge, behavior, and attitudes about childhood vaccines and reasons for vaccine refusal: A qualitative and quantitative research. *Ankara Medical Journal*, 20(1), 180-195.

Demiroğlu, Y. Z. (2021). *DTP Vaccination.* In Esin Şenol, Ali Acar, Selma Alp Çavuş, & Çiğdem Erol (Eds.), *Turkish Clinical Microbiology and Infectious Diseases Association Publications*, Konya. https://asi.klimik.org.tr/kutuphane. Accessed: 6.04.2024.

Durmaz, N., Ataş, E., & Ulukol, B. (2018). *Adolescence and immunization.* In Ü. Aydoğan (Ed.), *Adolescent Health and Problems -II* (pp. 23-33). Türkiye Klinikleri, Ankara.

Eskiocak, M., & Marangoz, B. (2019). *Status of immunization services in Turkey. Türk Tabipleri Birliği Yayınları*, Ankara. https://www.ttb.org.tr/kollar/_asi/userfiles/images/halk/turkiyede_bagisiklama.pdf. Accessed: 4.04.2024.

Etesamınıa, S., & Bağcı Derinpınar, K. (2021). The role of social media in vaccine hesitancy. *International Journal of Research in Health Management and Strategies*, 7(2), 377-390.

Gesser Eldesburg, A., Walter, N., Shir Raz, Y., Sassoni Barlev, O., & Rosenblat, S. (2017). The behind-the-scenes activity of parental decision-making discourse regarding childhood vaccination. *American Journal of Infection Control*. https://doi.org/10.1016/j.ajic.2016.10.009.

Göl, İ., & Açıkgöz, S. (2021). *Immunization*. In Özüm Erkin, Aslı Kalkım, & İlknur Göl (Eds.), *Public Health Nursing*. Çukuova Nobel Tıp Kitabevi, Ankara.

Kaçmaz, B., Tuna, A., Gül, S., Çalışkan, O., Ayvaz, G., Tuncel, B., Bulut, C., & Kandemir, S. (2019). Evaluation of the side effects of measles-mumps-rubella vaccine administered to healthcare personnel. *Anatolian Current Medical Journal*, 1(2), 23-25.

Karakuş, R. (2021). *Practical information on adult vaccination*. In Esin Şenol, Ali Acar, Selma Alp Çavuş, & Çiğdem Erol (Eds.), *Turkish Clinical Microbiology and Infectious Diseases Association Publications*, Konya. https://asi.klimik.org.tr/kutuphane. Accessed: 6.04.2024.

Keşli, R., Dünya, Y., Zaheer, A., Roudkoli, D. R., Bardak, M., Gün, R., Yücesan, E. Z., Demirayak, M. R., Dilcioğlu, F. Ö., Öztürk, F. B., Şener, B., Turhan, M., Özkan, E. C., Çetin, F. H., & Terzi, Y. (2021). Investigation of the knowledge levels of families with autistic children about vaccines, the frequency and reasons of vaccine refusal in different regions of Turkey. *Journal of General Medicine*, 31(3), 225-231.

Korkmaz, H. A. (2010). *Evaluation of the side effects of vaccines administered in the well-child clinic of Dokuz Eylül University Hospital* (Thesis No. 267028) [Expert thesis, Dokuz Eylül University]. YÖK Thesis Center. https://tez.yok.gov.tr/UlusalTezMerkezi/tezSorguSonucYeni.jsp.

Küçüktürkmen, B., & Bozkır, A. (2018). Evaluations in terms of drugs and applications that require special storage conditions or are subject to cold chain. *Turkish Journal of Hygiene and Experimental Biology*, 75(3), 305-322.

Kutlu, M. (2021). *HPV Vaccination*. In Esin Şenol, Ali Acar, Selma Alp Çavuş, & Çiğdem Erol (Eds.), *Turkish Clinical Microbiology and Infectious Diseases Association Publications*, Konya. https://asi.klimik.org.tr/kutuphane. Accessed: 6.04.2024.

Mackroth, M. S., Irwin, K., Vandelaer, J., Hombach, J., & Eckert, L. O. (2010). Immunizing school-age children and adolescents: Experience from low- and middle-income countries. *Vaccine*, 28(5), 1138-1147. https://doi.org/10.1016/j.vaccine.2009.11.008.

Ministry of Health. Vaccine. https://asi.saglik.gov.tr/asi-takvimi2. Accessed: 4.04.2024.

Mutlu, B. (2021). *HAV Vaccination*. In Esin Şenol, Ali Acar, Selma Alp Çavuş, & Çiğdem Erol (Eds.), *Turkish Clinical Microbiology and Infectious Diseases Association Publications*, Konya. https://asi.klimik.org.tr/kutuphane. Accessed: 6.04.2024.

Öneş, Ü., & Palanduz, A. (1996). Side effects of vaccines. *Flora Magazine*, 2, 102-106.

Özceylan, G., Toprak, D., & Esen, E. S. (2020). Vaccine rejection and hesitation in Turkey. *Human Vaccines & Immunotherapeutics*, 16(5), 1034-1039. https://doi.org/10.1080/21645515.2020.1717182.

Özer, M., Büyükçam, A., Bayhan, C., Özsürekçi, Y., & Kara, A. (2016). Attitudes towards varicella vaccine acceptance and vaccine-related side effects among Turkish medical students. *Journal of Pediatric Health and Diseases*, 59, 55-60.

Özmen, S., & Aksoy, N. (2022). Examining Covid-19 vaccine literacy and vaccine hesitancy levels: An application example on university students. *Gümüşhane University Journal of Health Sciences*, 11(2), 550-558.

Peretti-Watel, P., Larson, H. J., Ward, J. K., Schulz, W. S., & Verger, P. (2015). Vaccine hesitancy: Clarifying a theoretical framework for an ambiguous notion. *PLOS Currents*, 7.

Peretti-Watel, P., Ward, J. K., Vergelys, C., Bocquier, A., Raude, J., & Verger, P. (2019). 'I think I made the right decision…I hope I'm not wrong.' Vaccine hesitancy, commitment, and trust among parents of young children. *Sociology of Health & Illness*, 41(6), 1192-1206. https://doi.org/10.1111/1467-9566.12902.

Saada, A., Lieu, T. A., Morain, S. R., Zikmund-Fisher, B. J., & Wittenberg, E. (2015). Parents' choices and rationales for alternative vaccination schedules: A qualitative study. *Clinical Pediatrics*, 54(3), 236-243. https://doi.org/10.1177/0009922814548838.

Saltoğlu, N. (2021). *HBV Vaccination.* In Esin Şenol, Ali Acar, Selma Alp Çavuş, & Çiğdem Erol (Eds.), *Turkish Clinical Microbiology and Infectious Diseases Association Publications*, Konya. https://ası.klımık.org.tr/kutuphane. Accessed: 6.04.2024.

Sezen, B. (2022). *Evaluation of parents' knowledge, attitudes, and behaviors regarding childhood vaccinations* (Thesis No. 776863) [Master's thesis, Çankırı Karatekin University]. YÖK Thesis Center. https://tez.yok.gov.tr/UlusalTezMerkezi/tezSorguSonucYeni.jsp.

Shukla, V. V., & Shah, R. C. (2018). Vaccinations in primary care. *The Indian Journal of Pediatrics*, 85(12), 1118-1127. https://doi.org/10.1007/s12098-017-2555-2.

Smith, T. C. (2017). Vaccine rejection and hesitancy: A review and call to action. *Open Forum Infectious Diseases*, 4(3), 146. https://doi.org/10.1093/ofid/ofx146.

Song, B. J., & Katial, R. K. (2004). Update on side effects from common vaccines. *Current Allergy and Asthma Reports*, 4(6), 447-453.

Tanrıkulu, Y., & Tanrıkulu, G. (2021). Vaccine hesitancy and parents' attitudes. *Balıkesir Journal of Health Sciences*, 10(2), 199-204.

Tezol, Ö., Erkasa, F., & Çıtak, E. (2020). Trait anxiety levels and opposition to vaccination of parents of pediatric cancer patients. *Osman Gazi Medical Journal*, 42(2), 51-58.

Tunç, S., & Öztürk Çopur, E. (2022). Examining the vaccine hesitancy and vaccine opposition levels of parents applying to family health centers. *YBH Journal*, 3(3), 29-46.

Turhan, U., Ozkısa, T., Aydoğan, M., & Gümüş, S. (2017). A rare vaccine complication: BCG keloid. *Izmir Chest Hospital Journal*, 31(1), 57-59.

Uzun, E. (2007). *Cold chain, current situation, and practices in family health centers in Isparta province and district centers* (Thesis No. 203473) [Expert thesis, Süleyman Demirel University]. YÖK Thesis Center. https://tez.yok.gov.tr/UlusalTezMerkezi/tezSorguSonucYeni.jsp.

Vandelaer, J., & Olaniran, M. (2015). Using a school-based approach to deliver immunization—global update. *Vaccine*, 33(5), 719-725. https://doi.org/10.1016/j.vaccine.2014.11.037.

World Health Organization (WHO). (2015)a. *Immunization in practice: A practical guide for health staff – 2015 update.* https://www.who.int/publications/i/item/immunization-in-practice-a-practical-guide-for-health-staff. Accessed: 6.04.2024.

World Health Organization (WHO). (2015)b. https://www.who.int/news/item/18-08-2015-vaccine-hesitancy-a-growing-challenge-for-immunization-programmes Accessed: 6.04.2024.

World Health Organization (WHO). (2024a). *Vaccine-preventable diseases.* https://www.who.int/teams/immunization-vaccines-and-biologicals/diseases. Accessed: 4.04.2024.

World Health Organization. (2024b). *Immunization coverage.* Retrieved from https://www.who.int/news-room/fact-sheets/detail/immunization-coverage Accessed: 4.04.2024.

Wolfson, L. J., Gasse, F., Lee-Martin, S. P., Lydon, P., Magan, A., Tibouti, A., Johns, B., Hutubessy, R., Salama, P., & Okwo-Bele, J. M. (2008). Estimating the costs of achieving the WHO-UNICEF Global Immunization Vision and Strategy, 2006-2015. *Bulletin of the World Health Organization*, 86(1), 27-39. https://doi.org/10.2471/blt.07.045096.

Yiğit, T., Oktay, B. Ö., Özdemir, C. N., & Moustafa Pasa, S. (2020). Anti-vaccination and its intellectual development. *Journal of Social and Humanities Sciences Research*, 7(53), 1244-1261.

Yüksel, G. H., & Topuzoğlu, A. (2019). Increasing vaccine rejection and factors affecting anti-vaccination. *Estüdam Public Health Journal*, 4(2), 244-258. https://doi.org/10.35232/estudamhsd.525983.

Zerbo, O., Modaressi, S., Goddard, K., Levis, E., Fireman, B. H., Daley, M. F., Irving, S. A., Jackson, L. A., Donahue, J. G., Qian, L., Getahun, D., Destefano, F., McNeil, M. M., & Klein, N. P. (2018). Vaccination patterns in children after autism spectrum disorder diagnosis and in their younger siblings. *Jama Pediatrics*, 172(5), 469-475.

Chapter 11

Preventing Accidents and Injuries at School

Adem Sümen[1,*], PhD
and Selma Öncel[2], PhD

[1]Department of Public Health Nursing, Akdeniz University, Kumluca Faculty of Health Sciences, Antalya, Türkiye
[2]Department of Public Health Nursing, Akdeniz University, Faculty of Nursing, Antalya, Türkiye

Abstract

Schools are structured environments where children leave homes and spend the majority of the day engaging in community life. During this period, students are more at risk of various accidents. An important group in taking necessary precautions against accident risks is the school community. School accidents and injuries are unexpected and unintentional incidents involving students. Students may be exposed to various types of accidents not only within the school building but also in areas such as playgrounds, sports fields, stairs, corridors, laboratories, gardens, and around the school. Accidents such as falls, bumps, burns, etc., are more frequently observed among school-aged children. Children are more prone to accidents than adults. Because they have not yet completed their physical, social, and psychological development, for this reason, the risks that will cause injuries can be eliminated with protective measures to be taken before school accidents occur. In this respect, all kinds of measures should be taken to ensure that all public and private schools comply with the necessary health conditions, and these measures should be supervised. In this direction, in order to ensure effective school safety and prevent accidents, it is important to take protective measures in the pre-accident period, to provide effective training, to make multidisciplinary planning and preparation, to protect school-age children who constitute the future of society, to ensure safety in schools, and to create healthy generations and a healthy future. As a result of the school community receiving the necessary training and taking the necessary precautions, the rate of accidents or deaths decreases. It is the responsibility of nurses to recognize risk factors and take necessary precautions by evaluating the characteristics of the child and their environment. School nurses should assume the role of leadership and coordinator by playing a key role in determining the risks in the schools where they work, implementing health programs and policies for the prevention of accidents and injuries, and developing health education.

---

* Corresponding Author's Email: ademsumen@akdeniz.edu.tr

In: Health Promotion and Prevention
Editor: Eda Kılınç İşleyen
ISBN: 979-8-89530-758-8

Keywords: school accident, injury, prevention, school-age children, school nursing

Introduction

School age is the period of growth and development of children. A healthy individual, who has an important role in determining the level of development of countries, is possible only by raising individuals who are aware of their health from childhood, protect their health, and recognize when their health deteriorates. Therefore, the school health approach is very important in building future generations (Onis et al., 2007). This approach aims to protect and improve the health of students and school staff and to ensure that students continue their school life in a healthy way (Sprague and Walker, 2021).

Accidents are unintentional and preventable events that may lead to physical or emotional harm (Sleet, 2018). Accidents and injuries to school-age children are a growing global public health problem. For every area where child injuries occur, there are proven ways to reduce the likelihood and severity of injury, but awareness of the problem and its preventability is important, as well as interventions to prevent school-age children from being injured (World Health Organization, 2008).

Children's vulnerability to accidents is closely linked to their developmental stage. The more immature children are, the lower their risk perception and the higher their vulnerability to accidents and injuries. This vulnerability varies according to the level of coordination of the nervous system, motor skills, sense of risk perception, and the level of protection provided to the child by parents and school health services (Sprague and Walker, 2021). It is also noted that there are significant improvements in children's autonomous behavior upon admission to school and that this increased independence supports greater exposure to risks in schools. In schools, children can be protected from accidents through safe and protective behaviors and habits that prevent illness or death from accidents (Reis et al., 2021).

Dealing with accidents and preventing injuries in school environments is of great importance. It is necessary to determine how and why students are injured and to find out which situations in schools cause these injuries. Additionally, rapid, efficient, and effective emergency response to injuries in schools should be ensured. Collecting injury data, managing critical incident investigations, developing a school emergency plan, dealing with crisis situations and their consequences, and developing prevention programs are needed. Injury prevention should not be limited to sports, physical education, playgrounds, laboratories, and vocational classrooms. It should take into account the physical characteristics of the school, including transportation to the school. In addition, physical and emotional damage to school-age children can be caused by bullying, sexual harassment, and prejudice-based violence (Bhasin et al., 2020).

School Accidents

Accidents are physical and mental injuries resulting from careless, imprudent, irresponsible, and uninformed behavior caused by an external force (Kılınç and Gür, 2018). According to the definition of the World Health Organization, an accident is an unplanned, unexpected event that causes injury, loss of life, and property (World Health Organization, 2008). *Injury* is an intentional or unintentional condition caused by acute exposure of the human body to energy or removal of vital elements. *Intentional injuries* are those resulting from self-harm, interpersonal violence, conflict, and war. *Unintentional injuries* are those resulting from poisoning, drowning, burns, falls, and traffic accidents, depending on the underlying cause (Akçay and Yıldırımlar, 2018; Kılınç and Gür, 2018; World Health Organization, 2008).

Accidents and injuries have a high mortality and morbidity rate and are a global public health problem because they can be prevented (Kılınç and Gür, 2018). School is the area where students spend most of their day. During this time, the risk of students facing various accidents increases. These risks can be eliminated by the protection measures taken by the school before accidents occur (Orton et al., 2016). When accidents cannot be prevented, injuries occur. Most injuries are minor cuts and bruises that heal quickly, but there are also a significant number of serious cases. Some of these include the student's absence from school, limitation of activities, hospitalization, disability, and death (Bou-Karroum et al., 2022).

In order for accidents occurring in schools to be school accidents, they must occur within the school timeframe, they must occur during school activities (sports activities, excursions), or when students are sent out of school on duty, they must occur while traveling to and from a place where a job is being done on duty with a service provided by the school administration. In addition, the child must be sent to the infirmary, home, or hospital, a medical intervention must be made for the child, and the child's social life must be restricted (Gür and Yıldız, 2009).

Causes of School Accidents

Table 1. Factors affecting school accidents

Personal factors	Environmental factors
• Age • Gender • Growth and development related cabamotor movements • Physical characteristics (height, obesity, etc.) • Physical disabilities (vision, hearing, etc.) • Aggressive behavior • Indifference/not caring • Inattention/fatigue/insomnia • Lack of awareness of accident occurrence and risk • Dangerous behaviors for the purpose of joking • Lack of knowledge on accident prevention	• Socio-economic status and family factors • Season • Natural disasters • Location and surroundings of the school building • Ignoring dangerous situations in school buildings, classrooms, stairs, and school yard • Laboratories and workshops • Crowded classrooms • Games that encourage dangerous behavior • Inadequacy of legal regulations

Every day, school-age children face different risks in the classrooms, playgrounds, corridors, cafeterias, and gymnasiums of schools. Factors affecting school-age children's injuries on playgrounds depend on their psychomotor skills, balance and endurance, decision-making ability, and experience with hazards. Students are more likely to have accidents during break times (Dilek, 2018; Şengel et al., 2020). The frequency and severity of injuries in schools vary from school to school. It is reported that ½ of the injuries are caused by the child's own behavior, ¼ are caused by another child, and ¼ are caused by the environment (Dilek, 2018;

Özdemir et al., 2022). Age, gender, socioeconomic status, and physical condition affect the recurrence and severity of accidents. Each child's level of exposure is influenced by many factors, such as the child's level of development, individual attention, school supervision, school environment, and materials used at school (Salminen et al., 2014). The factors that cause accidents and injuries in schools are shown in Table 1 in two groups as personal and environmental factors in line with the literature (Brussoni et al., 2015; Kim et al., 2019; Kutsyuruba et al., 2015; Orton et al., 2016; Özdemir et al., 2022; Pierpoint et al., 2016; Salam et al., 2016; Salminen et al., 2014; Şengel et al., 2020; Watson and Errington, 2016).

Types of School Accidents

Table 2. Types of accidents that occur in schools

Accident	Description
Falling	Falls are the most common type of accident in school-age children. Children's age, behavior, and environment affect these accidents. Most falls occur while running, jumping, swimming, playing sports, climbing or descending stairs, and climbing.
Crash	At school, children can be injured by running, walking, playing, and colliding with various equipment (tables, boards, etc.), trees, or each other. Head injuries resulting from collisions can cause serious trauma.
Burns	A burn is a severe trauma that occurs due to various reasons and causes disruption of skin integrity and requires special and emergency care/treatment. Burns are mostly the result of scalding hot water; as the age increases, burns occur as the result of flame-fire, electricity, and chemical substances. Uninformed persons should not interfere with the electrical system, bare cables should be repaired, and flammable liquids should not be kept in schools.
Cuts	Cuts that occur for any reason are one of the less common types of accidents in school-age children. Furthermore, bleeding because of cuts can cause serious problems.
Sprain	Sprains occur mostly during play and sports activities. Falls, whether from the same plane or from a height, in organized sports such as athletics or in unorganized sports, are the most common causes of injuries.
Foreign body penetration	As a result of careless behavior, objects such as scissors, pencils, or cutlasses cause injuries to school-age children. This is less common than other types of injuries.
Poisoning	Children are more sensitive than adults in terms of their structural development characteristics. Ingestion, ingestion, or inhalation of drugs or other poisonous substances left in the open may lead to serious consequences or death. Poisoning is increased by school-age children putting everything they can get their hands on into their mouths, rummaging around to get to know the environment, being curious, lack of knowledge, and carelessness of the people providing education.
Electric shock	Unprotected sockets or frayed electrical cables pose a great threat to school-age children. Loss of consciousness, respiratory and cardiac arrest, electrical burns, head, spinal cord, chest, or abdominal injuries that occur as a result of the child jumping and falling due to the effect of electric shock can be seen in school-age children exposed to electric shock.
Fractures	Fractures are the most common type of injury due to falls. Fractures in children differ from those in adults in terms of mechanism of occurrence, fracture type, and treatment approaches. The incidence of fractures in childhood may vary depending on many epidemiological factors. These factors include age, gender, race, socioeconomic status, season, living area, time of day, risky sports and behaviors, and dietary patterns that affect bone health. Fractures seen in school-age children between the ages of 6 and 12 occur mostly in boys, in the summer season, in the street environment or in the schoolyard because of a fall. Fractures are seen most often in the distal radius region, and most fractures can be treated conservatively. The increasing trend of fractures in school-age children today makes it mandatory to take various precautions for our future.

School-age children and young people spend a significant part of the day at school. In addition to their own behavior, inadequate environmental regulations and negligence can lead to accidents and injuries. Children are always exposed to many hazards: at the entrance to the school, during recess, during lessons, during activities, at lunchtime, and after school (Bhasin et al., 2020; Senterre et al., 2014). Students face these hazards mostly in the schoolyard, classrooms, stairs, toilets, canteens, school corridors, school buses, school entrances, and exits, laboratories, and workshops (Sosnowska & Kostka, 2003). In order to examine the effect of security measures taken in basic education institutions on school accidents, a study was conducted with administrators and employees working in 48 institutions. The employees who participated in the study stated that most of the accidents occurring in schools (79.2%) were caused by the students themselves, the first place in all schools (84.9%) was accidents caused by falling, accidents occurred mostly outside the school building; mostly in the school yard (72.9%), and inside the building on the stairs (61.6%) and in the classrooms (58.8%). It was determined that more general security measures were determined in private schools compared to public schools (Akar & Doğan, 2021). Fractures are the most common type of severe accident in schools. Fractures follow falls and cause trauma in school-age children. The types of accidents and parts of the body affected by the accident differ according to age. While simple accidents (abrasions, swelling) occur in kindergarten, falls, fractures, dislocations, and traumas occur in primary and secondary school (Senterre et al., 2014; Sosnowska & Kostka, 2003). The most common types of accidents in schools are given in Table 2 in line with the literature (Akar & Doğan, 2021; Alvarez, 2017; Bhasin et al., 2020; Peyton et al., 2017; Senterre et al., 2014; Sosnowska & Kostka, 2003).

Prevention and First Aid in School Accidents

Children spend most of their days in school. Happy, healthy, social adaptation to social life is formed only with children growing up in a safe environment. Furthermore, children who grow up in a safe environment are more successful academically, have better relationships with friends, and use communication more effectively in the social environment. Most of the activities students do at school throughout the day are low-risk behaviors that can be observed, controlled, and restricted. This situation shows that information about accidents occurring in the school environment can be collected, and risks can be reduced by taking potential protection measures (Emerce et al., 2022; Karakütük et al., 2017).

It is very important for the school administration to determine the risk factors and necessary precautions by evaluating the characteristics of the students and the school environment in order to prevent school accidents (Alver et al., 2016). Some of the measures that can be taken in schools;

- Evaluating the physical environment in schools in terms of security risks,
- Restricting pupils from traveling in potentially risky areas around the school,
- Informing students to stay away from broken stairs, stair railings, broken windows, holes, and defective surfaces. Elimination of these faults or problems, safety precautions, and signs until they are removed,
- It can be listed as psychological and emotional safety against violence, disasters, health and cleanliness, physical, sexual abuse, psychological and emotional safety (Dilek, 2018; Wang and Degol, 2016).

Ensuring School Safety

The physical characteristics of schools, where children spend the most time outside their families, are very important in terms of safety. The physical location, organization, and equipment of the educational institution are some of the important elements that affect the quality of education provided. The characteristics of these elements should respond to children's need for healthy/safe growth (Emerce et al., 2022). School safety conceptually means that students, teachers, and other staff feel physically, psychologically, and emotionally safe. School safety includes all stages, starting from the moment the student and other school personnel leave their homes to go to school until they return home again (Kutsyuruba et al., 2015; Lundgren and McMakin, 2018). The security between home and school is more important, especially for schools with transported education. If school security is considered in terms of space,

- Security between school and home,
- Safety inside the school,
- It covers security in three main areas, including security in the classroom (Emerce et al., 2022; Karakütük et al., 2017).

It has been observed that problems related to school security arise in the dimensions of physical (building, transportation, hygiene factors, and infrastructure), psycho-social (violence, abuse, suicide, substance abuse, and neglect), and external threats (school environment events, school environment structure, and system, abuse, psychological attacks, terrorism, theft, and violence). Similarly, studies in which a single dimension is analyzed in more detail and in-depth may be useful for the solution to that security problem. Again, in some of the security incidents, demographic factors such as school type, the province/region where the school where the security incident occurred is located, and socio-economic level may be determinative (Kahraman et al., 2019).

Organization of the Structure and Physical Features of the School

The school environment is the second most important environment that is effective in the health and development of the child after the family environment. A healthy school environment should be an environment in which the school and the family are in cooperation, suitable for the child's education, conducive to physical and social development, and free from hazards. The safety of the school environment is of primary importance (Centers for Disease Control and Prevention, 2019). Problems in the physical and social environments of schools adversely affect the safety of students and cause accidents and injuries. The most basic parameters are that school buildings should be robust, non-slip floors should be used in classrooms and corridors, cleaning and repair works should be carried out during the hours when students are not in the areas where they are carried out, window heights should be adjusted according to the physical characteristics of the students, and classrooms should be adequately and appropriately illuminated. The risk of accidents increases with the increase in materials used for education in schools. Necessary safety precautions should be taken when using tools in laboratories and workshops. It is also important that the cables of the computers used in the lessons should not be exposed and care should be taken in terms of electrical leakages in order to reduce accidents. It is stated that long school hours, inadequate school staff, inexperience of school nurses, and extracurricular alternative activities have a significant effect on school accidents. The low number of students, the presence of extracurricular alternative activities, and the excess of playground equipment in the school affect the rate of injury. Factors such as the size of the school building, the old history of the building, and the increase in the number of vehicles increase the injury rates. It was revealed that there were fewer injuries in schools where there was fixed playground equipment on the playgrounds and recess hours were different for each class. All kinds of foodstuffs to be used in the kitchen should be inspected continuously and frequently by the school administration. All kinds of foodstuffs offered to students and staff in the canteen and kitchen must be kept in a cooler or cupboard that can keep these substances intact. There should be no fixed rubbish accumulation place in the school garden. Garbage containers must be lidded, stainless, and leak-proof. School rubbish must be removed daily (Cleveland and Fisher, 2014; Higgins et al., 2005).

First Aid Practices after School Accidents

Table 3. The most common types of violent accidents in schools

Accident result	Intervention
Hemorrhages	External hemorrhages or nosebleeds are the most common causes of school accidents. In external bleeding, direct pressure is applied on the wound; if the bleeding does not stop, the pressure is increased by placing a second cloth, pressure is applied to the pressure point closest to the bleeding area, the bleeding area is lifted up, if the bleeding is in the arms or legs and there is no suspicion of fracture, the bleeding area is kept above the heart level, shock position is given, life signs are checked frequently (2-3 min. intervals). In case of a nosebleed, the student's head is tilted forward, and the wings of the nose are squeezed with two fingers for five minutes each, if the bleeding does not stop, 112 is immediately notified.
Fractures	In fracture, the student is not moved, sudden movements are avoided, and no attempt is made to replace the fracture if the fracture is in the arm; since edema will occur, items such as watches, etc. are removed and movement of the area is prevented, if there is an open fracture; the wound is covered with a clean cloth before fixation, the fractured area is fixed with a hard object such as cardboard, wood, etc., including the upper and lower joints, the fixed area is kept above, the pulse and skin color in the fractured area is checked, kept warm, medical help is called.
Injuries	In the case of injuries, the student's vital signs should be evaluated, the wound should be evaluated by cutting the clothes covering the wound and removing them without damaging the injured tissue (mode of occurrence, duration, presence of a foreign body, bleeding, etc.). If there is bleeding, bleeding should be controlled by pressing the wound with sterile gauze or a clean piece of fabric. In open wounds, the wound should be covered with sterile gauze to prevent infection. Organs that come out as a result of injury should not be tried to be replaced. They should be covered with a clean cloth. In the presence of a stabbed object or a foreign body, it should never be tried to be removed. It should be ensured to remain fixed. Since there is a risk of increasing bleeding during wound cleaning, wound cleaning should be done in the hospital. The student should be covered to prevent heat loss. If there is a fracture, the fractured area should be splinted and immobilized. Nothing should be applied to the wound. In injuries with limb (organ) rupture, if the rupture is complete, the ruptured part should be wrapped with sterile gauze, placed in a clean bag, placed in another bag filled with ice, and delivered to the health institution within six hours. If the skin is still attached and not completely detached, the detached piece should be brought over the wound and covered with a clean cloth. It should be ensured that the student goes to a health institution as soon as possible.

Table 3. (Continued)

Accident result	Intervention
Low blood sugar	The student's vital signs should be evaluated, and he/she should be made to sit or lie down. If he/she is conscious, he/she should eat 2-3 sugar cubes and drink fruit juice by way of support. If he/she feels good after the application, stay with him/her until he/she feels completely well. However, if the student's condition worsens, 112 is called, and medical professional help is provided as soon as possible.
Foreign body in the eyes, ears, and nose	If the foreign body in the eye is a substance such as dust, eraser dust, pencil tip, etc., the eye is turned to the side where the light is intense and washed with plenty of water. Try to prevent the student from rubbing the eye. If the foreign body in the eye is metal (science, artwork, etc. during course activities), professional medical assistance should be called and waited for without any intervention. In the case of a foreign body in the ear, without intervening with a sharp and piercing object, without contact with water, emergency medical assistance should be called, and the student should wait until the emergency medical personnel arrive. In the case of a foreign body in the nostril (eraser dust, pencil accessory, marble, small educational materials, etc.), the student should be supported to expel the foreign body with a strong blowing motion by pressing on the nasal wall. If it cannot be removed, 112 should be called to benefit from emergency health services without repeating the application.

First aid is of great importance in accidents occurring in schools. First aid, when applied consciously to injuries and acute diseases, is lifesaving and has an important role in preventing disabilities. However, today, there are no infirmaries or school nurses in schools other than boarding and private schools (Akgün et al., 2023). In accidents that may occur in schools, the fact that school employees have sufficient knowledge about ensuring student safety and first aid intervention affects the achievement of the desired results in ensuring student safety. Assuming that teachers are the first people to reach the accident scene in schools, it is of great importance that these first responders have a high level of knowledge about first aid in terms of first intervention for the injured. Teachers should be informed about accidents and first aid with the help of experts (Aktaş et al., 2019). In a study, 81.0% of teachers had knowledge of first aid, while only 23.0% claimed to have sufficient knowledge. It was determined that teachers had knowledge about first aid, but they were not confident enough to apply it (Faydalı et al., 2019).

Falls are one of the most common causes of school injuries. Most of the falls occur while running, sliding, jumping, doing sports, swimming, and climbing. The most common types of severe accidents in schools are hemorrhages, fractures, injuries due to falls, and traumas caused by foreign objects in the eyes, ears, and nose and low blood sugar levels (Table 3) (Akgün et al., 2023; Aktaş et al., 2019; Dilek, 2018; Faydalı et al., 2019; Neto et al., 2016; Reveruzzi et al., 2016).

Roles and Responsibilities of School Nurses in School Accidents

It is very important to create a healthy environment to ensure student attendance in schools and to protect high-risk students in terms of bad habits (Meydanlıoğlu and Gözüm, 2019). The school building and the environment where the school is located should be evaluated in terms of risks that may adversely affect health, such as injuries, violence and abuse, smoking, alcohol, and drugs. It is important to organize health-promoting activities such as increasing the availability of healthy foods and sports areas, establishing school policies for health protection and promotion, and organizing existing policies in this direction (Akgül and Ergün, 2021; Şahinöz ve ark., 2017). Health education in schools focuses on strengthening both the physical and psychosocial environment and aims to create a school environment where students can establish positive relationships and develop self-efficacy (Akgül and Ergün, 2021; Dilek, 2018).

One of the main duties of school nurses is to prevent accidents and injuries. They also have an important role in solving possible or existing problems in this field. The results of the research show that students are less absent, their activities are less restricted, and they are referred to health institutions less if there is a school nurse in schools. Studies have shown that the first-aid interventions that nurses can perform are sufficient for most of the injuries caused by accidents in schools (Bou-Karroum et al., 2022; Orton et al., 2016; Salam et al., 2016). Pennington and Delaney (2008) reported that the presence of a full-time nurse at school reduces the number of students sent home when they become ill or injured. For this reason, nurses play an important role in taking the necessary precautions for the occurrence of accidents in preventive health services for school-age children and reducing the mortality and morbidity rates that may occur as a result of accidents (Kim et al., 2019). Nurses are the key human power in taking safety precautions inside and outside the school, preventing accidents and making necessary interventions as a result of accidents, and identifying and solving health problems of school-age children and young people (Akgül and Ergün, 2021; Bou-Karroum et al., 2022).

Conclusion

School is a living space where children face social life for the first time outside their homes, share socially with others, make new friends, and engage in more social activities. The school-age childhood period covers the development process of children. The incidence of accidents is higher in the school environment. School health is important in terms of developing positive health behaviors in school-age children and planning appropriate interventions. Accidents occurring in childhood are an important health problem in our country as well as in the whole world. Factors such as the increased physical activity of school-age children, lack of awareness of risk, lack of cautious behaviors, inability to recognize dangers in time, curiosity to explore, weakness in decision-making, increased emotional stress, ignorance, problems related to traffic in schools, pressure from peers, desire to achieve dangerous physical activities increase the susceptibility to accidents. It is of great importance to inform administrators, teachers, and other employees about the causes, times, and places of accidents in schools; to provide training for students to be protected from school accidents and to behave carefully; to organize and supervise the school and its surroundings in a way not to cause accidents.

Disclaimer

None.

References

Akar, S. G., & Doğan, A. K. (2021). Investigation of the effects of security measures taken in primary education institutions on school accidents. *Gümüşhane University Journal of Health Sciences*, 10(1), 114-122.

Akçay, D., & Yıldırımlar, A. (2018). Investigation of children's school accident and behavior of their parents safety measures. *E-Journal of Dokuz Eylul University Nursing Faculty*, 11(1), 48-55.

Akgül, E., & Ergün, A. (2021). School health nursing in promotion public health. *Journal of Public Health Nursing*, 3(2), 141-153.

Akgün, M., Sekerci, N., Demirdağ, H., & Doğan, R. (2023). Determining preschool teachers' basic first aid knowledge levels. *Halic University Journal of Health Sciences*, 6(3), 30-38.

Aktaş, B., Yılmaz, M., Dereli, F., & Sarı, H. Y. (2019). Level of first aid knowledge of primary and secondary school teachers. *Journal of Academic Research in Nursing*, 5(1), 17-22.

Alvarez, A. (2017). "Seeing their eyes in the rearview mirror": Identifying and responding to students' challenging experiences. *Equity & Excellence in Education*, 50(1), 53-67.

Alver, E., Adigüzel, T., & Öztürk, O. (2016). School safety study on 11 different schools in İstanbul. *International Journal of Eurasia Social Sciences*, 7(23), 274-298.

Bhasin, S., Gill, T. M., Reuben, D. B., Latham, N. K., Ganz, D. A., Greene, E. J., ... & Peduzzi, P. (2020). A randomized trial of a multifactorial strategy to prevent serious fall injuries. *New England Journal of Medicine*, 383(2), 129-140.

Bou-Karroum, L., El-Jardali, F., Jabbour, M., Harb, A., Fadlallah, R., Hemadi, N., & Al-Hajj, S. (2022). Preventing unintentional injuries in school-aged children: A systematic review. *Pediatrics*, 149(Suppl 6), e2021053852J.

Brussoni, M., Gibbons, R., Gray, C., Ishikawa, T., Sandseter, E. B. H., Bienenstock, A., ... & Tremblay, M. S. (2015). What is the relationship between risky outdoor play and health in children? A systematic review. *International Journal of Environmental Research and Public Health*, 12(6), 6423-6454.

Centers for Disease Control and Prevention. (2019). *Your guide to using the school health index*. Atlanta: US Dept of Health and Human Services.

Cleveland, B., & Fisher, K. (2014). The evaluation of physical learning environments: A critical review of the literature. *Learning Environments Research*, 17, 1-28.

Dilek, S. (2018). The effect on the knowledge and behavior of students of the education given on accident-free days training program to prevent school accidents [Unpublished master dissertation]. University of Akdeniz.

Emerce, A., Şahin, M. S., Telli, N., & Timur, Ş. (2022). School safety according to school managers and teacher perceptions. *Socrates Journal of Interdisciplinary Social Studies*, 16, 26-50.

Faydalı, S., Küçük, S., & Yeşilyurt, M. (2019). Incidents that require first aid in schools: Can teachers give first aid? *Disaster Medicine and Public Health Preparedness*, 13(3), 456-462.

Gür, K., & Yıldız, A. (2009). Development of scales of pupils' knowledge and attitude towards the security prevention against school accidents. *Maltepe University Journal of Nursing Science and Art*, 2(1), 10-21.

Higgins, S., Hall, E., Wall, K., Woolner, P., & McCaughey, C. (2005). *The impact of school environments: A literature review*. London: Design Council.

Kahraman, H., Şemin, F. K., & Uğurlu, C. T. (2019). School security: Reflected to the press in Turkey. *Journal of History Culture and Art Research*, 8(1), 392-408.

Karakütük, K., Özbal, E. Ö., & Sağlam, A. (2017). Teacher's and school manager's opinions on implementations made in school management to provide school security. *Mersin University Journal of the Faculty of Education*, 13(3), 1214-1232.

Kılınç, E., & Gür, K. (2018). Effect of health belief model in prevention of school injuries. *Journal of Health Science and Profession*, 5(3), 467-475.

Kim, S. S., Yu, M., Kim, S. S., & Yu, M. (2019). Factors affecting the practice of accident prevention behavior in middle-school students. *Child Health Nursing Research*, 25(4), 388-397.

Kutsyuruba, B., Klinger, D. A., & Hussain, A. (2015). Relationships among school climate, school safety, and student achievement and well-being: A review of the literature. *Review of Education*, 3(2), 103-135.

Lundgren, R. E., & McMakin, A. H. (2018). *Risk communication: A handbook for communicating environmental, safety, and health risks*. John Wiley & Sons.

Meydanlıoğlu, A., & Gözüm, S. (2019). Practices and programs developing school health in Turkey. *Turkiye Klinikleri Public Health Nursing-Special Topics*, 5(1), 16-23.
Neto, N. M. G., Pereira, J. D. C. N., Muniz, M. L. C., Gavião, D., de Souza, N. M. G., de Sena Neri, M. F., ... & de Vasconcelos, E. M. R. (2016). Health education intervention on first aid in school: Integrative review. *International Archives of Medicine*, 9(144), 1-7.
Onis, M. D., Onyango, A. W., Borghi, E., Siyam, A., Nishida, C., & Siekmann, J. (2007). Development of a WHO growth reference for school-aged children and adolescents. *Bulletin of the World Health Organization*, 85(9), 660-667.
Orton, E., Whitehead, J., Mhizha-Murira, J., Clarkson, M., Watson, M. C., Mulvaney, C. A., ... & Kendrick, D. (2016). School-based education programmes for the prevention of unintentional injuries in children and young people. *Cochrane Database of Systematic Reviews*, 12(12), CD010246.
Özdemir, S., Akça, H. Ş., Algın, A., Kokulu, K., & Özkan, A. (2022). Characteristics of school injuries presenting to the emergency department. *Avicenna Journal of Medicine*, 12(2), 61-66.
Pennington, N., & Delaney, E. (2008). The number of students sent home by school nurses compared to unlicensed personnel. *Journal of School Nursing*, 24(5), 290-297.
Peyton, R. P., Ranasinghe, S., & Jacobsen, K. H. (2017). Injuries, violence, and bullying among middle school students in Oman. *Oman Medical Journal*, 32(2), 98-104.
Pierpoint, L. A., Williams, C. M., Fields, S. K., & Comstock, R. D. (2016). Epidemiology of injuries in United States high school track and field: 2008-2009 through 2013-2014. *American Journal of Sports Medicine*, 44(6), 1463-1468.
Reis, T. D. S., Oliveira, I. D. S., Santos, J. M. D. J., Farre, A. G. M. D. C., Rodrigues, I. D. C. V., Leite, A. M., & Freitas, C. K. A. C. (2021). Knowledge and attitudes of schoolchildren about the prevention of accidents. *Ciência & Saúde Coletiva*, 26, 1077-1084.
Reveruzzi, B., Buckley, L., & Sheehan, M. (2016). School-based first aid training programs: A systematic review. *Journal of School Health*, 86(4), 266-272.
Salam, R. A., Arshad, A., Das, J. K., Khan, M. N., Mahmood, W., Freedman, S. B., & Bhutta, Z. A. (2016). Interventions to prevent unintentional injuries among adolescents: A systematic review and meta-analysis. *Journal of Adolescent Health*, 59(4), S76-S87.
Salminen, S., Kurenniemi, M., Råback, M., Markkula, J., & Lounamaa, A. (2014). School environment and school injuries. *Frontiers in Public Health*, 1, 76.
Senterre, C., Dramaix, M., & Levêque, A. (2014). Epidemiology of school-related injuries in Belgium. A better knowledge for a better prevention. *Open Journal of Preventive Medicine*, 4(06), 408-420.
Sleet, D. A. (2018). The global challenge of child injury prevention. *International Journal of Environmental Research and Public Health*, 15(9), 1921.
Sosnowska, S., & Kostka, T. (2003). Epidemiology of school accidents during a six school-year period in one region in Poland. *European Journal of Epidemiology*, 18, 977-982.
Şahinöz, T., Şahinöz, S., & Kıvanç, A. (2017). The easiest way to promote health: School health. *Gümüşhane University Journal of Health Sciences*, 6(4), 303-312.
Şengel, A., Gür, K., & Kılınç, E. (2020). The epidemiology of students' injuries in a private primary school in Turkey from 2012 to 2018. *Clinical and Experimental Health Sciences*, 10(4), 362-368.
Sprague, J. R., & Walker, H. M. (2021). *Safe and healthy schools: Practical prevention strategies*. Guilford Publications.
Wang, M. T., & Degol, J. L. (2016). School climate: A review of the construct, measurement, and impact on student outcomes. *Educational Psychology Review*, 28(2), 315-352.
Watson, M. C., & Errington, G. (2016). Preventing unintentional injuries in children: Successful approaches. *Paediatrics and Child Health*, 26(5), 194-199.
World Health Organization. (2008). *World report on child injury prevention*. Geneva, Switzerland.

Chapter 12

Sun Protection in School-Age Children

Özüm Erkin[1,*], PhD
and Ebru Konal Korkmaz[2], PhD
[1]İzmir Demokrasi University, Faculty of Health Sciences, Department of Public Health Nursing, Izmir, Türkiye
[2]Ege University, Faculty of Nursing, Department of Public Health Nursing, Izmir, Türkiye

Abstract

Skin cancers are becoming more prevalent worldwide, including in our country. Sun protection behaviors learned during childhood and adolescence can help reduce the harmful effects of the sun and risk factors for skin cancer. Efforts are being made globally to protect school-age children from the sun and raise awareness of sun protection from an early age. The growth of the young population in sunny countries as healthy individuals depends on acquiring the correct knowledge and habits at an early age. Developing positive sun protection behaviors is crucial in reducing the burden of skin cancers on public health. Research shows that acquiring knowledge of sun protection and behaviors during childhood and adolescence provides significant benefits in protecting against skin cancer. School nurses play a crucial role in raising awareness of sun protection. This section summarizes the literature on sun protection methods for school-age children.

Keywords: sun protection, school-age children, school health

Introduction

Skin cancer is a preventable disease, yet its incidence has been increasing globally (Brunssen et al., 2017). Among Caucasian populations, the most common types of skin cancer are non-melanoma skin cancers (NMSC) and malignant melanoma (MM) (American Cancer Society, 2024). Individuals with fair skin, many moles or skin spots, a history of prolonged sun exposure, and especially sunburn in childhood are at higher risk (Thoonen et al., 2020). The primary cause of skin cancer is exposure to ultraviolet (UV) radiation, which directly damages

* Corresponding Author's Email: ozum.erkin@idu.edu.tr

In: Health Promotion and Prevention
Editor: Eda Kılınç İşleyen
ISBN: 979-8-89530-758-8

Deoxyribonuclear Acid (DNA) (Lucas et al., 2018). In recent years, the depletion of the ozone layer has contributed to increased UV radiation reaching the Earth's surface, thereby heightening the risk of skin cancer development (NASA, 2021; WHO, 2021).

Risk factors for skin cancer include excessive exposure to sunlight, gender, phenotypic characteristics, family history, Fitzpatrick I-II skin type, childhood sunburn and sun exposure, environmental carcinogens, artificial light sources, nevi, and genetic syndromes (Gül, 2015; Hoel et al., 2016; Watson, 2016). The risk of malignant melanoma is twice as high in individuals with the Fitzpatrick skin type I-II phenotype. These individuals typically have light-colored eyes (blue or green), light-colored hair (blonde or red), and skin that burns easily, freckles readily, and does not tan (Gül, 2015; Watson, 2016). It is well-established that exposure to sunlight during childhood plays a significant role in the development of skin cancer. Therefore, protecting school-age children from the sun is a major concern for families, friends, and school staff (Tokur Kesgin and Çağlar, 2019). Schools have a crucial role in fostering and promoting positive health behaviors in school-age children (Mert and Aksayan, 2016). Programs designed to shield school-age children from the harmful effects of the sun play a critical role in fostering lifelong sun protection behaviors (Starfelt Sutton and White, 2016).

Sun Protection Strategies for School-Age Children

The aim of skin protection is to reduce UV exposure and prevent undesirable effects. Human skin has a natural defense mechanism against UV radiation. UV radiation exposure during childhood is one of the main significant risk factors for the development of skin cancer later in life. Correct sun protection behaviors should be made a habit starting from childhood (Walls and Weinstock, 2018). There are five sun protection methods recommended and accepted by the World Health Organization (World Health Organization, 2022).

- Protection with clothing
- Protection with sunscreen products
- Protection with a wide-brimmed hat
- Protection with sunglasses
- Protection by staying in the shade

Protection with Clothing

The most effective and simple way to protect oneself from the sun is to wear sun-protective clothing. Sun-protective clothing is defined as thick, tightly woven, double-layered clothing with long sleeves and legs that cover the body. It is worth noting that dark-colored clothing provides higher UV protection than light-colored clothing. However, it is important to keep in mind that dark-colored clothes absorb more UV rays, which can cause discomfort and warmth in the individual. For this reason, it is recommended to wear light-colored clothing. During the summer, it is advisable to wear non-synthetic, lightweight fabrics such as cotton, viscose, and linen. Clothes with a high collar that do not hug the body are preferable. Families should be advised to dress their children in long-sleeved clothes during summer (Downs and Harrison, 2018; Tripp et al., 2016; Skin Cancer Foundation, 2021a).

Table 1. Evaluation and classification of sun-protective clothing

UPF Rating	UV Blocking (%)	UPF Classification
UPF 15	93.3	Minimum Protection
UPF 30	96.7	Good Protection
UPF 50, 50+	98	Perfect Protection

Reference: SunSmart. (2022a). Sun-protective clothing. http://www.sunsmart.com.au/downloads/resources/info-sheets/sun-protective-clothing-info-sheet.pdf.

Ultraviolet Protection Factor (UPF) is used in UV protection of clothing. UFP is defined as the measure of how effectively a fabric blocks UV radiation from reaching the skin. While Sun Protection Factor (SPF) is used for sunscreens, UPF is specifically used for textile and clothing products, highlighting their protective capacity against the sun's harmful rays. The UPF is classified into three categories (Sunsmart, 2022a) (Table 1).

The protection of clothes from UV radiation depends on various factors, including the fibers and additives used in the fabrics, their structural properties, color, the use of optical bleaching agents, tension, and moisture content. Wool, silk, linen, and cotton are the fibers that offer the highest protection against UVR. However, linen and cotton fabrics provide lower protection compared to others. Among synthetic fibers, polyester offers the best protection against UVR (Gambichler et al., 2016; Gies et al., 2007). When selecting clothing, it is important to consider UV protection features. This is especially true when choosing holiday clothing, such as UV-protected clothing with a UPF rating of at least 40, beachwear, and surf vests for children (Sunsmart, 2022a).

Protection with Sunscreen Products

Sunscreen products can be classified as organic or inorganic depending on their form, such as cream, lotion, gel, or spray. It is important to use sunscreen products with a high sun protection factor before going out in the sun to ensure the absorption and reflection of UV rays, which can have negative effects on the skin (Sambandan and Ratner, 2011; Saray and Duman, 2015).

While sunscreen products containing UV filters are considered medicines in countries such as the United States (USA), they are considered cosmetic products in European Union countries. UV filters are divided into two groups: organic (chemical) and inorganic (physical). Sunscreen products should protect against ultraviolet A (UVA) and ultraviolet B (UVB) rays, but a single filter cannot provide sufficient protection. UV filters are used in combination to provide complete protection against UV rays. Inorganic UV filters Titanium dioxide and zinc oxide, which have large particles, are considered more reliable than chemical UV filters because they are not absorbed through the skin (AAD, 2022; AAD, 2023).

SPF is an index that indicates the ability of a sunscreen product to filter UV rays (Gül, 2015). The higher the SPF, the more effective the product is. It is recommended to use sunscreen products with an SPF of 30 or higher. It is advisable to choose sunscreen products that protect against both UVA and UVB rays, are odorless and colorless, have a high SPF, and are effective against water, sweat, evaporation, and friction (AAD, 2022; AAD, 2023; Linden, 2018).

When applying the sunscreen product,

- It should be applied to every part of the body at a rate of 2 mg/2 cm^2.
- It should be applied 15-30 minutes before going out and repeated every 2 hours.
- Most sunscreen products may not have water resistance features and may not provide water resistance. Therefore, it should be reapplied immediately after swimming and sweating.
- A lip balm with at least 15 SPF can be used to protect the lips.
- The skin is exposed to the sun's harmful UV rays, even in winter or on cloudy days. Sunscreen products should be used in all seasons but should be used more frequently and intensively in the summer.
- It is more beneficial to keep babies away from the sun and use protective clothing, hats, and sunshades instead of using sunscreen for the first six months. Babies under six months should not be exposed to direct sunlight due to their sensitive skin structure. The use of sunscreen products is not recommended for babies under six months of age (AAD, 2022; AAD, 2023; Linden, 2018; Skin Cancer Foundation, 2021b).

Protection with a Wide-Brimmed Hat

Hats offer effective protection by shading the face, neck, and nape of the neck. It is recommended to wear a wide-brimmed hat that covers the face, neck, ears, forehead, and eyes, with a circumference of at least 10 cm (Backes et al., 2018a). Wearing a wide-brimmed hat can reduce ultraviolet radiation by 50%, providing a protection level of around 3-5 GPF. When selecting a hat, it is advisable to consider the UPF of the fabric, whether it is made of cotton or a tightly woven material, its design (such as surfer style), and its effectiveness, affordability, and safety. When choosing a hat for children, it is important to consider factors such as age, head circumference, size, hat type, and brim length (SunSmart, 2022b) (Table 2).

Table 2. Brim lengths specific to hat style

Age group	Head circumference measurement	Minimum edge length with wide brim	Surfer style minimum side length
Newborn-12 months	41-43 cm	5 cm	5 cm
1-2 years old	49-52 cm	5 cm	5 cm
3-8 years old	50-54 cm	5 cm	5 cm
9-12 years old	55-57 cm	6 cm	6 cm

*Reference: SunSmart (2022b). Sun protective hats. http://www.sunsmart.com.au/downloads/resources/info-sheets/sun-protective-hats-info-sheet.pdf.

Protection with Sunglasses

UV radiation causes serious damage to the eyes and the eye area. Harmful UV rays and invisible wavelengths from the sun cause skin cancers on the eyelids. The use of glasses or contact lenses that block UV radiation is an effective method to protect the eyes (Backes et al., 2018b). Sunglasses that filter UVA and UVB radiation and completely cover the edges of the eyes should be used. When choosing sunglasses, care should be taken to choose glasses with 99-100% UV protection (Backes et al., 2018b; Chen et al., 2021).

Protection by Staying in the Shade

The level of UV radiation fluctuates depending on factors such as the season, ozone layer density, latitude, angle of incidence, and environmental pollution (Opene et al., 2017). The most intense UV radiation occurs between 10:00 and 16:00 when the sun is directly overhead. The most effective and economical way to protect oneself from UV radiation is to avoid outdoor activities during peak hours or to minimize exposure. Staying in the shade can reduce ultraviolet exposure by approximately 75% (Cancer Institute NSW, 2023). To understand safe hours in terms of UV exposure, a simple method is to observe that a person's shadow is longer than their own height (SunSmart, 2024; United States Environmental Protection Agency, 2024). It is recommended that they seek shade, such as under trees, throughout the year and carry an umbrella with them (Cancer Institute NSW, 2023; SunSmart, 2024).

Research

School-age children and adolescents spend the majority of their time outdoors; therefore, they are more exposed to the sun than adults. It is known that an individual who reaches the age of nineteen has received more than 50% of the UV radiation they will be exposed to throughout their lifetime (Şendur, 2010). Studies in the literature indicate that children are exposed to three times more UV radiation than adults and receive most of their UV exposure during childhood (Raymond-Lezman et al., 2023; Reyes et al., 2021). The relationship between childhood sun exposure and skin cancer can be reduced with appropriate protective measures taken from an early age (Walker, 2012). Therefore, students constitute an important target group for skin cancer prevention programs and have frequently been the sample group for descriptive and experimental studies (Walker, 2012; Thoonen et al., 2020).

Descriptive studies examining the knowledge, attitudes, and behaviors of students and families regarding sun protection in Turkey have shown that children exhibit low levels of sun protection behavior, such as staying in the shade during peak sun hours and wearing light-colored clothing, while families have low levels of knowledge about the harmful effects of the sun and exhibit low rates of appropriate sun protection behavior. It has been determined that parents prefer light-colored clothing for their children and that the use of sunscreen is low. They only place importance on sun protection during infancy (Altınkürek and Kaya, 2020; Ergin et al., 2011; Ergül and Özeren, 2011; Kaptanoğlu et al., 2012). International studies have shown that children have a low rate of sun protection use. It has been observed that staying in the shade and choosing appropriate clothing are less frequently practiced (Glenn et al., 2015; Kruzel et al., 2022; Mortier et al., 2015; Wan et al., 2016). It has been found that girls use sunscreen more than boys and that parental influence is crucial in sun protection behavior (Patel et al., 2019; Stockfleth and Revol, 2022).

In semi-experimental and experimental studies, it has been found that awareness of skin cancer risk factors and sun protection behaviors increases among students and families after education and initiatives, parents acquire sun protection behaviors for themselves and their children, and the frequency of using sun protective products increases (Aygün and Ergün, 2014; Balyacı et al., 2012; Erkin and Temel, 2017; Horvath et al., 2021; Reynolds et al., 2020).

Conclusion

School-based programs can help children learn healthy sun protection practices, reducing their risk of skin cancer. School nurses play a crucial role in this effort. Nurses should offer consultation regarding the early diagnosis and risk factors of skin cancer. They should also strive to maintain the highest level of function for diagnosed patients throughout the disease process. It is important for nurses to take advantage of training opportunities for early diagnosis and prevention measures, particularly when dealing with at-risk groups. The aim is to improve sun protection behaviors among students and families through public awareness campaigns and intervention-based follow-up studies with children, families, and teachers.

Disclaimer

None.

References

Altunkürek, Ş. Z., & Kaya, E. (2020). The effect of sun protection self-efficacy on the sun protection behavior of 8th grade students in a secondary school in Ankara. *Health Sciences University Nursing Journal*, 2(3), 137-144.

American Academy of Dermatology Association (AAD). (2022). Is sunscreen safe? https://www.aad.org/public/everyday-care/sun-protection/shade-clothing-sunscreen/is-sunscreen-safe.

American Academy of Dermatology Association (AAD). (2023). SUNSCREEN FAQS. https://www.aad.org/media/stats-sunscreen.

American Cancer Society. (2024). *Cancer Facts & Figures 2024*. Atlanta: American Cancer Society. https://www.cancer.org/research/acs-research-news/facts-and-figures-2024.html.

Aygün, O., & Ergün, A. (2014). Decisional balance and self-efficacy for sun protection: Measurement among Turkish adolescents. *Nursing Research*, 63(5), 309-319.

Backes, C., Religi, A., Moccozet, L., Vuilleumier, L., Vernez, D., & Bulliard, J. L. (2018a). Facial exposure to ultraviolet radiation: Predicted sun protection effectiveness of various hat styles. *Photodermatology, Photoimmunology & Photomedicine*, 34(5), 330-337.

Backes, C., Religi, A., Moccozet, L., Behar-Cohen, F., Vuilleumier, L., Bulliard, J. L., & Vernez, D. (2018b). Sun exposure to the eyes: Predicted UV protection effectiveness of various sunglasses. *Journal of Exposure Science and Environmental Epidemiology*, 29, 753-764. https://doi.org/10.1038/s41370-018-0087-0.

Balyacı, Ö. E., Koştu, N., & Bayık Temel, A. (2012). Training program to raise consciousness among adolescents for protection against skin cancer through performance of skin self-examination. *Asian Pacific Journal of Cancer Prevention*, 13(10), 5011-5017. https://doi.org/10.7314/APJCP.2012.13.10.5011.

Brunssen, A., Waldmann, A., Eisemann, N., & Katalinic, A. (2017). Impact of skin cancer screening and secondary prevention campaigns on skin cancer incidence and mortality: A systematic review. *Journal of the American Academy of Dermatology*, 76(1), 129-139.e10.

Cancer Institute NSW. (2023). Why is shade important for UV protection? *Cancer Institute NSW*. https://www.cancer.nsw.gov.au/prevention-and-screening/preventing-cancer/preventing-skin-cancer/shade-and-uv-protection/why-is-shade-important-for-uv-protection.

Chen, L. J., Chang, Y. J., Shieh, C. F., Yu, J. H., & Yang, M. C. (2021). Relationship between practices of eye protection against solar ultraviolet radiation and cataract in a rural area. *PLOS ONE*, 16(7), e0255136.

Downs, N. J., & Harrison, S. L. (2018). A comprehensive approach to evaluating and classifying sun-protective clothing. *British Journal of Dermatology*, 178(4), 958-964.

Ergin, A., Bozkurt, A. İ., Bostancı, M., & Önal, Ö. (2011). Assessment of knowledge and behaviors of mothers with small children on the effects of the sun on health. *Pamukkale Medical Journal*, 4(2), 72-78.

Ergül, S., & Özeren, E. (2011). Sun protection behavior and individual risk factors of Turkish primary school students associated with skin cancer: A questionnaire-based study. *Asian Pacific Journal of Cancer Prevention*, 12(3), 765-770.

Erkin, Ö., & Temel, A. B. (2017). A nurse-led school-based sun protection programme in Turkey. *Central European Journal of Public Health*, 25(4), 287-292.

Gambichler, T., Rooms, I., & Scholl, L. (2016). Photoprotection by clothing and fabric. In *Principles and Practice of Photoprotection* (pp. 417-428). Adis, Cham.

Gies, P. (2007). Photoprotection by clothing. *Photodermatology, Photoimmunology & Photomedicine*, 23, 264-274.

Glenn, B. A., Lin, T., Chang, L. C., Okada, A., Wong, W. K., Glanz, K., & Bastani, R. (2015). Sun protection practices and sun exposure among children with a parental history of melanoma. *Cancer Epidemiology, Biomarkers & Prevention*, 24, 169-177. https://doi.org/10.1158/1055-9965.EPI-14-0650.

Gül, Ü. (2015). Sun, heat and our skin. *Ankara Medical Journal*, 15(3), 145-152.

Hoel, D. G., Berwick, M., de Gruijl, F. R., & Holick, M. F. (2016). The risks and benefits of sun exposure 2016. *Dermato-Endocrinology*, 8(1), e1248325.

Horváth, Z., Evelin, C. A., Oláh, P., Gyulai, R., & Lengyel, Z. (2021). Results of a primary skin-cancer-prevention campaign in early childhood on sun-related knowledge and attitudes in Southern Hungary. *Cancers*, 13(15), 3873.

International Commission on Illumination-CIE. (2006). *Technical report. UV protection and clothing*. CIE Central Bureau, Vienna, Austria.

Kaptanoğlu, A. F., Dalkan, C., & Hıncal, E. (2012). [Sun protection in the North Cyprus Turkish population: Knowledge, attitude and behaviors of elementary school children and their families]. *Türkderm*, 46(3), 121-129.

Kruzel, M., Tobiasz, A., Łyko, M., Szepietowski, J., & Jankowska-Konsur, A. (2022). Photoprotection among young children: Assessment of mothers' awareness and health behaviors. *Advances in Dermatology and Allergology/Postępy Dermatologii i Alergologii*, 39(2), 392-396.

Linden, K. G. (2018). Sunscreen sun protection factor (SPF): Is higher better? *Journal of the American Academy of Dermatology*, 78(5), 911-912.

Lucas, R. M., Neale, R. E., Madronich, S., & McKenzie, R. L. (2018). Are current guidelines for sun protection optimal for health? Exploring the evidence. *Photochemical & Photobiological Sciences*, 17, 1956-1963. https://doi.org/10.1039/c7pp00374a.

Mert, K., & Aksayan, S. (2016). [School nursing interventions that promote positive health behavior]. *Turkiye Klinikleri Journal of Public Health Nursing-Special Topics*, 2(1), 1-6.

Mortier, L., Lepesant, P., Saiag, P., Robert, C., Sassolas, B., Grange, F., & Lebbe, C. (2015). Comparison of sun protection modalities in parents and children. *Journal of the European Academy of Dermatology and Venereology*, 29(2), 16-19. https://doi.org/10.1111/JDV.12897.

NASA. (2021). Ozone hole watch. https://ozonewatch.gsfc.nasa.gov.

Opene, C., Chren, M. M., & Linos, E. (2017). Types of shade vary in protection just like sunscreens. *JAMA Dermatology*, 153(10), 1070-1071.

Patel, A. R., Zaslow, T. L., Wren, T. A. L., Daoud, A. K., Campbell, K., Nagle, K., & Coel, R. A. (2019). A characterization of sun protection attitudes and behaviors among children and adolescents in the United States. *Preventive Medicine Reports*, 16, 100988.

Raymond-Lezman, J. R., Riskin, S., & Riskin, S. I. (2023). Attitudes, behaviors, and risks of sun protection to prevent skin cancer amongst children, adolescents, and adults. *Cureus*, 15(2).

Reyes-Marcelino, G., Wang, R., Gultekin, S., Humphreys, L., Smit, A. K., Sharman, A. R., Laurent, A. G., Evaquarta, R., & Dobbinson, S. J. (2021). School-based interventions to improve sun-safe knowledge, attitudes and behaviors in childhood and adolescence: A systematic review. *Preventive Medicine*, 146, 106459. https://doi.org/10.1016/j.ypmed.2021.106459.

Reynolds, K. D., Buller, D. B., Buller, M. K., Massie, K., Berteletti, J., Ashley, J., & Meenan, R. (2020). Randomized controlled trial evaluating an intervention supporting implementation of sun safety policies in California public elementary schools. *Preventive Medicine*, 137, 106125.

Sambandan, D. R., & Ratner, D. (2011). Sunscreens: An overview and update. *Journal of the American Academy of Dermatology*, 64(4), 748-758.

Saray, Y., & Duman, D. (2015). [Current information and developments about sunscreens]. *Turkiye Klinikleri Journal of Dermatology-Special Topics*, 8(4), 21-27.

Skin Cancer Foundation. (2021a). What is safe clothing? https://www.skincancer.org/skin-cancer-prevention/sun-protection/sun-protective-clothing/.

Skin Cancer Foundation. (2021b). Sun protection. https://www.skincancer.org/skin-cancer-prevention/sun-protection/#:~:text=The%20Skin%20Cancer%20Foundation%20advises,or%20after%20swimming%20or%20sweating.

Starfelt Sutton, L. C., & White, K. M. (2016). Predicting sun-protective intentions and behaviours using the theory of planned behaviour: A systematic review and meta-analysis. *Psychology & Health*, 31(11), 1272-1292.

Stockfleth, E., & Revol, O. (2022). Encouraging sun protection early in life: From a successful prevention programme in children to the identification of psychological barriers in adolescents. *Journal of the European Academy of Dermatology and Venereology*, 36, 12-21.

SunSmart. (2022a). Sun-protective clothing. http://www.sunsmart.com.au/downloads/resources/info-sheets/sun-protective-clothing-info-sheet.pdf.

SunSmart. (2022b). Sun protective hats. http://www.sunsmart.com.au/downloads/resources/info-sheets/sun-protective-hats-info-sheet.pdf.

SunSmart. (2024). SunSmart shade assessment. https://www.sunsmart.com.au/downloads/schools-early-childhood/vels/shade-audit.pdf.

Şendur, N. (2010). Sun protection in childhood. *Turkiye Klinikleri Journal of Cosm Dermatology-Special Topics*, 3(2), 76-80.

Thoonen, K., van Osch, L., Crutzen, R., de Vries, H., & Schneider, F. (2022). Identification of relevant sociocognitive determinants explaining multiple parental sun protection behaviors. *Health Education & Behavior*, 49, 392-404. https://doi.org/10.1177/10901981211010434.

Tokur Kesgin, M., & Çağlar, S. (2019). [Development of school nursing in the World and Turkey]. *HEAD*, 16(4), 343-352.

Tripp, M. K., Watson, M., Balk, S. J., Swetter, S. M., & Gershenwald, J. E. (2016). State of the science on prevention and screening to reduce melanoma incidence and mortality: The time is now. *CA: A Cancer Journal for Clinicians*, 66(6), 460-480.

United States Environmental Protection Agency. (2024). UV index. https://www.epa.gov/sunsafety/learn-about-uv-index.

Walker, D. K. (2012). Skin protection for (SPF) kids program. *Journal of Pediatric Nursing*, 27(3), 233-242.

Walls, A. C., & Weinstock, M. A. (2018). Sun protection. In *The American Cancer Society's Principles of Oncology: Prevention to Survivorship* (pp. 99-109). Wiley-Blackwell.

Wan, M., Hu, R., Li, Y., Wang, Y., Xie, X., Yue, P., & Lai, W. (2016). Attitudes, beliefs, and measures taken by parents to protect their children from the sun in Guangzhou City, China. *Photochemistry and Photobiology*, 92(5), 753-759.

Watson, M., Holman, D. M., & Maguire-Eisen, M. (2016). Ultraviolet radiation exposure and its impact on skin cancer risk. *Seminars in Oncology Nursing*, 32(3), 241-254.

World Health Organization (WHO). (2021). Ultraviolet (UV) radiation and skin cancer. https://www.who.int/news-room/q-a-detail/ultraviolet-(uv)-radiation-and-skin-cancer.

World Health Organization (WHO). (2022). Ultraviolet radiation. https://www.who.int/news-room/fact-sheets/detail/ultraviolet-radiation.

Chapter 13

The Fundamentals and Features of Health Education in Schools

Ayla Tuzcu İnce, PhD
and Habibe Ozcelik*, PhD
Department of Public Health Nursing, Akdeniz University, Faculty of Nursing, Antalya, Turkiye

Abstract

Health education is the organization of all activities and actions used for the health of individuals and society for learning purposes. As a tool for health promotion, this education is critical to improving the health of populations and supporting health capital. Health education in schools is carried out to support positive health knowledge, attitudes, and behaviors acquired by the child in the pre-school period or to change the inadequate ones. The most frequently taught health-related topics in schools are healthy nutrition, physical activity, tobacco and substance use prevention, mental health, sexually transmitted diseases prevention, and safety. School nurses must demonstrate their professional performance in the field of health education, and they must take their initiatives by considering the general characteristics of children's developmental period and teaching strategies when planning health education for school-age children. Ensuring the continuity of health education will increase behavior change and help improve public health.

Keywords: health education, school health, school nursing

Introduction

Health education can be thought of as a set of experiences that affect health knowledge and attitudes toward health (Gözüm, 2016). Another definition is the organization of all activities and actions used for the health of the individual and society for learning purposes. In a more comprehensive definition, health education is defined as any learning experience aimed at creating health-related thoughts, concepts, beliefs, attitudes, behaviors, and lifestyle changes in people through their own experiences (Köksal and Attila, 2015).

---

* Corresponding Author's Email: hozcelik@akdeniz.edu.tr

In: Health Promotion and Prevention
Editor: Eda Kılınç İşleyen
ISBN: 979-8-89530-758-8

Health education, as a tool for health promotion, is critical to improving the health of populations. Health education that protects against ill health includes educational efforts to influence lifestyles, as well as increasing participation in disease prevention services. Effective health education focuses on improving individuals' capacity through educational, motivational, skill development, and awareness-raising techniques (World Health Organization [WHO], 2012). The WHO evaluates health education as a tool that enables individuals to take responsibility for their own and then each other's health (WHO, 2012). In this way, health education becomes an intervention that will enable the public to participate directly in health services and is one of the significant practices in health promotion (Tulchinsky and Varavikova, 2018). Health education is important for school-age children because it helps them develop lifelong healthy habits and make informed decisions about their well-being (Pelen and Günay, 2013).

Objectives of Health Education

The main goal of health education is to make health a social value, equip society and individuals with the knowledge and skills they can use to overcome their own health problems, and ensure the development of health services. These purposes vary by national and social needs. Since health is determined by behavioral patterns and the individual's environment, it will not be right to limit health education to solely "provision of information" about health. Today, different models and theories are emphasized regarding health education and communication. These are approaches used alone and sometimes in combination to create behavioral change (Köksal and Attila, 2015).

The objective of health education in schools is to support the beneficial health knowledge, attitudes, and behaviors that the child acquired in the pre-school period or to improve the inadequate ones (Gözüm, 2016). Health education should aim to create a healthy society by providing students with "behavior change for a lifelong healthy life" (Özcebe et al., 2008). Since health-related behavioral patterns are established during childhood and adolescence, acquiring healthy habits early in life plays a crucial role in protecting individual health and reducing future health risks (Gözüm, 2016). In health education, students should first be taught to acquire responsibility for improving and maintaining their own health and also to share responsibility for protecting other people's health (Özcebe et al., 2008). It has been stated that healthy behaviors gained through health education given in schools in childhood continue into adulthood. It is important to address the physical, mental, and social health needs of school-age children at an early age, as they spend most of their developmentally critical years in school. Promoting healthy behaviors during this period lays the foundation for healthier individuals and societies in the future (Akgül and Ergün, 2021; Yurttutan and Altay, 2018).

The WHO carries out many health education activities in schools throughout the Eastern Mediterranean Region. They cover a wide range of topics, such as healthy nutrition, physical activity, tobacco use prevention, mental health, sexually transmitted diseases prevention, and safety. Although "health educators" often work with limited budgets and receive less appreciation than those in other areas of the health care system, they perform their duties in a hard-working, enthusiastic, and dedicated manner. There are many success stories with health education, particularly with the setting approach, including health-promoting schools, workplaces, clinics, and communities (WHO, 2012).

Health Education Curriculum in Schools

It is more useful to implement continuous and comprehensive programs instead of intermittent health courses to teach healthy lifestyle behaviors. Therefore, it is recommended that comprehensive health education be implemented in schools. A school health education curriculum should be structured and continuous to develop students' life skills to improve health, prevent diseases, and reduce health-related risky behaviors.

- Ideally, a comprehensive health education curriculum should address the physical, mental, emotional, and social dimensions of health.
- It should improve health knowledge, attitudes, and skills,
- It should take into account all age levels.
- It should motivate and help students protect and improve health and prevent diseases (Gözüm, 2016).

The Role of the School Nurse in Health Education

According to the WHO, nurses constitute the highest number of occupational groups in the health sector in the world (WHO, 2020). The International Council of Nurses (ICN) has stated that nurses should take an active role in improving health, preventing diseases, providing holistic care during the disease process, and healthcare training, as well as research (ICN, 2022). The American Nurses Association (ANA) has mentioned the role of the nurse as an educator in Standards 5 and 5B, which are among the nursing practice standards, and has stated that all nurses should use health education to support health in their professional practices (ANA, 2015). The educator role of the nurse includes planned education practices aimed at protecting and improving individual, family, and community health, healing in case of illness, and promoting appropriate health behavior (Gedük, 2018). The American National Association of School Nurses (NASN) has defined the performance of school nurses in the field of health education within professional performance standards. According to these standards, the expectations of school nurses are the following:

- School nurses participate in the assessment of health education needs for students and the school community,
- Provide formal health education appropriate for the development of students by using the course curriculum based on reliable learning theory,
- Offer individual/group education and consultancy,
- Participate in the planning and development of the health curriculum,
- Contribute to the evaluation of health curricula, health education materials, and other health education activities,

- Act as a resource person for other school staff regarding health education and health education materials,
- Help implement health promotion principles in other areas of school life, such as nutrition and security services and
- Promote self-care and safety by educating school staff about their own and students' health (Selekman and Coates, 2012).

The ten areas of general health education identified by the American School Health Association (public health, consumer health, environmental health, personal health and wellness, family life education, healthy nutrition, disease prevention and control, safety and prevention of injury, prevention of substance use and abuse, and growth and development) may shed light on nurses (ANA, 2015). When planning health education for school-age children in schools, they must determine interventions that consider the general characteristics of school-age children's developmental periods and teaching strategies (Gözüm, 2016).

For nurses to effectively fulfill their role as educators, they must be experts in their field, have the ability to communicate effectively, empathize, cope with stress, and have knowledge, skills, and experience in the field of education. Undoubtedly, considering changes and developments and the abundance of resources to be used in acquiring and maintaining these characteristics, individual and professional continuous development and lifelong learning are important professional responsibilities (Bastable, 2023).

According to the nursing regulation published in Turkey, school nursing is a subfield of public health nursing. In the regulation, there are statements about the school nurse's role as an educator among their duties and responsibilities. In addition to the role of educator, their role as a consultant, advocate, and change agent has also been defined (Nursing Regulation in Turkey, 2010).

Examples of School Health Education

Health Workforce and Health Education in Schools

Although schools are important places to support health, shortcomings in the health workforce still prevail. According to the National School Nurse Workforce Study conducted in the United States, the rate of health education provided in schools ranged between 8% and 12%, depending on the license model of the school nurse. The demographic profile and activities of nurses working in schools were examined, and it was determined that the nurses mostly engaged in activities such as medication management, acute care, chronic conditions, health care plans, and direct care (Willgerodt et al., 2018). In another study conducted in the United States, the perspectives of experienced community health workers on how community health workers could be integrated and used in schools due to an inadequate number of school nurses were examined. One of the seven main themes created in this qualitative study was education. The participants recommended education about health and medical conditions. The topics recommended for schools were childhood development periods, chronic diseases, nutrition, mental health, cardiopulmonary resuscitation, and first aid (Yao et al., 2023). As seen from the studies, there is inadequate school nurse employment, and students have an unmet need for health education in a variety of subjects.

Models Created for School Nursing Practices

There are many methodological studies in the literature aimed at developing a model to create a standardized health promotion program or evidence-based guidelines for school nurses' practices. In a methodological study conducted in the USA, an evidence-based clinical practice guide model was created for school nurses to provide quality care to students with special health needs. The model was established to provide a professional structure, a standardized process, and a strong methodology by creating evidence-based guidelines. Professional school nurses develop individualized health care, emergency response, and individual education plans, as well as implement and evaluate educational plans (Shannon and Maughan, 2020). In a methodological study conducted to improve student health, a guide was created to develop school nursing practices. Focusing on health promotion, the guide was based on Pender's Health Promotion Model. In the guide, nurses' health promotion strategies included physical activity, healthy nutrition, mental health, stress management, and social support (Muniz et al., 2022). In a methodological study conducted in Colombia, a school nursing vocational practice model was created. Education and health were summarized as a bond of care, and experts were consulted on this subject. In the model, nurses act as educators and offer programs to promote health and prevent diseases. These programs include topics such as health education, vaccination, promotion of a healthy lifestyle, and information and communication about health services. Additionally, the school nurse takes care of not only students but also the teaching staff, principals, administrative staff, and those in the general services. Parents, and other family members are also within the scope of the duty of the school nurse (Ferro Carvajalino et al., 2020).

Different studies have been performed to standardize school nursing education in Türkiye, as in the world. The Delphi technique was used in a doctoral thesis study to develop a curriculum for the national school nursing certificate program. Academic nurses and school nurses were consulted about the topic. At the end of the study, consensus was reached on nine main headings, 255 sub-headings, and 167 learning outcomes. The main identified topics were school nursing, knowing the school community, assessment of health and making nursing diagnoses, the promotion of health and prevention of diseases, health problems and nursing management, school environment, and safety, disaster and emergency management, sensitive/vulnerable/disadvantaged groups, risk assessment, and nursing interventions, school health services management, and evidence-based practices. The content of the education program included subjects aimed at ensuring the competence of nurses to provide health education in schools and topics to improve health, such as sexual health, mental health, addiction and substance use, exercise, nutrition, hygiene, and sleep. Chronic diseases that are common in childhood, such as diabetes, obesity, cancer, epilepsy, chronic kidney disease, cystic fibrosis, and heart failure, and mental health problems, such as anxiety, depression, attention deficit, and hyperactivity, were also among other subjects of the education program (Özdemir and Kadıoğlu, 2022).

The Content of the Education Provided by School Nurses

Nurses provide health education on various subjects in schools. According to the literature, these subjects are mostly about health-promoting behaviors such as physical activity and nutrition. In a cross-sectional study conducted in Brazil, some health promotion activities were carried out by family health teams under the school health program. The most common educational topics given to students by school nurses were reproduction, sexual health, and sexually transmitted diseases prevention, as well as healthy nutrition, and prevention of the use of alcohol, tobacco, and other addictive substances. Additionally, an increase was detected in the education provided to teachers working in schools to promote health education and physical activity (Silva et al., 2021). In a qualitative study performed in England, the role of the school nurse in providing health education was examined. The function of the school nurse in health education was one of the main themes of the study. Hygiene, sexual health, tobacco use, obesity, healthy nutrition, oral health, alcohol and substance use, and mental health were the priority health education topics (Hoekstra et al., 2016). In a systematic review of school nurses and their experiences with the Human Papilloma Virus (HPV) vaccine, it was emphasized that school nurses provided education as HPV vaccine educators (McNally et al., 2024).

A randomized controlled study was performed in Turkey to detect the effect of health literacy education for school-age children with asthma and their parents on disease self-management. Following the planned education given to the intervention and control groups, it was observed that the health literacy of parents and children did not change, while the symptoms of asthma decreased. The number of school-age children experiencing attacks after physical activity, presenting to the emergency department, and complaining of cough, wheezing, phlegm, and shortness of breath decreased (Güney Kızıl, 2022). In an intervention study, the effect of health education given to primary school students on their health-related behaviors was evaluated. There was an increase in the rate of the following behaviors in the intervention group compared to the control group following education: washing hands when getting up in the morning, before and after meals, and in the toilet; having breakfast regularly; and having knowledge about various infectious diseases and harmful habits such as smoking and alcohol (Pelen and Günay, 2013). In another intervention study, secondary school students were given health education, and changes in their health-related knowledge and behaviors were determined. Following the intervention, there was an increase in the following areas compared to before taking a bath every three days: brushing teeth for 2-3 minutes; knowing who is authorized to give first aid, the factors that cause noise pollution, the importance of minerals for our body, and the awareness about consuming pulp and fibrous foods (Coşgun and Kara, 2015). In a review, it was emphasized that the school nurse was in a key position in preventing peer bullying. It was stated that the school nurse fulfilled the role of an educator by providing education to school staff and students about peer bullying (Avşar and Ayaz Alkaya, 2018). In another review, it was stated that adolescents needed education on sexual health, the education given within the scope of health courses in schools was inadequate, and that the school nurse could meet this need (Yücesan and Ayaz Alkaya, 2018).

The nursing regulation published in Turkey involves some statements about the health education to be provided by the school nurse. The health education areas in the regulation are as follows:

"g) The school nurse plans and carries out health education activities (importance of cleanliness, protection from accidents and diseases, first aid, harms of smoking and alcohol, and sexual education, etc.) to convey correct health information to students at school and to impart positive health behaviors.
h) The school nurse plans, carries out, and supervises the health education of the personnel working in the school canteen on issues such as personal hygiene, canteen hygiene, and food safety.
i) The school nurse provides health education for school cleaners on issues such as toilet hygiene and classroom hygiene and supervise them.
"i) The school nurse plans, carries out, and supervises health training for personnel working in the school kitchen on personal hygiene, kitchen hygiene, and purchasing, storing, processing, and storing food after processing" (Nursing Regulation in Turkey, 2010).

To Whom Does the School Nurse Provide Health Education?

It is already known that the school nurse should provide health education to students within the scope of their responsibilities. In addition to students, school nurses serve school staff and students' families and educate them on various health-related issues. A cross-sectional study was conducted to investigate school nurses' perceptions of the nurse-family relationship in the care of elementary school students with asthma and attention-deficit hyperactivity disorder in Minnesota. The results showed that school nurses performed positive evaluations of family nursing practices but that overall scores were lower in the context of attention deficit hyperactivity disorder compared to asthma. It was recommended in the study that nurses who provided care for students with chronic health problems needed to carry out interventions to increase their family nursing practices (Brown et al., 2019). In a study performed in Brazil, it was emphasized that health education needed to be given not only to students but also to teachers (Silva et al., 2021). In a study conducted in Colombia, students, parents, other family members, teachers, and administrative staff were within the scope of the school nurse's responsibilities as an educator (Ferro Carvajalino et al., 2020). In a qualitative study performed in the USA, it was stated that the roles and responsibilities of community health workers in schools included providing health education. It was explained that education needed to be provided not only for students but also for families and school staff (Yao et al., 2023). The nursing regulation published in Turkey lists the individuals for whom the school nurse provide health education. The list includes students, school canteen staff, school cleaners, and those working in the school kitchen (Nursing Regulation in Turkey, 2010).

Conclusion

Health education is a fundamental component in shaping individuals' knowledge, attitudes, and behaviors related to health from an early age. Schools, where children spend a significant portion of their developmental years, provide an optimal setting for implementing structured and continuous health education programs. These programs are essential in fostering lifelong healthy behaviors and supporting informed decision-making. Effective health education addresses physical, mental, emotional, and social dimensions of health, aiming to empower students to take responsibility for their own well-being and contribute to the health of others. In this context, school nurses play a critical role not only in delivering health education but also in acting as consultants, advocates, and role models. Their professional expertise, communication skills, and holistic approach enhance the quality and reach of health education efforts within the school environment. In conclusion, evidence-based and developmentally appropriate health education, supported by multidisciplinary collaboration and led by competent school health professionals, contributes significantly to the promotion of lifelong health. Initiating such efforts during childhood is essential for the development of healthier individuals and communities.

Disclaimer

None.

References

Akgül, E., & Ergün, A. (2021). School health nursing in promoting community health. Journal of Public Health Nursing, *3*(2), 141-153.

American Nurses Association (ANA). (2015). *Nursing: Scope and Standards of Practice, 3rd Ed.* American Nurses Association.

Avşar, F., & Ayaz Alkaya, S. (2018). The Role of School Health Nurses in the Prevention of Peer Bullying. *Journal of Hacettepe University Faculty of Nursing*, *5*(1), 78-84.

Bastable, S. (2023). The Nurse as an Educator. Nobel Medical Bookstores.

Brown, C., Looman, W. S., & Garwick, A. E. (2019). School Nurse Perceptions of Nurse-Family Relationships in the Care of Elementary Students with Chronic Conditions. *J Sch Nurs*, *35*(2), 96-106. https://doi.org/10.1177/1059840517741944.

Coşgun, M., & Kara, F. (2015). Evaluation of the Impact of Health Education Given to Students on Knowledge and Attitudes. *Journal of Continuing Medical Education*, *24*(2), 55-63.

Ferro Carvajalino, M. C., Fuentes Ramirez, A., Chinchilla Salcedo, T. C., & Sanchez Herrera, B. (2020). Education and Health: A Care Bond. School-Nursing Model for Colombia. *Invest Educ Enferm*, *38*(2). https://doi.org/10.17533/udea.iee.v38n2e05.

Gedük, A. (2018). Evolving Roles of the Nursing Profession. Journal of Health Sciences and Professions, *5*(2), 253-258. https://doi.org/https://doi.org/10.17681/hsp.358458.

Gözüm, S. (2016). Improving the health of school-age children. Vize Publishing.

Güney Kızıl, E. (2022). *The Effect of Education Given to Asthmatic School Children and Their Parents, Considering Health Literacy, on the Self-Management of Asthma* Ege University]. Izmir.

Hoekstra, B. A., Young, V. L., Eley, C. V., Hawking, M. K., & McNulty, C. A. (2016). School Nurses' perspectives on the role of the school nurse in health education and health promotion in England: a qualitative study. *BMC Nurs*, *15*, 73. https://doi.org/10.1186/s12912-016-0194-y.

ICN. (2022). *Nursing Definitions*. Retrieved 10 Ağustos 2022 from https://www.icn.ch/resources/nursing-definitions.

Köksal, O., & Attila, S. (2015). Community Nutrition. In Ç. Güler & L. Akın (Eds.), Basic Information on Public Health 3 (pp. 1210-1215). Hacettepe University Publications.

McNally, K., Roess, A., Weinstein, A., Lindley, L., & Wallin, R. (2024). School Nurses' Experiences and Roles in Promoting and Administering the HPV Vaccine: A Systematic Review Using the Socioecological Framework. *J Sch Nurs*, *40*(1), 43-57. https://doi.org/10.1177/10598405231206109.

Muniz, E. A., Queiroz, M. V. O., Pinheiro, P., Silva, M., Moreira, T. M. M., Oliveira, E. N., Almeida, I., & Barbosa Filho, V. C. (2022). School Nursing Guide for student health promotion: construction and validity. *Rev Bras Enferm*, *76*(1), e20220260. https://doi.org/10.1590/0034-7167-2022-0260.

Nursing Regulation in Turkey. (2010). https://www.mevzuat.gov.tr/mevzuat?MevzuatNo=13830&MevzuatTur=7&MevzuatTertip=5.

Özcebe, H., Ulukol, B., Mollahaliloğlu, S., Yardım, N., & Karaman, F. (2008). School Health Book in Health Services. Yücel Ofset Printing Tourism Industry Trade Ltd. Co.

Özdemir, İ., & Kadıoğlu, H. (2022). *A Curriculum Development Project for a National School Nursing Certification Program: A Delphi Study* Marmara University]. Istanbul.

Pelen, K., & Günay, O. (2013). The Impact of Health Education Given to Primary School Students on Their Knowledge, Attitude and Behaviours. *(Journal of Health Sciences*, *22*(1), 52-63.

Selekman, J., & Coates, J. (2012). Disease Prevention In J. Selekman (Ed.), *School nursing: A comprehensive text* (pp. 473-515). FA Davis Company.

Shannon, R. A., & Maughan, E. D. (2020). A Model for Developing Evidence-Based Clinical Practice Guidelines for School Nursing. *J Sch Nurs*, *36*(6), 415-422. https://doi.org/10.1177/1059840519880938.

Silva, A. A., Gubert, F. D. A., Barbosa Filho, V. C., Freitas, R., Vieira-Meyer, A., Pinheiro, M. T. M., & Reboucas, L. N. (2021). Health promotion actions in the School Health Program in Ceara: nursing contributions. *Rev Bras Enferm*, *74*(1), e20190769. https://doi.org/10.1590/0034-7167-2019-0769.

Tulchinsky, T., & Varavikova, E. (2018). The New Public Health. Palme Publishing.

WHO. (2012). *Health education: theoretical concepts, effective strategies and core competencies: a foundation document to guide capacity development of health educators*. WHO Regional Office for the Eastern Mediterranean, Cairo. Retrieved 25.12.2023 from.

WHO. (2020). *State of the world's nursing 2020: investing in education, jobs and leadership* Retrieved 01 Aralık 2023 from https://www.who.int/publications/i/item/9789240003279.

Willgerodt, M. A., Brock, D. M., & Maughan, E. D. (2018). Public School Nursing Practice in the United States. *J Sch Nurs*, *34*(3), 232-244. https://doi.org/10.1177/1059840517752456.

Yao, N., Kowalczyk, M., Gregory, L., Cheatham, J., DeClemente, T., Fox, K., Ignoffo, S., & Volerman, A. (2023). Community health workers' perspectives on integrating into school settings to support student health. *Front Public Health*, *11*, 1187855. https://doi.org/10.3389/fpubh.2023.1187855.

Yurttutan, S., & Altay, N. (2018). The Roles of School Health Nurses in Children Receiving Inclusive Education. *Contemporary Medical Journal, 8*(1), 78-84.

Yücesan, A., & Ayaz Alkaya, S. (2018). Ignored Issue at Schools: Sexual Health Education. *Med J SDU*, *25*(2), 200-209. https://doi.org/10.17343/sdutfd.342828

Chapter 14

Health Promotion Theories and Models in School Health

Aslı Kalkım*, PhD
and Zuhal Emlek Sert, PhD
Department of Public Health Nursing, Ege University Faculty of Nursing, İzmir, Türkiye

Abstract

The primary purpose of nursing theories is to ensure the development of nursing science and to demonstrate the autonomy of nursing through the use of theories and models specific to the nursing discipline. Practice guided by nursing theory helps improve the quality of nursing care as it allows nurses to articulate what they do for individuals/patients and why they do it. One of the work areas where nurses can use theories and models is the school. Considering that children are influenced by their environment and the people who care for them and that health promotion principles and health behaviors are shaped during childhood, schools can play a critical role in improving the health of children and young people. Understanding these effects around a theoretical model can help develop interventions that effectively promote healthy behaviors. In this section, models and theories frequently used in nursing research on improving school health are included.

Keywords: health promotion, school health, theories and models, school nurses

Introduction

The primary purpose of nursing theories is to ensure the development of nursing science and to demonstrate the autonomy of nursing through the use of theories and models specific to the nursing discipline (Şengün İnan et al., 2013; Göçmen Baykara et al., 2019). Nurse researchers use theories as a guide to conceptualize the research problem and investigate the accuracy of propositions. At the same time, the use of theory and models guides the development and testing of interventions and enables the findings and study results to be explained within a scientific framework (Şengün İnan et al., 2013). Moreover, theoretical frameworks enable nurses to

* Corresponding Author's Email: aslikalkim@gmail.com

In: Health Promotion and Prevention
Editor: Eda Kılınç İşleyen
ISBN: 979-8-89530-758-8

assess the health status of individuals receiving care and to systematically organize, interpret, and analyze data collected throughout the care process (Koç and Yumru, 2019).

The use of theory and models in nursing research guides the systematic implementation of research, testing theories, and presenting research results. In addition, the use of theories and models in nursing research and practice is necessary to increase the quality of nursing care, professionalize the nursing profession, and increase nursing scientific knowledge (Koç and Yumru, 2019).

It is vital for nurses to have a theoretical understanding of people's behavior so that they can improve the health of the individual, family, group, or community (Raingruber, 2015). When working with individuals, groups, or communities, models and theories can be used to guide this process (Simpson, 2015). When determining a theory or model to guide health promotion or disease prevention programs, it is important to consider several factors, such as the specific health problem being addressed, the population(s) served, and the contexts in which the program is engaged (Çetinkaya, 2021).

Given the complexity of health promotion practice, multilevel, comprehensive interventions are needed to develop effective programs (Raingruber, 2015). Researchers have predicted that multifactorial programs will have a greater impact than narrow approaches that focus on a single risk factor (Domitrovich et al., 2009). Interventions that target unhealthy lifestyles by focusing on multiple factors simultaneously are more likely to be effective (Simpson, 2015).

The use of models in nursing;

a. allows for the addressing and recognition of people in all their dimensions,
b. enables understanding and revealing problematic situations,
c. ensures that nursing services are provided with a certain logic and systematically,
d. enables the development of professional perspective and professional communication (Gigliotti, 2008; Dağhan et al., 2022).

Nursing theory-guided practice improves the quality of nursing care because it allows nurses to articulate what they do for patients and why they do it (Younas and Quennell, 2019). Theories and models help transform nursing practices from implicit knowledge into clear and structured information. This supports better decision-making, helps predict how environmental factors affect care, and makes it easier to organize nursing knowledge and practices (Göçmen Baykara et al., 2019; Koç and Yumru, 2019).

Definitions of Theory and Model Terms

Health Promotion Model

The Health Promotion Model (HPM) was created by Pender in 1982 and was revised in 1987, 1996, and 2002 (Aqtam and Darawwad, 2018). The model states that an individual's health behavior is affected by past experiences (Çalık and Kapucu, 2017). Pender's background in nursing, human development, experimental psychology, and education has led her to use a holistic nursing perspective, social psychology, and education. HPM provides a framework for explaining and predicting specific health behaviors. The HPM consists of three core domains that nurses can use to assess health promotion behaviors:

1. Personal characteristics and experiences
2. Behavior-specific cognition and affect
3. Behavioral outcome

Additionally, HPM includes elements of the change process, including commitment to a plan of action and acceptance of competing demands. The end result is participation in health promotion behaviors. Pender's model guides nurses who focus on health promotion strategies for patients and research aimed at predicting health-promoting behaviors (Aqtam and Darawwad, 2018). The model consists of components including individual characteristics and experiences, behavior-specific domains, and behavioral outcomes (Figure 1);

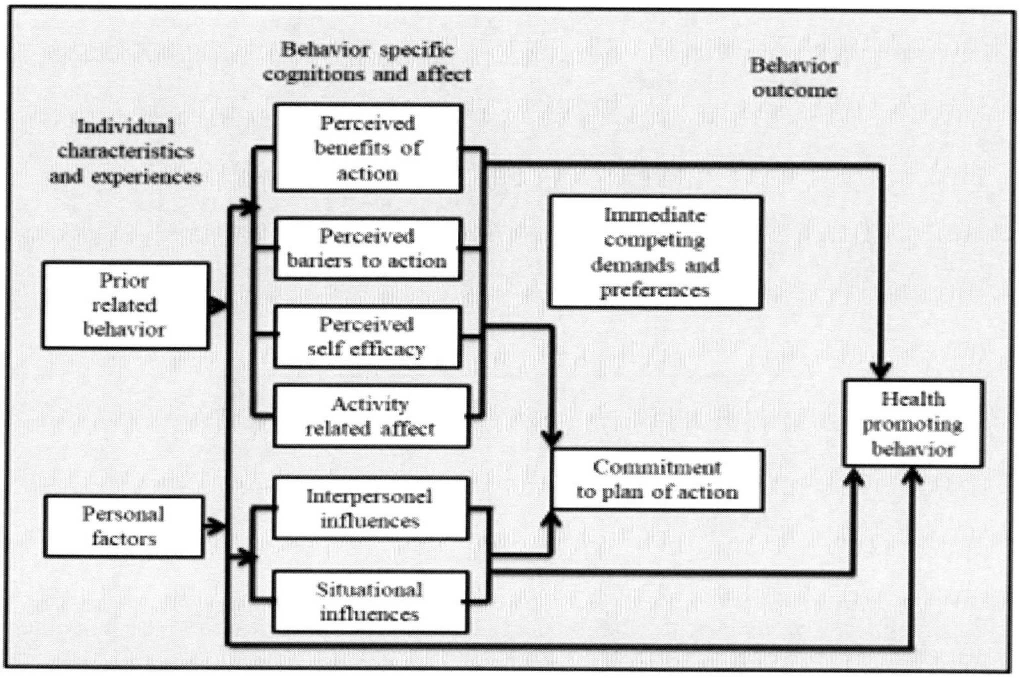

Figure 1. Diagram of Pender's health promotion model (Khoshnood et al., 2018).

Health Belief Model

In the 1950s in America, public health researchers noticed that demographic factors such as age, gender, socio-economic status, and ethnicity were effective in preventive health behaviors, and even if health services were provided free of charge, individuals with low socio-economic status used the service less. To explain the reason for this situation, Rosenstock developed the Health Belief Model in a usable form for the first time in 1966. The model was expanded in subsequent years through the work of Becker et al., The Health Belief Model (HBM) argues that individuals' health behaviors will be affected by their beliefs, values, and attitudes. If these beliefs and attitudes are detected, which are seen as problems, the health education to be given or the treatment methods to be applied can be determined to be more suitable for that person. If individuals are sensitive that a health problem will seriously harm them, they think that the harm to them will decrease if they take action. Eight components have been reported for HBM. These are perceived sensitivity/sensitivity, seriousness, benefit, motivation, obstacle, threat, effectiveness of behavior, and likelihood of taking action. Self-efficacy/sufficiency was added to the model later (Gözüm and Çapık, 2014). The model is presented in Figure 2.

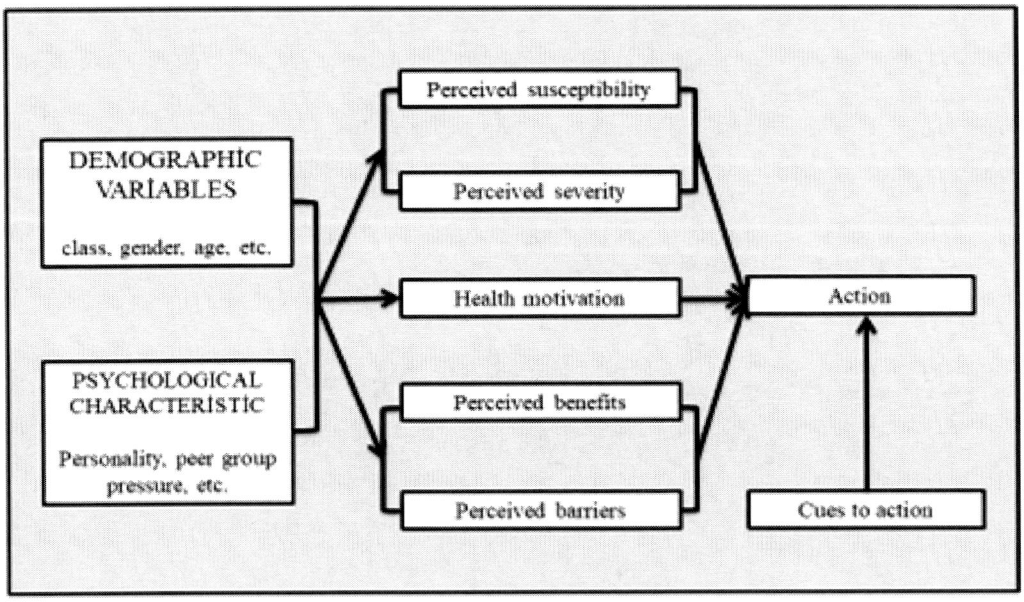

Figure 2. The health belief model (Abraham and Sheeran, 2005).

Transtheoretical Model (TTM)

The Transtheoretical Model (TTM), developed by James Prochaska and Carlo DiClemente in 1982, is an integrative biopsychosocial model that describes the stages of which individuals progress, from recognizing an unhealthy behavior to adopting a healthier one. The most important feature of this model that distinguishes it from other models used for behavior change is that it advocates that behavior change is a process. In other words, it classifies individuals not only according to whether they can perform a certain behavior or not but also according to the stages that passed in the behavioral change process. In TTM, behavioral change is defined as a gradual, continuous, and dynamic structure. The model focuses on helping individuals make intentional behavioral changes and understanding the change process. TTM evaluates the accurate evaluation of results, measurement of progress, and the effectiveness of initiatives (Ünver, 2019). The main components of the TTM are seen in Figure 3.

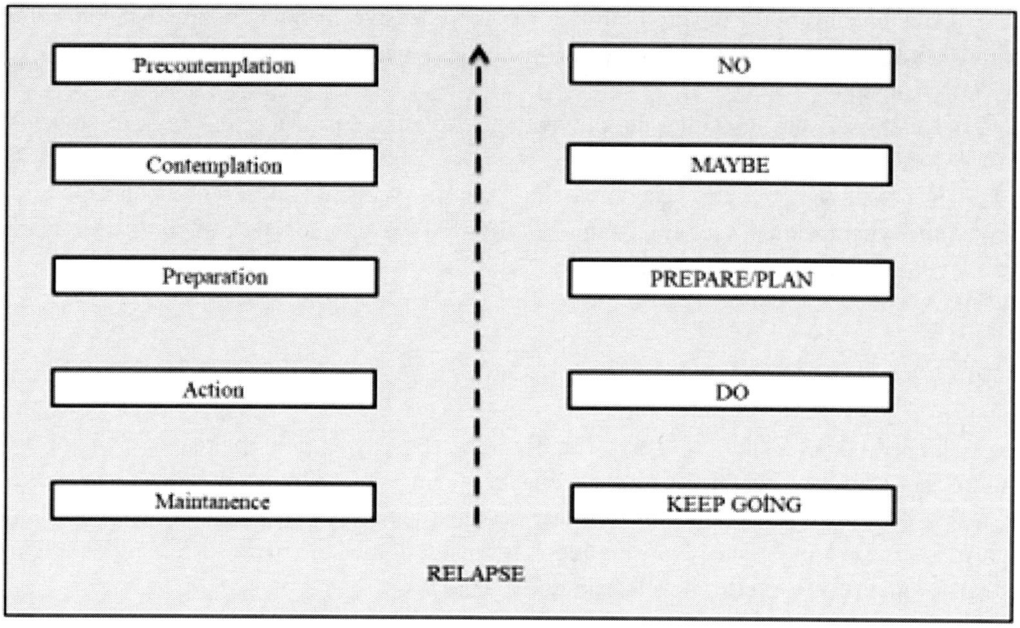

Figure 3. The transtheoretical model. (Prochaska and Diclemente, 2025).

Three-Component Model

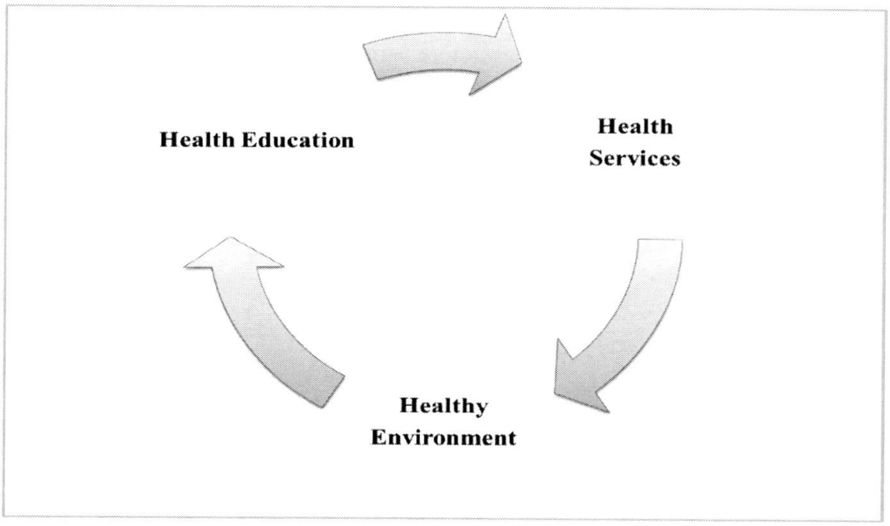

Figure 4. The three component model (Allensworth et al., 1997).

The three-component model is considered the traditional model of school health programs (Figure 4). This model, which emerged in the early 1900s and developed until the 1980s, defines the school health program as consisting of the following three basic components:

1. Health education, delivered through a comprehensive curriculum aimed at enhancing students' understanding of health principles and health promotion for behavioral change.
2. Health services including the prevention, early diagnosis, and treatment of students' health problems.
3. A healthy environment, encompassing both the physical and psychosocial aspects of the school setting, including safety, nutrition, food service, and a supportive learning atmosphere (Allensworth et al., 1997).

Eight-Component Model

A coordinated school health program (CSHP) model consists of eight interactive components (Figure 5). Families, healthcare professionals, the media, religious organizations, social organizations serving students, and young people themselves need to be systematically involved in the process. Schools are an important institution where many different institutions can work together to protect the well-being of students.

- Health education: Classroom-based health education that encompasses physical, emotional, mental, and social dimensions is designed to enhance students' overall well-being, prevent illness, and reduce engagement in risky behaviors.
- Physical education: Physical education is a planned and sequential curriculum that promotes lifelong physical activity while fostering fundamental movement and sports skills. It provides a structured environment in which students can learn, practice, and assess developmentally appropriate motor abilities, social competencies, and health-related knowledge to support their overall well-being.
- Health services: Health services encompass preventive care, health education, emergency interventions, referrals, and the management of both acute and chronic conditions, all aimed at preventing illness and injury while supporting student health.
- Nutrition services: Nutrition services involve nutrition education and an environment that promotes healthy eating habits.
- Health promotion for staff: Health promotion for staff provides opportunities that encourage school personnel to adopt a healthy lifestyle, leading to improved health, higher morale, and a stronger commitment to the school's overall coordinated health program. It has been found that productivity increases, and health insurance costs decrease with health promotion activities.
- Counseling and psychological services: Counseling and psychological services include individual and group assessments, interventions, and referrals, all aimed at preventing issues early and fostering healthy development.
- Healthy school environment: A healthy school environment encompasses the physical and aesthetic surroundings, as well as the psychosocial climate and culture of the school. Factors affecting the physical environment include the school building and the area surrounding it, biological/chemical factors harmful to health, and physical conditions such as temperature, noise, and lighting. The psychological environment

includes the physical, emotional, and social conditions that affect the well-being of students and staff.

- Parent/community engagement: Parent and community engagement involves a collaborative approach between schools, parents, and the community to enhance the health and well-being of students. School health advisory councils, coalitions, and broad-based school health groups can provide valuable support for school health program efforts (Allensworth et al., 1997).

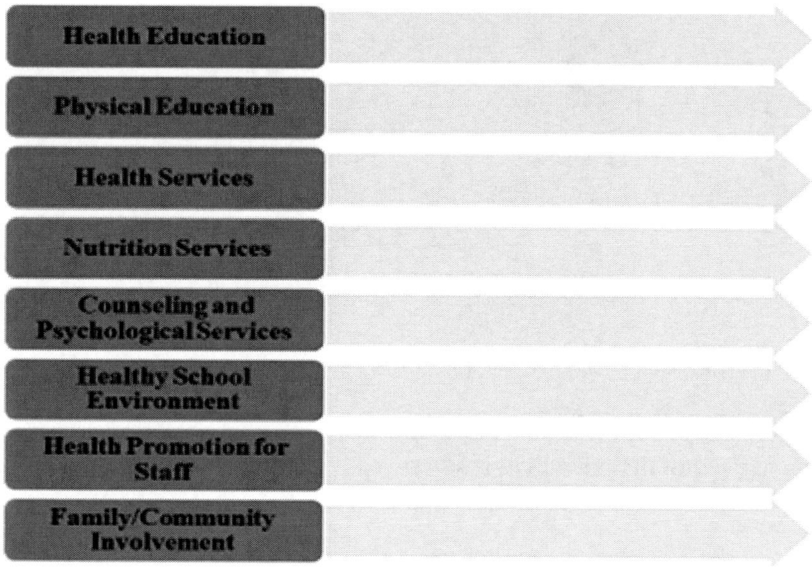

Figure 5. Coordinated school health eight component model.

Coordinated School Health Program (CSHP) Ecological Model

A complementary ecological model of the coordinated school health program (CSHP) that reflects 20 years of evolutionary changes is proposed. Ecology refers to the complex relationship between personal factors, interpersonal processes and primary groups, institutional factors, community factors, and public policy. Public health and child development theories, which include the impact of the personal and social environment on health behavior, as well as models that include the impact of ecology, have been used. The concepts of various models were combined with the eight components of the CSHP. It formulates an ecological model that includes six program and service components within an inner circle surrounded by four concentric rings representing the healthy school environment, the core structures of the CSHP, local school district management, and family and community involvement. This complementary ecological model is intended to serve as an additional conceptual approach to CSHP implementation, evaluation, and research and should prove particularly useful for practitioners and researchers who have a basic understanding of CSHP (Lohrmann, 2008). The model is presented in Figure 6.

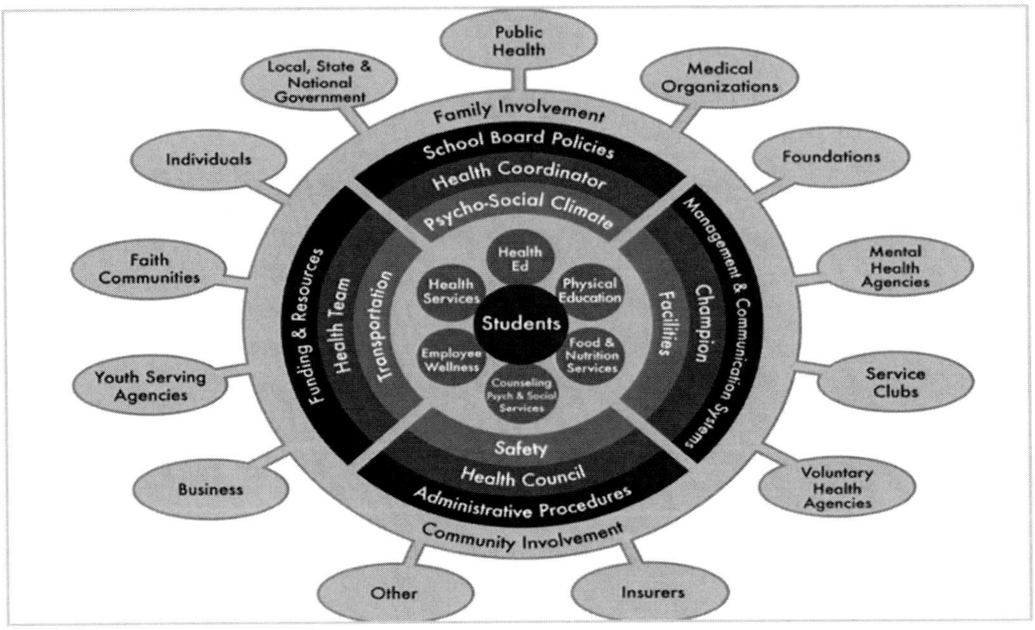

Figure 6. Coordinated school health program (CSHP) ecological model. (Lohrmann, 2008).

Comprehensive School Health Program

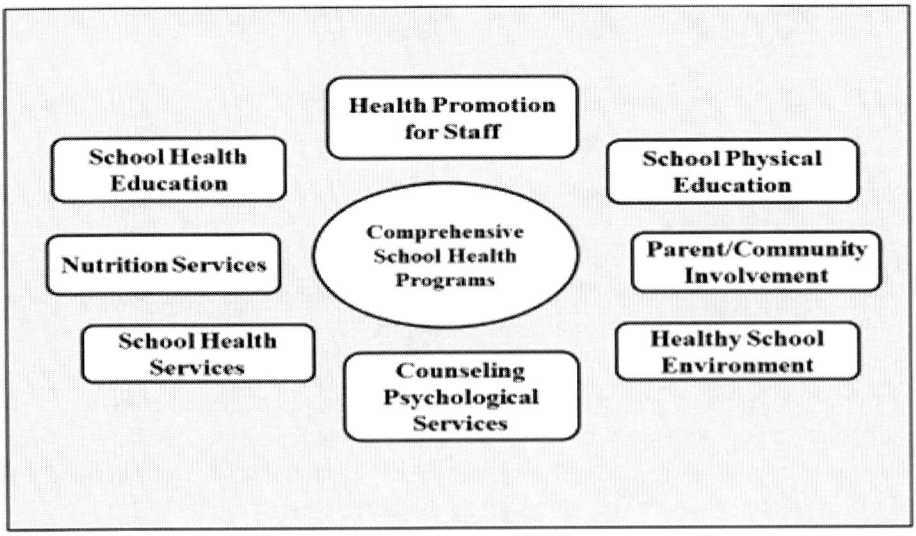

Figure 7. Comprehensive school health program (Torabi and Yang, 2020).

Allensworth and Kolbe (1987) proposed a model called the Comprehensive School Health Program (CSHP), which expands the classical triad of health education, health services, and a healthy school environment to include physical education, counseling and psychological services, and nutrition services (Institute of Medicine (US) Committee on Comprehensive School Health Programs, 1995). This model (Figure 7) consists of an organized set of policies and procedures. It consists of activities designed to protect and improve the health, safety, and well-being of students and school staff. The CSHP model requires systematic coordination among eight components to magnify the benefits available in each component. To protect the well-being of young people, families, health professionals, the media, religious and social organizations should cooperate (Torabi and Yang, 2000).

Health Behavior Interaction Model

The Health Behavior Interaction Model is a nursing-based, individual-centered, holistic health behavior model that enables learning the latest information about health behaviors by examining individual characteristics along with environmental factors (Figure 8) (Cox, 2003). The main purpose of the model is;

1. Describe the individual's autonomy regarding health behavior, the interaction style of clinicians that support health behavior, and the impact of individual-specific dynamic variables on health outcomes,
2. To guide the identification of individual characteristics that affect health behaviors and outcomes in research and
3. To lead the planning of initiatives by targeting these defined variables.

The conceptual framework of the model combines health behavior with physical, social, cognitive, motivational, affective, and environmental components. The model gives nurses a prominent conceptual role in influencing health outcomes.

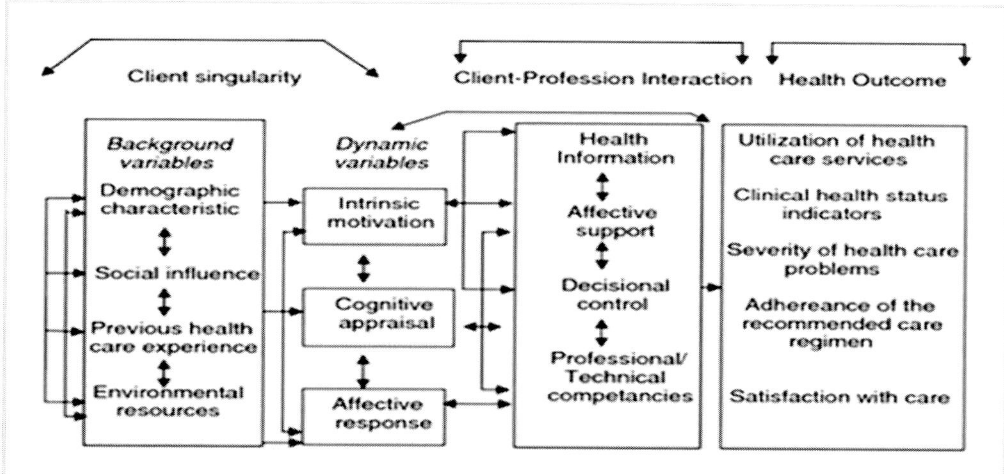

Figure 8. Health behavior interaction model (Johnson, 2019; Öztürk Haney and Erdoğan, 2013).

The model advocates the hypothesis that "if care professionals plan interventions according to the individual characteristics of the individual/patient, that person's health outcomes will be positive." The model recognizes that an individual's needs and emotions influence behavior. In the model, it is accepted that the individual's internal and external resources affect decisions regarding health behaviors. The Health Behavior Interaction Model (HBIM) recognizes the concept of intrinsic motivation as an important determinant of behavior. To determine and maintain health, the individual must be given maximum control within the limits of the internal and external environment. The model focuses on the individual's internal responsibility for positive health behaviors. The core of the model is the idea that the individual can make independent, informed, and competent choices about health behaviors (Öztürk Haney and Erdoğan, 2013).

Cognitive Development Theory

Piaget's theory focuses on theories of development and learning. Development focuses on the abilities of the learner, and learning focuses on the realization of such abilities, and education. Cognitive theory reflects the emergence of various psychological structures, organized units, or thought patterns that influence how behavior is interpreted by children. Cognitive development theories describe how children's reasoning abilities evolve as they acquire new ways of understanding and interpreting the world around them. Piaget's theory of inference assumes that all children go through the same developmental sequence, but they do so at different rates. The assessment should be based on individual progress rather than the normal standards of same-aged peers.

Piaget, J. (1983) An important consequence of Piaget's theory is the adaptation of teaching to the developmental level of the student. The teacher's role is to facilitate learning by providing various experiences (Lefa, 2014). The model is presented in Figure 9.

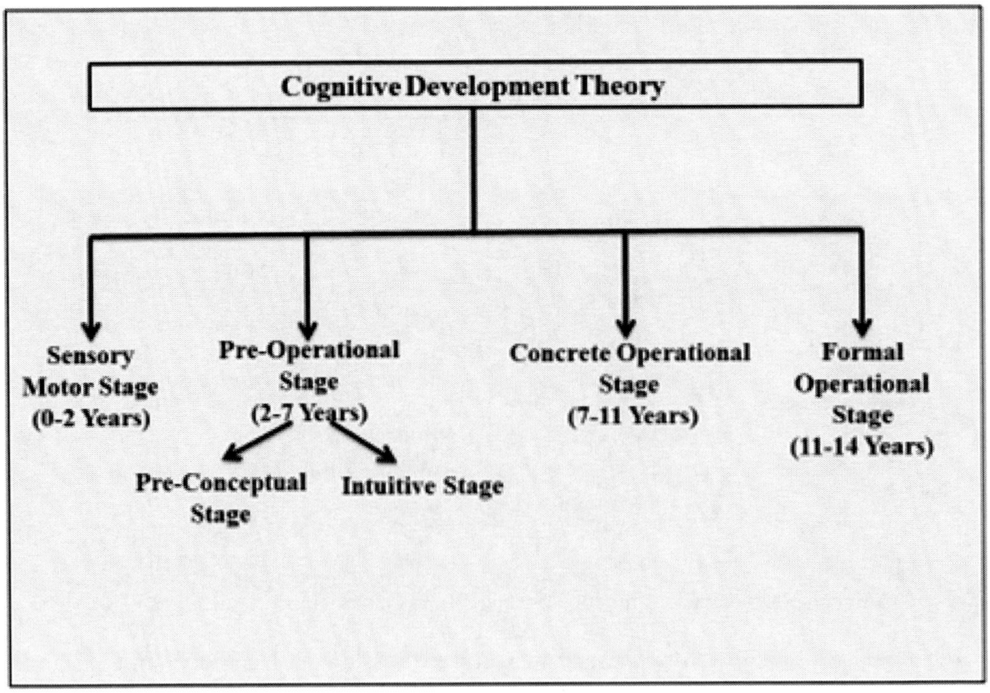

Figure 9. Cognitive development theory (Piaget, 1983).

Social Cognitive Learning Theory

Social Cognitive Learning Theory (SCLT) was explained by Bandura in 1986. SCLT, as a branch of social psychology, is often used to explain health behaviors. It focuses on behavioral change and the cognitive processes that affect it. SCLT has developed as a result of the interaction of environment and individual differences, and it is argued that people are in constant communication with their environment. This theory includes many dynamic relationships that express the effects of the environment on people and the effects of people on the environment and focuses on interpersonal communication. The purpose of the theory is to define methods that understand and predict individual or group behavior and reshape or change behavior (Bandura, 1989). The basic assumptions of SCLT are given below.

- People can learn about others' behavior through observation.
- Learning is an internal process that may or may not lead to behavioral change.
- Behavior is goal-directed.
- People can self-regulate their own behavior. They can learn to control their behavior and take responsibility.
- Reward and punishment affect behavior indirectly as well as directly.
- Behavior is more influenced by rewards or reinforcements received from previous experiences (Bandura, 1999).

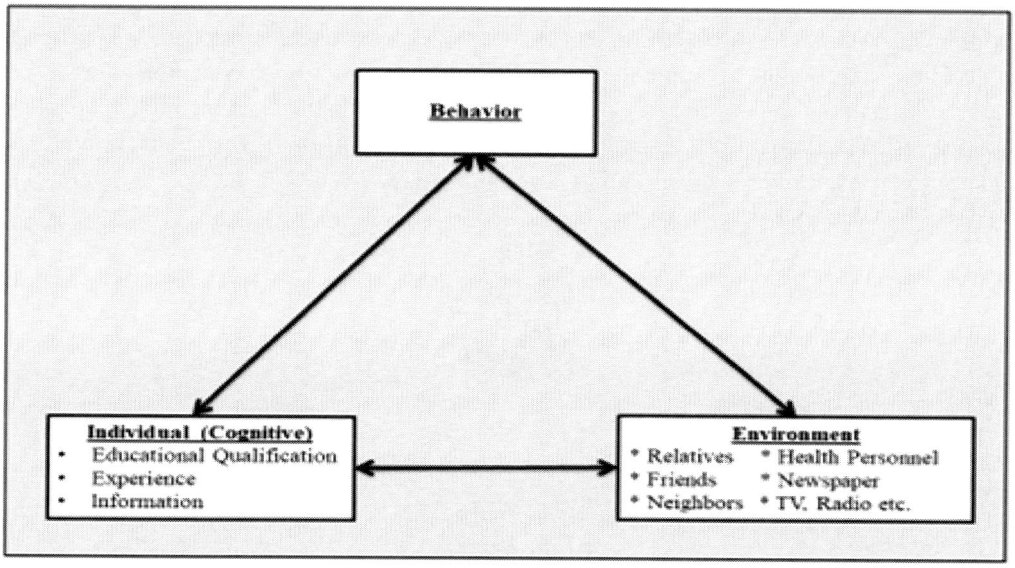

Figure 10. Social cognitive learning theory (Bandura, 1991).

In this model, cognitive, affective, and biological events, behavioral patterns, and environmental factors are interactional determinants that affect each other bidirectionally (Bandura, 2001). Based on the individual, the model states that characteristics such as the individual's thoughts, beliefs, attitudes, intentions, genetic history, gender, and age affect behavioral options. The development of behavioral skills, behavioral successes, and failures influence beliefs, attitudes, and intentions. Environmental influences—both social and physical—affect individuals by shaping their emotions, thoughts, and behaviors, especially when these influences are modified through modeling, instruction, and persuasion.

The individual also affects the environment through their interactions and behaviors. The way individuals interpret their social and physical environment plays a crucial role in shaping their responses within that environment. This model consists of three dimensions (environmental, behavioral, and cognitive) that form the basis of SCLT. The model is presented in Figure 10 (Bandura, 1999).

Model of Student Well-Being

Although there is no widespread consensus on the definition of well-being, it is generally characterized as including physical and mental health, as well as other elements or aspects of life (Nelson et al., 2015). Since its establishment in 1948, the World Health Organization has defined health as a state of complete physical, mental, and social well-being and not merely the absence of disease or infirmity (WHO, 2024). Although there is no consensus on the definition of well-being, it is clearly seen that it characterizes success in general and includes concepts such as well-being, happiness, and life satisfaction. Well-being is defined as a concept consisting of well-being, happiness, and satisfaction/success, which are elements of interpersonal/intrapersonal dimensions and internal and external systems. Internationally, the concept of well-being is used to define global health, quality of life, and general sustainability and is closely related to life satisfaction, happiness, and quality of life. It often includes people, environments, natural resources, communities, nations, etc., used to characterize. In the context of education, it is possible to define student well-being as the student's perception of quality of life, success, and life satisfaction. Well-being consists of five distinct and interactive domains: physical, affective, cognitive, economic, and social (PACES). These areas provide an organizational framework that is useful in program delivery (Nelson et al., 2015) (Figure 11).

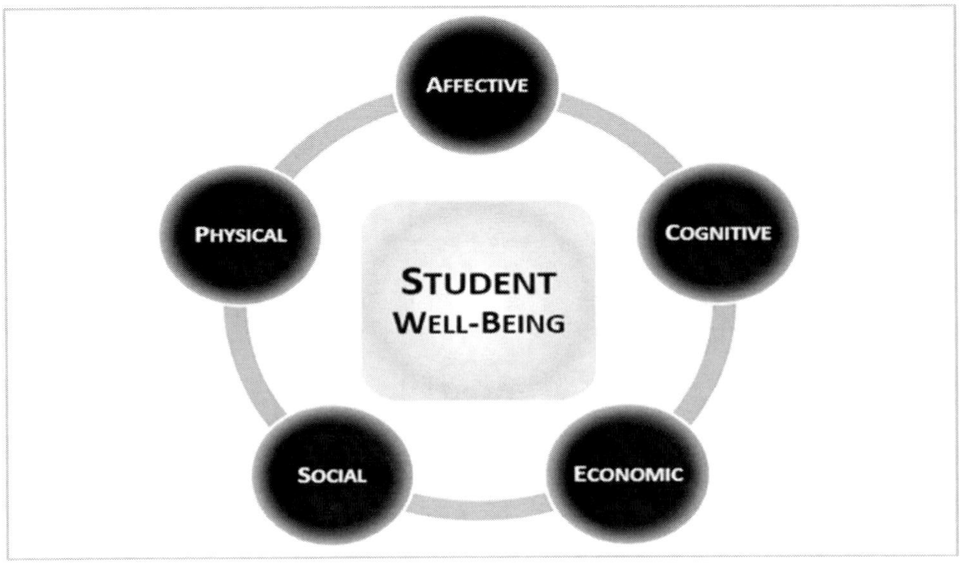

Figure 11. Model of student well-being (Nelson et al., 2015).

Importance of Health Promotion Models/Theories Usefulness for School Nursing

One of the work areas where nurses can use theories and models is the school. Children are influenced by their environment and the people who care for them. Health promotion principles and health behaviors are actually shaped while child, and therefore, schools can play a critical role in improving the health of young people (Jackson, 2022; Tancred et al., 2018). For example, school has many effects on physical activity patterns and healthy eating in adolescence. Understanding these effects in the context of a theoretical model can help develop interventions that effectively promote healthy behaviors (Kelly et al., 2012).

Scientific evidence shows that school can be an ideal environment for implementing health-related interventions (Pulimeno et al., 2020; Iudici, 2015). Today, young people face many health problems, and these health problems negatively affect the education of school-age students (Pulimeno et al., 2020; Glewwe, 2005).

The school is uniquely positioned to address students' basic needs in health education (Gillies et al., 2011; Torabi and Yang, 2000). Through a specific revision of the curriculum, schools can integrate the promotion of students' health into their usual teaching and learning practices (Pulimeno et al., 2020). Intervention strategies within schools are effective in reducing a range of risky behaviors, as well as strengthening and maintaining positive health behaviors for many students (Gillies et al., 2011). This means that programs or policies that improve children's health will also improve children's educational outcomes (Glewwe, 2005; Gillies et al., 2011). Given the importance of education for economic development, this link can be an important mechanism to improve the quality of life of people, especially in developing countries (Glewwe, 2005).

Improving students' well-being can reduce the prevalence of diseases and increase their academic achievement. At least 80% of cases of heart disease, type 2 diabetes, and one-third of all cancers can be prevented through health education (Pulimeno et al., 2020). At the same time, health education can improve the well-being of teachers and parents (Bada et al., 2019). From this perspective, primary prevention and health promotion should start as early as possible, and the ideal action environment should be found at school (Pulimeno et al., 2020).

Students are prone to many risky lifestyle behaviors such as physical inactivity, unhealthy diet, smoking, and stress. To prevent these risks, programs must address not only the behavior but also the factors surrounding it. Models and theories can provide a framework for program planners to build upon when developing health promotion programs (Simpson, 2015).

There are fundamental similarities, common values, and principles in health-promoting school models. It highlights three key principles that apply across different models of health-promoting schools (Whitman and Aldinger, 2009).

These include:

1. Integrating health education topics into the school curriculum;
2. Promoting student well-being through supportive school values and a positive social and physical environment;
3. Establishing connections with the community to enhance children's health, including active involvement of parents in community health intervention (Bada et al., 2019).

Table 1. School nursing studies based on theory and model

Author	Year		
Greening et al.	2011	Social Cognitive Learning Theory	A decrease in body fat percentage, an increase in physical activity level, and a decrease in fatty nutrition were detected.
Erkin Ö & Bayık Temel	2017	Transtheoretical Model	In students, it was found that sun protection behaviors such as using sunscreen products and clothing, wearing hats and sunglasses, and staying in the shade increased, and the perception of self-efficacy and decision balance improved positively.
Akcan & Ergün	2018	Social Cognitive Learning Theory	As a result of the research, it was seen that the Aggressive Behavior Prevention Program developed in line with Social Cognitive Theory was effective in reducing children's aggression.
Böyükbaş	2019	Health Promotion Model	It was determined that school nurses' practices at school and student levels to prevent obesity, self-efficacy, benefit, and social barrier perception scores were above average.
Can	2019	Stages of Change Model	It has been found that the trainings, organized according to the Pick Klop game and the Stages of Change Model, are effective in helping adolescents move away from nicotine addiction, both individually and together.
Başçı	2020	Health Behavior Interaction Model	Healthy nutrition education based on the Health Behavior Interaction Model has improved children's nutrition self-efficacy and nutrition attitudes.
Emlek Sert Z. & Bayık Temel	2020	Precede-Proceed Model and Social Cognitive Learning Theory	As a result of the program developed based on the Precede-Proceed Model and Social Cognitive Learning Theory, a positive change was achieved in healthy nutrition and physical activity behaviors and therefore weight management in the experimental group compared to the control group.

Researchers have shown that the most effective school health education programs follow comprehensive school health program models, are theory-based, and include family and community involvement (Torabi and Yang, 2000).

School-based health promotion programs and the models used in these programs are considered a cost-effective intervention for early diagnosis, reduction of lifelong chronic diseases, and prevention of obesity (Ekwaru et al., 2017; Denke and Winkleblack, 2020; Emlek Sert et al., 2023). Theory- and model-based school nursing studies are presented in Table 1.

Conclusion

The use of theory and models ensures coordination among nurse professionals. Thus, differences in the execution of applications are reduced, and the success rate in application results increases. In school nursing practice, it is vital for nurses to have a theoretical understanding of people's behavior so that they can improve the health status of the individual, family, group, or community. Theories and models used in school-based health promotion programsare considered a cost-effective intervention to reduce lifelong chronic diseases and prevent obesity.

Disclaimer

None.

References

Akcan, A., & Ergün, A. (2019). The effect of an aggressive behavior prevention program on kindergarten students. *Public Health Nursing, 36*(3), 330-340.

Allensworth, D., Lawson, E., Nicholson, L., & Wyche, J. (1997). Evolution of school health programs. In *Schools & Health: Our Nation's Investment*. National Academies Press (US).

Aqtam, I., & Darawwad, M. (2018). Health promotion model: An integrative literature review. *Open Journal of Nursing, 8*, 485-503. https://doi.org/10.4236/ojn.2018.87037.

Bada, E., Darlington, E., Masson, J., & Santos, R. M. (2019). *European Standards & Indicators for Health Promoting Schools*. ISBN 978-87-971891-3-9. https://www.schoolsforhealth.org/sites/default/files/editor/Teachers%20resources/european_standards_and_indicators_on_hps_en.pdf.

Bandura, A. (1989). Social cognitive theory. In R. Vasta (Ed.), *Annuals of child development* (Vol. 6, pp. 1-60). Greenwich, CT: Jai Press LTD.

Bandura, A. (1991). Social cognitive theory of self-regulation. *Organizational Behavior and Human Decision Processes, 50*, 248-287.

Bandura, A. (1999). Social cognitive theory: An agentic perspective. *Asian Journal of Social Psychology, 2*(1), 21-41.

Bandura, A. (2001). A cognitive theory: An agentic perspective. *Annual Review of Psychology, 52*, 1-26.

Başçı, A. B. (2020). [The effect of healthy nutrition program based on health behavior interaction model on nutritional attitudes and behaviors of primary school students] [Doctoral dissertation, Hacettepe University, Department of Public Health Nursing].

Bergh, I. H., Stralen, M. M., Grydeland, M., Bjelland, M., Lien, N., Andersen, L. F., Anderssen, S. A., & Ommundsen, Y. (2012). Exploring mediators of accelerometer assessed physical activity in young adolescents in the Health in Adolescents study – A group randomized controlled trial. *BMC Public Health, 12*, 814. https://doi.org/10.1186/1471-2458-12-814.

Böyükbaş, Z. (2019). [School nurses' practices for preventing childhood obesity based on health promotion model, their self-efficacy levels, perceived benefits and barriers] [Master's thesis, Marmara University, Department of Nursing].

Can, R. (2019). [Effects of training based on the pickklop game and the dam model on adolescents' nicotine addiction] [Doctoral dissertation, Eskisehir Osmangazi University, Department of Nursing].

Cox, C. L. (2003). A model of health behavior to guide studies of childhood cancer survivors. *Oncology Nursing Forum, 30*, 92-99.

Çalık, A., & Kapucu, S. (2017). Developing healthy lifestyle behaviors in diabetic patients: Pender's health promotion model. *Hacettepe University Faculty of Nursing Journal, 4*(2), 62-75.

Çetinkaya, A. (2021). [Theories and Models in Public Health Nursing] [Chapter 2, pp. 55-85]. In Ö. Erkin, A. Kalkım, & İ. Göl (Eds.), Public Health Nursing. Çukurova Nobel Medical Bookstore. ISBN: 978-605-2369-37-1.

Dağhan, Ş., Toraman, A. U., & Özsezer, G. (2022). Investigation of postgraduate theses conducted using model in school health nursing in Turkey: A systematic review. *Sağ Aka Derg, 9*(2), 177-185. https://doi.org/10.52880/sagakaderg.988866.

Institute of Medicine (US) Committee on Comprehensive School Health Programs. (1995). Defining a Comprehensive School Health Program: An Interim Statement. Allensworth D, Wyche J, Lawson E, Nicholson L, editors. Washington (DC): National Academies Press (US).

Denke, N. J., & Winkleblack, L. K. (2020). Challenges and opportunities in population health: The role of school nurses as complexity leaders. *Nursing Administration Quarterly, 44*(2), 136-141.

Domitrovich, C., Bradshaw, C., Greenberg, M. T., Embry, D. D., Poduska, J. M., & Ialongo, N. (2009). Integrated models of school-based prevention: Logic and theory. *Psychology in the Schools, 47*(1), 71-88. https://doi.org/10.1002/pits.20452.

Ekwaru, J. P., Ohinmaa, A., Tran, B. X., Setayeshgar, S., Johnson, J. A., & Veugelers, P. J. (2017). Cost-effectiveness of a school-based health promotion program in Canada: A life-course modeling approach. *PLOS One, 12*(5), e0177848. https://doi.org/10.1371/journal.pone.0177848.

Emlek Sert, Z., & Bayık Temel, A. (2020). The effects of the training program to improve healthy nutrition and physical activity behaviors of school children on weight management. *Progress in Health Sciences, 10*(2), 29-38. https://doi.org/10.5604/01.3001.0014.6584.

Emlek Sert, Z., Altuğ Özsoy, S., & Kalkım, A. (2023). School health nursing based on intersectoral collaboration: A proposal for developing a cost-effective model. *Progress in Health Sciences, 13*(2), 63-71. https://doi.org/10.5604/01.3001.0054.2477.

Erkin, Ö., & Bayık Temel, A. (2017). A nurse-led school-based sun protection programme in Turkey. *Central European Journal of Public Health, 25*(4), 287-292.

Gigliotti, E. (2008). The value of nursing models in practice. *Dokuz Eylul University School of Nursing Electronic Journal, 1*, 42-50.

Gillies, S., Dimitrijevich, S., & Lambert, M. (2011). What is a health promoting school? https://wahpsa.org.au/wp-content/uploads/2015/09/What-is-a-HPS-2011.pdf.

Glewwe, P. (2005). The impact of child health and nutrition on education in developing countries: Theory, econometric issues, and recent empirical evidence. *Food and Nutrition Bulletin, 2*(26), 235-250.

Göçmen Baykara, Z., Çalışkan, N., Öztürk, D., & Karadağ, A. (2019). The use of nursing theories and models: A qualitative study. *Cukurova Medical Journal, 44*(1), 281-289. https://doi.org/10.17826/cumj.562393

Gözüm, S., & Çapık, C. (2014). [A guide to developing health behaviors: The health belief model]. Dokuz Eylul University School of Nursing Electronic Journal, *7*(3), 230-237.

Greening, L., Harrell, K. T., Low, A. K., & Fielder, S. E. (2011). Efficacy of a school-based childhood obesity intervention program in a rural southern community: TEAM Mississippi project. *Obesity, 19*(6), 1213-1219.

Iudici, A. (2015). Health promotion in school: Conceptual assumptions. In *Health promotion in school: Theory, practice, and clinical implications* (pp. 28). https://www.researchgate.net/publication/271552439.

Jackson, A. (2022). Health promotion for nursing associates: The principles of health promotion. *Chapter 1*. https://uk.sagepub.com/sites/default/files/upm-assets/121805_book_item_121805.pdf.

Johnson, C. (2019). Telephone advice nursing: Communication, patient satisfaction, and tool development. https://doi.org/10.3384/lic.diva-153620.

Kelly, S., Melnyk, B. M., & Belyea, M. (2012). Predicting physical activity and fruit and vegetable intake in adolescents: A test of the information, motivation, behavioral skills model. *Nursing Research, 35*(2), 146-163. https://doi.org/10.1002/nur.21462.

Koç, Ş., & Yumru, H. (2019). [Theory/Model usage in nursing research related to child health in Turkey: A systematic review]. *Dokuz Eylul University School of Nursing Electronic Journal, 21*(3), 85-103.

Lefa, B. (2014). The Piaget theory of cognitive development: An educational implication. *Educational Psychology, 1*(1), 9.

Lohrmann, D. K. (2008). A complementary ecological model of the coordinated school health program. *Public health reports, 123*(6), 695-703.

National Academies Press. https://nap.nationalacademies.org/.

Nelson, M., Tarabochia, D., & Koltz, R. (2015). PACES: A model of student well-being. https://www.researchgate.net/publication/290436780.

Öztürk Haney, M., & Erdoğan, S. (2013). [Sağlık davranışı etkileşim modeli: Çocukların beslenme alışkanlıklarını belirlenmek için bir rehber]. *DEUHYO ED, 6*(4), 218-223.

Pulimeno, M., Piscitelli, P., Colazzo, S., Colao, A., & Miani, A. (2020). School as an ideal setting to promote health and wellbeing among young people. *Health Promotion Perspectives, 10*(4), 316-324. https://doi.org/10.34172/hpp.2020.50.

Prochaska, J. O. & Diclemente, C. C. (Access Date 2025). The Transtheoretical Model (Stages of Change). https://www.habitweekly.com/models-frameworks/the-transtheoretical-model-stages-of-change.

Raingruber, B. *Health promotion theories*. Chapter 3. https://samples.jbpub.com/9781284094749/Chapter_3.pdf.

Simpson, V. (2015). Models and theories to support health behavior intervention and program planning. *Health and Human Sciences, Purdue Extension*. https://extension.purdue.edu/extmedia/hhs/hhs-792-w.pdf.

Şengün İnan, F., Üstün, B., & Bademli, K. (2013). [Review of theory/model based nursing research in Turkey]. Anatolian Journal of Nursing and Health Sciences, *16*(2), 132-139.

Tancred, T., Paparini, S., Torres, G. J. M., Thomas, J., Fletcher, A., Campbell, R., & Bonell, C. (2012). A systematic review and synthesis of theories of change of school-based interventions integrating health and academic education as a novel means of preventing violence and substance use among students. *BMC Systematic Reviews, 7*(190). https://doi.org/10.1186/s13643-018-0862-y.

Torabi, M. R., & Yang, J. Z. (2000). Comprehensive school health model: An integrated school health education and physical education program. https://www.eduhk.hk/icpe2004/English%20Sample.pdf.

Ünver, Z. (2019). The use of transteorethic model in changing health behaviors. Inonu University Health Services Vocational School Journal, 7(2), 218-228. https://doi.org/10.33715/inonusaglik.643162.

World Health Organization (WHO). (2024). *Constitution.* https://www.who.int/about/governance/constitution.

Younas, A., & Quennell, S. (2019). Usefulness of nursing theory-guided practice: An integrative review. *Scandinavian Journal of Caring Sciences, 33*, 540-555.

Whitman, C. V., & Aldinger, C. E. (Eds.). (2009). *Case studies in global school health promotion: from research to practice.* Springer Science & Business Media. ISBN 978-0-387-92268-3 e-ISBN 978-0-387-92269-0 DOI: 10.1007/978-0-387-92269-0.

Chapter 15

Health Promotion Programs in Schools

Yasemin Demir Avcı*, **PhD**
Department of Public Health Nursing, Akdeniz University, Faculty of Nursing, Antalya, Türkiye

Abstract

Health promotion programs in school health encompass all practices to help students, their families, and school staff lead healthier lives. These programs are supported by international organizations such as WHO, UNESCO, and UNICEF. The aim of school health programs is to improve the living conditions and lifestyles of students. The main goals of school health promotion programs are to promote equity and inclusion in the school community, to create a greater sense of ownership in school life, and to create an environment that fosters social relationships and academic success. Health promotion programs around the world vary according to the cultural, economic, and educational systems of the countries. Healthy school programs have been implemented in countries such as Europe, Turkey, the USA, Canada, Finland, Asia, and Brazil and have resulted in significant improvements in various health areas. School nurses are actively involved in health promotion programs. These programs and initiatives aim to improve the quality of education, the health of students and school staff, and the health of future generations.

Keywords: health promotion program, school health, school nurse

Introduction

The term "school health" encompasses all efforts aimed at assessing and improving the health of school-age children, fostering and maintaining a healthy school environment (Meydanlıoğlu and Gözüm, 2019). The *Health Promoting Schools* initiative encourages the development of positive behaviors and supports overall well-being through activities such as physical activity, recreation and play, balanced nutrition, physical fitness, tobacco use prevention, and bullying prevention. The concept of Health Promoting Schools was introduced in 1992 by the World Health Organization (WHO), the United Nations Educational, Scientific and Cultural

---

* Corresponding Author's Email: ydemir@akdeniz.edu.tr

In: Health Promotion and Prevention
Editor: Eda Kılınç İşleyen
ISBN: 979-8-89530-758-8

Organization (UNESCO), and the United Nations International Children's Emergency Fund (UNICEF) (WHO, 2024).

Health-promoting school programs include ensuring and maintaining a healthy school environment, assessing and improving the health status of school-age children and school staff, and providing health education to school-age children (Meydanlıoğlu and Gözüm, 2019) (Table 1). In the field of school health, many programs and projects are actively carried out by different institutions and organizations. In the field of school health, many programs and projects are actively carried out by different institutions and organizations.

Table 1. Key components of a whole school approach to health promotion programs (Vilaça et al., 2019)

Component 1	Well-defined documents or established procedures aimed at enhancing health and wellness are known as healthy school policies. These guidelines might specify what foods are permitted to be provided in schools or provide guidance on how to stop bullying there. A policy is a component of the curriculum.
Component 2	A school's grounds, buildings, and surroundings make up its physical environment. Making school grounds more appealing for leisure and physical exercise, for instance, could contribute to the formation of a healthy physical environment.
Component 3	The quality of relationships among members of the school community, such as those between students and staff, is a key component of the school's social environment. In addition to ties with parents and the larger community, social competencies within the school community can have an impact on the social environment.
Component 4	The curriculum and activities that foster the information and abilities necessary for learners to construct competencies support the development of individual health skills and action competencies. Take steps to improve your well-being, health, and academic performance. Activities should be a part of the school's everyday routine. The goals should include things like social skill development, physical activity on a daily basis, health literacy, and a balanced diet.
Component 5	Community linkages are those that exist between the school and important individuals or groups in the neighborhood, as well as between the school and the families of its pupils. Supporting the school community in its health promotion efforts and consulting and working together with community stakeholders in the school's health promotion initiatives.
Component 6	Health services are school-related or school-based local and regional services that directly assist kids in order to promote and maintain their health. Students with special needs are included in this. Healthcare professionals may collaborate with educators on particular topics such as sex education and hygiene.

Several factors have been identified as contributing to effective school programs that promote health.

- Fostering and maintaining involvement and democracy in the school community (Vilaça et al., 2019).
- Active ownership of school life by all members of the school community—including students, staff, and parents—fosters a sense of shared responsibility and engagement, which is essential for the success of health promotion initiatives within schools (Svanbjörnsdóttir et al., 2016).
- Pursuing a whole-school approach to health promotion rather than the traditional classroom-only approach (Warren et al., 2019).
- Creating a school climate with high expectations for students' social relationships and academic achievement (Gietz et al., 2014).
- Knowledge of a variety of learning and teaching strategies to use different educational management (El-Sabagh, 2021).

- Exploring health issues in the context of students' lives and society (Vilaça et al., 2019).

Teachers can use this holistic understanding of health to design their lesson plans in a way that enhances mental well-being and fosters academic success (by improving students' social skills). Therefore, health promotion in schools can support significantly to achieving educational, social, and staff-related goals, while also positively influencing the overall health and well-being of the entire school community (Kwon et al., 2021; Vilaça et al., 2019; Warren et al., 2019).

Health Promotion Programs in Schools at National and International Levels

There are many programs and projects actively carried out by different institutions and organizations in the field of school health. Although these programs vary according to the country, they basically aim to improve health in schools. The strategies adopted by each country are shaped according to the cultural, socioeconomic, and education system-specific dynamics of that country. Institutions such as the European Union (EU) and the WHO provide guidance by promoting standardized health education frameworks and registries. Interventions such as the European Union's 'Education for Health' program and the World Health Organization's 'Health in Schools' initiative serve as valuable resources for advancing health promotion efforts within school settings (WHO, 2024). The Schools for Health in Europe Network Foundation mapping (SHE mapping) report is an international effort to map the level of implementation of health promotion in schools in SHE member countries and how this implementation is carried out. Such programs and interventions show that health education is sustained in education systems across Europe (Vilaça et al., 2019).

It is aimed to establish a school health model in Turkey where a holistic approach is adopted. In order for the school health approach in Turkey to be more comprehensive and holistic, a Scientific Board and Steering Committee were established with the participation of the Ministries of National Education and Health, academics, public institutions, and organizations. The "School Health Services Cooperation Protocol" was signed between the Ministry of National Education (MoNE) and the Ministry of Health (MoH) in 2016. The name of the program is "Health Prevention and Promotion Program in Schools " which was launched. This program is intended to form the framework of all programs and projects that have been and will be carried out in schools within the scope of school health and to create the school health model of the country. There are six key components in this program: health services, physical activity, family and community involvement, balanced nutrition, a safe and healthy school environment, and health education (General Directorate of Public Health, 2023a). Several projects have been implemented to health promotion in schools, including 'Projects for Adolescents,' the 'Bright Smiles, Bright Futures Project,' the 'Oral and Dental Health Education Project,' and the 'First Step to First Aid Project (Meydanlıoğlu and Gözüm, 2019). In addition, hearing and vision screening programs are among the ongoing health initiatives implemented in schools (General Directorate of Public Health, 2023b). Annual periodic screening and examinations for school-age children were initiated by Family Medicine Units at the end of 2016. In line with new legislation, structured workflows were established for school health services, and an Implementation Guide was published. Within the scope of the School Health Prevention and Promotion Program, annual periodic follow-ups of all school-age children are carried out by family physicians in line with protocols (General Directorate of Public Health, 2023a).

In the United States, there are a variety of federal, state, and local programs for health education in schools and for students to adopt healthy living habits. A wide range of health issues are addressed, including nutrition, physical activity, mental health, and sexual health education. The programs aim to teach students about healthy eating, regular exercise, emotional well-being, and healthy sexual behaviors. These health programs also include education to prevent smoking and substance use (US Department of Education, 2021).

In Canada, a healthy school approach is a program where school communities come together to create an environment where health and well-being are valued and promoted throughout the school. The healthy school program covers a wide range of subjects, such as academic achievement, fruit and vegetable consumption, bullying, absenteeism, tobacco and substance use, and sedentary behavior. It also addresses topics such as mental health, resilience, self-esteem and confidence, school staff well-being, physical activity, sense of belonging, engagement, and a deeper connection with the school community (Canadian Healthy Schools Alliance, 2021).

Finland pioneers health promotion programs in schools. The School Health Promotion (SHP) study monitors the well-being and health of Finnish children and adolescents and their work at school. The aim of the SHP study is to strengthen the planning and evaluation of health promotion activities at school, municipal, and national levels. The questions about well-being, involvement and leisure, health and functional ability, lifestyle, family and housing conditions, school attendance and studies, the safety of the growing environment, and access to services and help are all included in the SHP study. The resulting statistics are utilized to enhance social welfare, health services, educational methods, and the health and well-being of children, adolescents, and their families (School Health Promotion Study, 2024). The Finnish Institute for Health and Welfare has implemented several initiatives, including action plans addressing drugs, alcohol, tobacco, and gambling; the National Mental Health Strategy 2020–2030; the Non-Violent Childhoods Action Plan; the Suicide Prevention Program; the Technology Supporting Smart Aging and Home Care Program (SOLID); and the Finnish Indoor Air and Health Program 2018–2028 (The Finnish Institute for Health and Welfare, 2024).

The framework for health-promoting schools in Asia is characterized by six key factors. The school's health and well-being policies, the school's physically and socially healthy learning environment, the school's community connections, the inclusion of healthy living action competencies in both formal and informal curricula, and regional variations in the availability of health and health promotion services are among them (Ogasawara et al., 2022).

School health promotion programs in Southeast Asia have gained momentum in recent years, and Japan has been one of the countries that has made significant contributions to school health promotion in the region. Countries such as Lao PDR, Cambodia, the Philippines, and Thailand have established and implemented school health programs on nutrition, sanitation, and deworming, among others, through strengthened collaboration with international organizations (Estrada et al., 2020).

Table 2. The systematic reviews and meta-analysis of health promotion programs implemented in schools

Author, Year Country	Subject	Type of Research	Age group	Number of studies	Results
Wright et al., 2023, Austria	Digital tools for mental health promotion	Systematic Review and Meta-Analysis	11 to 18 Year	27	Digital intervention has been found to have the potential to improve adolescents' mental health. Digital tools have been found to have small but promising effects on health, alleviating anxiety and increasing protective factors. Some factors that influence the digital intervention include the setting, the level of guidance and support, and adherence to the intervention.
Dodd ve ark., 2022, UK	Peer education in schools	Systematic Review	11 to 18-years	73	Most of the publications reviewed treatments that addressed drinking, smoking, and substance use (n = 16), promotion of healthy lifestyles (n = 17), and sex education/HIV prevention (n = 23). The majority of the publications (67/73, 91.8%) reported the outcomes of the peer learners. Evidence of the efficacy of the interventions pointed to peer education as a possible beneficial tactic for enhancing school health.
Bramantoro et al., 2021, USA	School-based oral health promotion programs	Systematic Review	3 to 7 years	31	Seven of the articles involved students in kindergarten, seventeen studies involved students in primary school, and seven studies involved students in high school. School-based oral health promotion programs improved children and adolescents' oral health knowledge, behaviors, attitudes, status, and quality of life.
Lameiras-Fernández et a., 2021, Spain	Sexual and reproductive health	Systematic Review	10 to 19 years	20	A total of 20 studies (10 in school settings, 9 using digital platforms, and 1 blended learning program). The effectiveness of sex education programs has mostly focused on reducing risky behaviors (e.g., Sexually transmitted diseases, or unintended pregnancies) as public health outcomes.
Mansfield et al., 2021, USA	Human papillomavirus vaccination	Systematic Review	adolescents	57	Age at vaccination, awareness, and understanding of HPV vaccination, socioeconomic status, insurance status, race/ethnicity, and individual-level preventive care practices are the most consistent impacts of HPV vaccination. The consequences of immunization at the relationship level of parental health habits and family/peer support are what providers advocate.
Salamet al., 2020, Canada	Obesity	Systematic Review and Meta-Analysis	0 to 19 years	654	A total of 359 studies targeted obesity prevention, 280 studies targeted obesity management, and 15 studies targeted both prevention and management. According to these studies, diet and exercise for obesity prevention and a combination of interventions such as diet, exercise, and behavioral therapy for obesity management are most appropriate.
Cadenas-Sanchez et al., 2020, USA	Association between physical fitness and mental health	Systematic Review and Meta-Analysis	2 to 18 years	58	There was a significant positive overall relationship between physical fitness and mental health in children and adolescents. No relevant study focusing on preschool children was identified.
Chaves Costa et a., 2020, Brazil	Educational technologies for cardiovascular health promotion	Systematic Review	3 to 14 years	8	Technology-based games developed and evaluated for cardiovascular health promotion in children have been found to provide important diversity in health education.
Prescott et al., 2020, USA	Farm to school activities	Systematic Review	School age	21	The results from farm-to-school studies show positive impacts on food and nutrition-related knowledge; most studies also show a positive relationship between school meals in the farm-to-school program and healthy food choices and nutrition self-efficacy.

In Brazil, school-based health promotion programs include the promotion of healthy eating and physical activity, oral hygiene, health screening, reduction of morbidity and mortality related to accidents and violence, monitoring and updating of vaccination program, psychosocial assessments for mental health, prevention of alcohol consumption, drug use, and smoking (Silva et al., 2017).

School Nurses Roles in School Health Promotion Programs

Countries have given various roles and authorities to school nurses in accordance with their laws and requirements. School health is another area of public health nursing. Public health nurses significantly improve the health of schools through school visits, routine check-ups, and health records. In countries where school health services are developed, nurses come to the forefront in the creation and execution of programs to improve public health (Kesgin and Çağlar, 2019). School nurses have early diagnosis, screening, health promotion, and health education programs to protect and improve the health of students and school staff (Ulutaşdemir et al., 2016).

School nurses play a key role in delivering health education both individually and within classroom settings, addressing a broad spectrum of topics related to health, growth, and development. These topics include healtly eating, physical activity, communicable diseases, growth and development, and school safety. In addition to health education, school nurses provide direct medical care to school-age children. Their responsibilities include managing minor sports injuries, performing basic wound care, and assessing and treating common medical conditions and injuries within the school environment (Brown et al., 2024).

In school health promotion programs, the responsibilities of school nurses in primary prevention include providing health education, promoting healthy lifestyle behaviors, offering guidance, organizing environmental and school health policies, and supporting immunization efforts. Within the scope of secondary prevention, school nurses are responsible for conducting health screenings, addressing existing health issues through early intervention, and preventing potential complications. In the context of tertiary prevention, their roles involve preventing secondary complications in students with chronic illnesses or disabilities, supporting the development of life skills, and facilitating rehabilitation services (Akgül and Ergün, 2021).

As a result, school nurses are actively involved in health promotion programs. These responsibilities are in line with the laws and requirements of the countries. In addition to health education, early diagnosis, and intervention methods, they provide support in protecting and improving the health of students and school staff. School nurses make the school environment a healthy environment by providing training on various health-related issues. These efforts of nurses are important in raising healthy generations and implementing health promotion programs.

Summary of Literature on Health Promotion Programs in Schools

There are many systematic reviews on school health programs (Wright et al., 2023; Dodd et al., 2022; Bramantoro et al., 2021; Lameiras-Fernández et al., 2021; Mansfield et al., 2021;

Salam et al., 2020; Cadenas-Sanchez et al., 2020; Chaves Costa et al., 2020; Prescott et al., 2020). These systematic reviews or meta-analyses have addressed a variety of topics in the literature, including oral and dental health education, sexual and reproductive health programs, the promotion of Human Papillomavirus (HPV) vaccination, obesity prevention strategies, the mental health benefits of physical activity, and healthy eating education. According to research, there are promising ways to improve health in schools. These approaches can improve the quality of life and overall health of school-age children (Table 2).

Conclusion

Although school-based health promotion programs are implemented across different cultural and economic contexts worldwide, their common objective is to support students in building a healthier future. Supported by major organizations such as UNESCO, UNICEF, and WHO, these activities contribute to academic success as well as health promotion in school communities. These programs are important in improving the overall health of the community by improving the quality of the education system through the efforts of school nurses and school staff.

The literature shows that school-based health promotion programs address various topics, including oral and dental health education, sexual and reproductive health programs, the promotion of HPV vaccination, obesity prevention strategies, the mental health benefits of physical activity, and healthy eating education. Although school-based health promotion programs are similar in issues such as obesity and physical activity, they vary according to the needs of countries.

- As in Finland, which is exemplary in its education system, national screenings can be conducted every year based on the results of knowledge tests that will improve the health and well-being of students according to their level.
- School community members, including students, school staff, and parents, should be active in school setting.
- A whole-school approach should be followed instead of the traditional classroom-only approach to health promotion.
- A school climate with high expectations for students' social relationships and academic achievement should be created.
- Develop a variety of learning and teaching strategies using different learning methods.
- Research should be conducted on health issues in the context of students' lives and society.
- School nurses should be encouraged to take part in health promotion programs.
- The multidisciplinary team (students, teachers, parents, and school nurses) involved in school health programs should actively participate in these programs and provide information about the programs.

Disclaimer

None.

References

Akgül, E., & Ergün, A. (2021). School health nursing in promotion public health. *Journal of Public Health Nursing*, 3(2), 141-153.

Bramantoro, T., Santoso, C. M. A., Hariyani, N., Setyowati, D., Zulfiana, A. A., Nor, N. A. M., Nagy, A., Pratamawari, D. N. P., & Irmalia, W. R. (2021). Effectiveness of the school-based oral health promotion programmes from preschool to high school: A systematic review. *PLOS ONE*, 16(8), e0256007. https://doi.org/10.1371/journal.pone.0256007.

Brown, H., Rose-Wright, J., & Bailey, C. (2024). The role of nurses in the school health program. *Pan American Health Organization*. https://www.paho.org/en/role-nurses-school-health-program.

Cadenas-Sanchez, C., Mena-Molina, A., Torres-Lopez, L. V., Migueles, J. H., Rodriguez-Ayllon, M., Lubans, D. R., & Ortega, F. B. (2021). Healthier minds in fitter bodies: A systematic review and meta-analysis of the association between physical fitness and mental health in youth. *Sports Medicine (Auckland, N.Z.)*, 51(12), 2571–2605. https://doi.org/10.1007/s40279-021-01520-y.

Canadian Healthy Schools Alliance. (2021). *Canadian Healthy School Standards*. Ottawa, Ontario. https://static1.squarespace.com/static/5fa5d3a995cc5537744e8b52/t/60f1aab61673b2086a3ba52b/1626450621787/2021.07.16+CHSS_Final+v2-EN.pdf.

Chaves Costa, F. B., Catrib, A. M. F., Branco, J. G. O., de Sales, R. O., da Silva Junior, G. B., Abdon, A. P. V., & de Almeida, L. P. C. M. (2020). Use of educational technologies in the promotion of children's cardiovascular health: A systematic review. *Global Health Promotion*, 27(4), 32–41. https://doi.org/10.1177/1757975920909119.

Dodd, S., Widnall, E., Russell, A. E., Curtin, E. L., Simmonds, R., Limmer, M., & Kidger, J. (2022). School-based peer education interventions to improve health: A global systematic review of effectiveness. *BMC Public Health*, 22(1), 2247. https://doi.org/10.1186/s12889-022-14688-3.

El-Sabagh, H. A. (2021). Adaptive e-learning environment based on learning styles and its impact on development students' engagement. *International Journal of Educational Technology in Higher Education*, 18(1), 53.

Estrada, C. A. M., Gregorio, E. R., Jr, Kanyasan, K., Hun, J., Tomokawa, S., Dumlao, M. C., & Kobayashi, J. (2020). School health promotion in South-East Asia by Japan and partners. *Pediatrics International: Official Journal of the Japan Pediatric Society*, 62(9), 1029–1038. https://doi.org/10.1111/ped.14284.

Gietz, C., & McIntosh, K. (2014). Relations between student perceptions of their school environment and academic achievement. *Canadian Journal of School Psychology*, 29(3), 161-176.

General Directorate of Public Health. (2023a). *School health protection and promotion program*. Ministry of Health. https://hsgm.saglik.gov.tr/tr/sagligin-gelistirilmesi-programlari/okulda-sagligin-korunmasi-gelistirilmesi-programi.html.

General Directorate of Public Health. (2023b). *Screening programs*. https://hsgm.saglik.gov.tr/tr/programlar/tarama-programlari.html.

Kwon, K. A., Ford, T. G., Jeon, L., Malek-Lasater, A., Ellis, N., Randall, K., ... & Salvatore, A. L. (2021). Testing a holistic conceptual framework for early childhood teacher well-being. *Journal of School Psychology*, 86, 178-197.

Kesgin, M. T., & Çağlar, S. (2019). The development of school nursing around the world and in Turkey. *HEAD*, 16(4), 343-352.

Lameiras-Fernández, M., Martínez-Román, R., Carrera-Fernández, M. V., & Rodríguez-Castro, Y. (2021). Sex education in the spotlight: What is working? Systematic review. *International Journal of Environmental Research and Public Health*, 18(5), 2555. https://doi.org/10.3390/ijerph18052555.

Mansfield, L. N., Vance, A., Nikpour, J. A., & Gonzalez-Guarda, R. M. (2021). A systematic review of human papillomavirus vaccination among US adolescents. *Research in Nursing & Health*, 44(3), 473–489. https://doi.org/10.1002/nur.22135.

Meydanlıoğlu, A., & Gözüm, S. (2019). [Türkiye'de okul sağlığını geliştiren uygulama ve programlar]. In Z. Bahar (Ed.), *Yaşam döngüsünde sağlığı geliştirme: Hemşirelik uygulamaları* (1st ed., pp. 16-23). Türkiye Klinikleri.

Ogasawara, R., Yamanaka, H., Kobayashi, J., Tomokawa, S., Sugita, E., Hirano, T., Kigawa, M., Nishio, A., Akiyama, T., Nam, E. W., Gregorio, E. R., Jr, Estrada, C. A. M., Thongthien, P., Kanyasan, K., Devkota, B., Hun, J., Ma, Y., & Yamamoto, B. A. (2022). Status of school health programs in Asia: National policy and implementation. *Pediatrics International: Official Journal of the Japan Pediatric Society*, 64(1), e15146. https://doi.org/10.1111/ped.15146.

Prescott, M. P., Cleary, R., Bonanno, A., Costanigro, M., Jablonski, B. B. R., & Long, A. B. (2020). Farm to school activities and student outcomes: A systematic review. *Advances in Nutrition (Bethesda, Md.)*, 11(2), 357–374. https://doi.org/10.1093/advances/nmz094.

Salam, R. A., Padhani, Z. A., Das, J. K., Shaikh, A. Y., Hoodbhoy, Z., Jeelani, S. M., ... & Bhutta, Z. A. (2020). Effects of lifestyle modification interventions to prevent and manage child and adolescent obesity: A systematic review and meta-analysis. *Nutrients*, 12(8), 2208.

School Health Promotion Study. (2024). *Wellbeing at school.* https://www.globaleducationparkfinland.fi/future-skills/wellbeing-at-school.

Silva, U. O. A., Nascimento, G. L., Santos, I. K., Azevedo, K. P. M., Santos, C. F., Knackfuss, M. I., & Medeiros, H. J. (2017). Health program in a Brazilian school. *Salud Publica de Mexico*, 59(1), 28–33. https://doi.org/10.21149/8412.

Svanbjörnsdóttir, B. M., Macdonald, A., & Frímannsson, G. H. (2016). Views of learning and a sense of community among students, paraprofessionals and parents in developing a school culture towards a professional learning community. *Professional Development in Education*, 42(4), 589-609.

The Finnish Institute for Health and Welfare. (2024). *Programmes.* https://thl.fi/en/research-and-development/programmes.

Ulutaşdemir, N., Balsak, H., Çopur, E. Ö., & Demiroğlu, N. (2016). [Halk sağlığı hemşireliğinin bir dalı: okul sağlığı hemşireliği]. *Türkiye Klinikleri J Public Health Nurs-Special Topics*, 2(1), 121-124.

US Department of Education. (2021). *Supporting child and student social, emotional, behavioral, and mental health needs.* https://www2.ed.gov/documents/students/supporting-child-student-social-emotional-behavioral-mental-health.pdf.

Vilaça, T., Darlington, E., Velasco, M. J. M., Martinis, O., & Masson, J. (2019). *SHE school manual 2.0: A methodological guidebook to become a health promoting school.* Schools for Health in Europe Network Foundation (SHE).

Warren, E., Bevilacqua, L., Opondo, C., Allen, E., Mathiot, A., West, G., ... & Bonell, C. (2019). Action groups as a participative strategy for leading whole-school health promotion: Results on implementation from the INCLUSIVE trial in English secondary schools. *British Educational Research Journal*, 45(5), 979-1000.

World Health Organization (WHO). (2024). *Making every school a health-promoting school.* https://www.who.int/initiatives/making-every-school-a-health-promoting-school.

Wright, M., Reitegger, F., Cela, H., Papst, A., & Gasteiger-Klicpera, B. (2023). Interventions with digital tools for mental health promotion among 11-18 year olds: A systematic review and meta-analysis. *Journal of Youth and Adolescence*, 52(4), 754–779. https://doi.org/10.1007/s10964-023-01735-4.

Chapter 16

Health Literacy in School-Age Children

Adile Tümer[1,*], PhD
and Fehime Nida Kürklüoğlu[2], MSc
[1]Muğla Sıtkı Koçman University/Faculty of Health Sciences/Department of Public Health Nursing, Muğla, Türkiye
[2]Denizli Provincial Health Directorate/Beyağaç Community Health Center, Emergency Nurse, Denizli, Türkiye

Abstract

Health literacy is an important requirement for individuals to access health-related information throughout their lives, to make the right decisions, and to make this a lifestyle. Meeting this need requires having the competence to receive, understand, and use basic health information and services. In the case of inadequate health literacy, both individual and community health are negatively affected. Therefore, health literacy is an issue that is closely concerned with public health. In order to understand health-related information correctly and to achieve better health outcomes, health literacy skills should be provided to school-age children starting from an early age. There are a limited number of studies to determine the level of health literacy in school-age children. The health literacy measurement tools for children and adolescents are also limited. It has been reported that inadequate or limited health literacy leads to poor nutrition, inadequate physical activity, poor hygiene, substance abuse, and home accidents and negatively affects the quality of life in children. School nurses, who have the opportunity to reach all groups in the community, are in an important position to intervene to improve health literacy for children and adolescents. The level of health literacy in school-age children can be improved with a holistic approach that includes school nurses, teachers, and parents. School nurses play a key role in planning, implementing, and evaluating programs to improve health literacy in schools.

Keywords: health literacy, school-age children, school nursing

---

* Corresponding Author's Email: tadile@mu.edu.tr

In: Health Promotion and Prevention
Editor: Eda Kılınç İşleyen
ISBN: 979-8-89530-758-8

Introduction

Health literacy, a concept that began to emerge in the 1970s, has since become an important topic on the public health agenda (Liu et al., 2020). Health literacy is defined as an individual's ability to access, understand, and use health information to prevent illness, promote well-being, and maintain health. It is related to a person's capacity to make informed, health-related decisions in daily life (Guo et al., 2022; Liu et al., 2020). Health literacy plays an important role in individuals' ability to accurately comprehend health professionals' guidance regarding disease prevention, disease management, appropriate medication use and adherence, as well as interpreting written health information and numerical data (Çınar et al., 2018). When the literature is examined, it is seen that different approaches and models are used regarding the concept of health literacy. The most frequently used of these are Nutbeum's Conceptual Model and Integrated Model. Nutbeam (2000) discussed the concept of health literacy under three subheadings: basic/functional, communicative/interactive, and critical health literacy. Basic/functional literacy is the ability of individuals to use basic reading and writing skills effectively in daily life. Health risks or how to use the health system show how to realize the ability to read actively. Communicative/interactive literacy includes highly developed cognitive and literacy skills, together with social skills, obtaining and using information, making sense of different ways of communication, and applying this information to new situations. Critical literacy, together with social skills, is more advanced cognitive skills that enable a critical approach to health-related information, critical thinking, and controlled use of health information in daily life (Nutbeam, 2000; Türkoğlu and Kılıç 2021). The Integrated Model developed by Sørensen et al., (2012) is summarized under four headings: access, understanding, evaluation, and implementation (Sørensen et al., 2012). In short, these models highligt importance of individuals' ability to critically analyze health messages and make informed decisions regarding their own health. Health literacy is an important indicator of an individual's ability to make informed decisions about lifestyle, nutrition, and health services, therefore serving as a foundation for improving individual and public health, preventing disease, and improving quality of life (de Buhr et al., 2020).

When health literacy is insufficient or limited, it leads to an increase in chronic diseases and subsequent unnecessary hospitalization costs (Liu et al., 2020). Furthermore, it is observed that hospitalization periods are prolonged, unnecessary tests are performed at higher rates, and unnecessary emergency room use is also increasing (Çopurlar and Kartal, 2016). Inadequate health literacy of individuals is not only limited to personal health but also affects the school-age children in their care. It has been determined that health literacy is associated with undesirable conditions for school-age children, such as malnutrition, obesity, higher injury rates, poor oral health, faulty medication use, or unnecessary visits to emergency services (de Buhr et al., 2020). An inadequate level of health literacy has been found to be associated with problems in accessing preventive health services, delays in early diagnosis, poor health practices, and adverse health outcomes (Brega et al., 2016; Tözün and Sönmez, 2015). It is important that health literacy, which is an important determinant of health, is given to school-age children starting at an early age with family and school-based education and developed throughout life.

Health Literacy in School-Age Children

During childhood, health-related behaviors and skills are acquired alongside fundamental cognitive, physical, and emotional development. The competencies developed during these formative years are crucial not only for healthy development but also for maintaining personal health and well-being into adulthood. Health literacy is a learning process that begins in childhood and continues throughout life as a multifaceted socio-cultural construct. Therefore, engaging school-age children with health literacy interventions can help promote healthy behaviors and reduce future health risks (Bröder et al., 2017). Health literacy in school-age children encompasses the ability to engage in physical and psychosocial activities at appropriate standards, interact effectively with others, adapt to changes, and support comprehensive physical, mental, and social development (Çoban and Özcebe, 2019). School-age children's health literacy is a multidimensional concept consisting of three domains: functional, interactive, and critical health literacy, as in adults (Guo et al., 2022).

Functional health literacy refers to having basic skills in reading and understanding health information, such as having knowledge of basic health issues such as healthy eating and exercising. Interactive health literacy refers to advanced communication and interaction skills that allow individuals to obtain and understand health information from various forms of communication. An example of this would be when an individual starts exercising regularly using their knowledge of exercise. Critical health literacy represents more advanced skills that can be used to critique and evaluate health information and gain control over the determinants of health. An example is individuals demanding safe spaces for exercise (Akça and Ayaz Alkaya, 2021; Guo et al., 2022).

Health literacy is affected by individuals' environmental, cultural, and social characteristics. It is known that parents, the living environment, culture background, and school experiences are effective in the development of health literacy in school-age children (Güler, 2022). Bröder et al., (2019) developed the "6D Model" that addresses the health literacy of school-age children. According to this model, it is argued that children not only make sense of the world around them but also make sense of their own health, experience, and develop ideas. Items of the model;

1) Different epidemiology and health perspectives: Concepts such as health, illness, and well-being are open to interpretation and cultural meaning. School-age children may assess what it means to be healthy or well based on their personal experiences and the interpretation or adoption of health-related beliefs and attitudes in their social environment.
2) Demographic variables and inequalities: School-age children are vulnerable to social and health inequalities. Factors such as low family socioeconomic status, poor living conditions, limited access to social support structures, as well as having a migration background are associated with an increased risk of educational disadvantage.
3) Developmental change and socialization process: Childhood and adolescence are life stages in which biological, psychological, cognitive, emotional, and social development processes take place. In order to improve the health literacy of school-age children, it is important to recognize the processes of sociological and psychosocial development, as well as the skills for cognitive development.

4) Power structures and interdependence within intergenerational relationships: School-age children due to their developmental dependency, rely on their parents' support, competencies, economic resources, and social networks. However, they also actively shape their own social environments. Within child-adult interactions, intergenerational power dynamics and conflicts emerge, often resulting in power imbalances.
5) Democratic approach and active participation: School-age children have the right to receive and access health information and make decisions about their health. The role of active participation of children and adolescents can be defined depending on the social structure and opportunities in the community.
6) Digitalization/growing digital worlds: School-age children grow up in highly digital and media-interactive environments, where they frequently encounter health information. These interactions present both opportunities and challenges that must be addressed when considering the health literacy of school-age children (Bröder et al., 2019).

Some health literacy skills that children need to acquire at different stages of life according to their development should be included in health education programs. For example, a 10-year-old child should know the importance of wearing a helmet while riding a bicycle, pay attention to personal hygiene behaviors, read the labels of foods, and decide whether they are healthy or not (Çoban and Özcebe, 2019). Hygiene and personal care skills, adequate and balanced nutrition, physical activity, sexual education, reducing technology addiction, avoiding smoking, alcohol, and substance use, protection from accidents and injuries, and protection from neglect and abuse are expressed as basic health behaviors that should be acquired and recommended for children. Therefore, the acquisition of health literacy skills should not only be considered as prevention of diseases, but also as access to health services. It should not be forgotten that this concept is a skill that should be acquired in childhood and covers a lifelong process (Üstündağ, 2020).

Health Literacy Measurement Tools and Research on Health Literacy in School-Age Children

Although there are many measurement tools developed to measure health literacy for adults in the literature, there are very few scales used to measure children's health literacy (Güler, 2022). Most of the tools used to measure health literacy in research are considered inadequate because they only measure the ability to recognize or read health-related vocabulary. The Rapid Estimate of Adolescent Literacy in Medicine (REALM Teen), a health literacy measurement tool developed for adolescents, is administered to children and adolescents aged 10-19 years. The test uses a vocabulary test to measure children's reading skills and level (Çınar et al., 2018; Davis et al., 2006). Paakkari et al., (2016) developed the health literacy for school-aged children scale for children aged 13-15 years. The scale was developed to measure children's health-related knowledge by using clear, simple, and clear language. The scale has five components consisting of theoretical knowledge, practical knowledge, critical thinking, self-awareness, and citizenship concepts. It is a 10-item scale with two items in each component (Güler, 2022; Paakkari et al., 2016). The European Health Literacy Survey Questionnaire (HLS-Child-Q15) was developed by Bollweg et al., (2020) for children aged 9-10 years. This scale is an adaptation of the European Health Literacy Scale for adults and children. The scale was developed to assess children's personal health literacy, being healthy, disease prevention, and health promotion. The scale has 15 items and measures the perceived difficulty in accessing, understanding, evaluating, and applying health-related information for the definition of health literacy (Bollweg et al., 2020).

In a study covering 10 European countries using the Health Literacy for School-Age Children scale, it was determined that 13% of the participants had low health literacy, 67% had moderate health literacy, and 20% had high health literacy (Paakkari et al., 2020). According to the Health Behaviour in School-aged Children study, among 12 countries, Turkey had the highest rate of low health literacy (18.4%), followed by Czechia (17.7%) and Austria (16.6%) (Health Literacy in Schools, 2020). In a study conducted in Germany with children aged 9-10 years using the European Children's Health Literacy Scale, it was reported that children's health literacy was at a high level (Fretian et al., 2020). In a study conducted by Ran et al., (2018) in China, it was determined that 25.5% of children's health literacy was low level and 48.3% was medium level. In a study conducted with children and adolescents in China, it was determined that the level of health literacy was high and increased with age. In the same study, it was determined that there was a significant positive relationship between health literacy and quality of life (Qiao et al., 2021). In a study conducted on adolescents, it was noted that those with high health literacy participated more in sports activities (Paakkari et al., 2017). Again, in a study conducted with this age group, it was emphasized that alcohol and cigarette use decreased as the level of health literacy increased (Hoffman et al., 2017). In a study conducted with 1044 participants in Turkey with 10-year-old children, it was noted that the level of health literacy was at a medium level (Üstündağ, 2020). In another study conducted in Turkey, the health literacy of adolescents was found to be at a medium level. In the same study, it was found that as the health literacy of adolescents increased, their hygiene behavior scores also increased (Kocataş et al., 2023).

Health Literacy in School-Age Children and the Role of the School

Considering that the first and most critical years of an individual's life are spent in the school environment, the most appropriate period for protecting and improving health is the school period (Kocataş et al., 2023). Based on the Shanghai Declaration on health promotion, most professionals around the world agree that the role of education in schools is important for health promotion. Reaching all school-age children and adolescents through schools provides an opportunity to create favorable conditions for long-term interventions aimed at developing and strengthening their health literacy capacities (Vamos et al., 2020).

A key foundation of health literacy is individuals' engagement in lifelong learning regarding their health; thus, a broad range of complementary and reinforcing learning opportunities—particularly through key social institutions such as schools and the healthcare system—is essential. Health education can be adapted according to age and added to the curriculum in a basic, understandable, and easy language Kickbusch et al., 2013). Health education in schools provides important opportunities to improve health literacy, make positive decisions about one's own health, identify factors affecting health, and work on health literacy.

Some techniques can help improve health literacy. These can be listed as didactic teaching, experiential teaching, workshops, small group exercises, role-playing activities, video reviews, and simulation applications (Akça and Ayaz Alkaya, 2021). In this direction, schools offer the necessary educational environments through curricula and cooperation with institutions and organizations (Kickbusch et al., 2013). The education system and the interaction model that will enable health literacy to become stronger are shown in Figure 1.

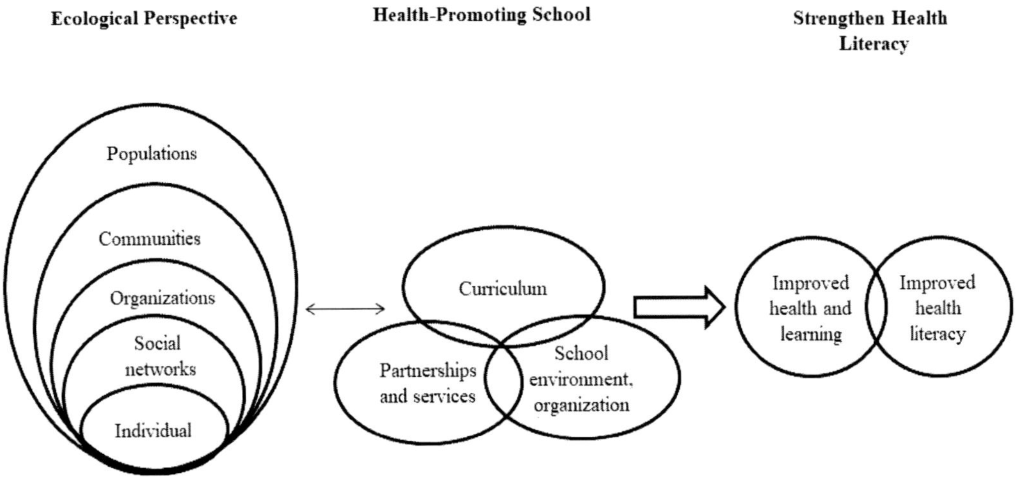

Figure 1. Education system and ınteraction model to enable stronger health literacy (Kickbusch et al., 2013.

Health Literacy and School Nursing

In recent years, the role of the school nurse has been expanded to include important components such as surveillance, chronic disease management, emergency preparedness, health education, behavioral health assessment, and multifaceted case management (Akça and Ayaz Alkaya, 2021). The school nurse is a professional who provides education and counseling services to students, student groups, and classes, in short, to the whole school community in direct health-related issues in line with the needs in order to improve health. By assuming the role of education and counseling play a critical role in providing and maintaining a healthy school life for school-age children, developing desired health behaviors, and creating permanent behavioral change for undesirable behaviors (Kocataş et al., 2023). The school nurse should determine the level of health literacy of children and adolescents and direct them to where and how to find the right resources for this. The development of health literacy skills is possible with a complete and comprehensive curriculum and educational environments for the protection of individual and social health (Şenyurt, 2021). School nurses should create understandable, continuous, and repetitive education programs to improve health literacy and plan health education for this purpose. The subject content should be framed and limited in health education programs to improve health literacy (Akça and Ayaz Alkaya, 2021). Education topics can be listed as personal health, hygiene, first aid, habits harmful to health and substance abuse, nutrition, physical activity, etc. (Şenyurt, 2021).

In developing health literacy, school nurses should work on health literacy with parents as well as working with children and adolescents. In recent studies, parents' health literacy levels have been associated with important health outcomes for child health. It has been determined that the health outcomes of the children of parents with low health literacy levels are worse (Muslu and Kolutek, 2018). While creating awareness of health literacy, the example of parents to their children is effective in their children's behaviors. It has been stated that children of parents with inadequate health literacy have similar behaviors, such as not knowing and accessing preventive and preventive health services, malnutrition, obesity, poor oral health, and addictions such as smoking (Üstündağ, 2020).

In the literature, there are significant relationships between parents' health literacy level and child health and literacy. In a study conducted with 1016 parent-child participants in the America, it was found that parents with inadequate health literacy had significantly worse oral and dental health status and similarly poor oral health of their children (Brega et al., 2016). In a study conducted with mothers, it was found that children of those with low health literacy were at high risk of having home accidents (Demirköse et al., 2021). In a study examining the relationship between parents' level of health literacy and utilization of pediatric services, it was determined that parents with high health literacy benefited more from the services (Alp and Oral Kaya, 2023).

School nurses should also cooperate with teachers. They should regularly conduct the health training included in the curriculum together with teachers and complete the deficiencies in health-related issues (Güler, 2022). When looking at the literature, there are studies showing that teachers have insufficient or limited health literacy (Deniz et al., 2020; Güner et al., 2020; Yilmazel and Cetinkaya, 2015). Considering that teachers are role models for school-age children, studies that determine and improve the health literacy levels of teachers should be conducted.

Conclusion

In terms of public health, school-age children are an important target group for health literacy research and practices. Health literacy has an impact on individuals' lifestyles, increases living standards, and improves health. Considering that health behaviors acquired during childhood and adolescence are maintained in adulthood, it is understood that it is important to develop health literacy during the school-age period. Schools enable children to develop health literacy through the supportive environments and curricula they provide. It is necessary to adopt an approach to improving health literacy within the scope of health education and integrate some health literacy skills that children need to acquire at various life stages according to their development into health education programs. The school nurse plays an important role in the planning, implementation, and evaluation of programs to improve health literacy in schools. Culturally appropriate scales need to be developed for a sensitive assessment of health literacy in children and adolescents. Health literacy measurement tools and research in this field are limited to children and adolescents. The research conducted serves as a guide for initiatives that aim to improve health literacy. In this way, school-age children develop the skills to gain accurate information, positive attitudes, and behaviors about health. The level of taking responsibility for lifelong health increases, health inequalities decrease, individuals' health levels improve, and a better quality of life is ensured.

References

Akça, A., & Ayaz Alkaya, S. (2021). *Health Literacy in School-Aged Children and the Role of the School Health Nurse. Hacettepe University Faculty of Nursing Journal*, 8(3), 328-334. https://doi.org/10.31125/hunhemsire.1050438.

Alp, S., & Oral Kara, N. (2023). A Study on Parental Health Literacy and Utilization of Pediatric Services. *Selcuk University Social Sciences Institute Journal* (50), 1-19. https://doi.org/10.52642/susbed.1153216.

Bollweg, T. M., Okan, O., Freţian, A. M., Bröder, J., Domanska, O. M., Jordan, S., Bruland, D., Pinheiro, P., & Bauer, U. (2019). Adapting the European Health Literacy Survey Questionnaire for Fourth-Grade Students in Germany: Validation and Psychometric Analysis. *Health Literacy Research and Practice*, 4(3), e144–e159. https://doi.org/10.3928/24748307-20200428-01.

Brega, A. G., Thomas, J. F., Henderson, W. G., Batliner, T. S., Quissell, D. O., Braun, P. A., Wilson, A., Bryant, L. L., Nadeau, K. J., & Albino, J. (2016). Association of Parental Health Literacy with Oral Health of Navajo Nation Preschoolers. *Health Education Research*, 31(1), 70–81. https://doi.org/10.1093/her/cyv055.

Bröder, J., Okan, O., Bauer, U., Bruland, D., Schlupp, S., Bollweg, T. M., Saboga-Nunes, L., Bond, E., Sørensen, K., Bitzer, E. M., Jordan, S., Domanska, O., Firnges, C., Carvalho, G. S., Bittlingmayer, U. H., Levin-Zamir, D., Pelikan, J., Sahrai, D., Lenz, A., Wahl, P., … Pinheiro, P. (2017). Health Literacy in Childhood and Youth: A Systematic Review of Definitions and Models. *BMC Public Health*, 17(1), 361. https://doi.org/10.1186/s12889-017-4267-y.

Bröder, J., Okan, O., Bollweg, T. M., Bruland, D., Pinheiro, P., & Bauer, U. (2019). Child and Youth Health Literacy: A Conceptual Analysis and Proposed Target-Group-Centred Definition. *International Journal of Environmental Research and Public Health*, 16(18), 3417. https://doi.org/10.3390/ijerph16183417.

Çınar, S., Ay, A., & Boztepe, H. (2018). *Çocuk Sağlığı ve Sağlık Okuryazarlığı* [Children's Health and Health Literacy]. *Sağlıkta Performans ve Kalite Dergisi*, 14(2), 25-39.

Çoban, T., & Özcebe, H. (2019). The Role of Health Literacy in Improving Health in Children. *Turkish Journal of Public Health,* 17(3), 337-349. https://doi.org/10.20518/tjph.464542.

Çopurlar, C. K., & Kartal, M. (2016). What is Health Literacy? How to Assess? Why is it Important?. *Turkish Journal of Family Medicine and Primary Care*, 10(1).

Davis, T. C., Wolf, M. S., Arnold, C. L., Byrd, R. S., Long, S. W., Springer, T., Kennen, E., & Bocchini, J. A. (2006). Development and Validation of the Rapid Estimate of Adolescent Literacy in Medicine (REALM-Teen): A Tool to Screen Adolescents for Below-Grade Reading in Health Care Settings. *Pediatrics*, 118(6), e1707–e1714. https://doi.org/10.1542/peds.2006-1139.

de Buhr, E., Ewers, M., & Tannen, A. (2020). Potentials of School Nursing for Strengthening the Health Literacy of Children, Parents, and Teachers. *International Journal of Environmental Research and Public Health*, 17(7), 2577. https://doi.org/10.3390/ijerph17072577.

Demirköse, H., Yapar, D., & Özkan, S. (2021). The Health Literacy Levels of Mothers with 0-6 Year Old Children and Their Relationship with the Incidence of Home Accidents in Children. *ESTÜDAM Journal of Public Health*, 31(2), 74-82.

Deniz, S., Bentli, R., Kalkanlı, M. T., Fırıncı, B., Yalınız, F., Demir, E., ... & Akbaba, M. (2020). Determination of the Health Literacy Levels and Related Factors of Teachers Working in Malatya Province. *Sakarya Medical Journal*, 10(1), 28-36.

Fretian, A., Bollweg, T. M., Okan, O., Pinheiro, P., & Bauer, U. (2020). Exploring Associated Factors of Subjective Health Literacy in School-Aged Children. *International Journal of Environmental Research and Public Health*, 17(5), 1720. https://doi.org/10.3390/ijerph17051720.

Guo, S., Yu, X., Davis, E., Armstrong, R., & Naccarella, L. (2022). Comparison of Health Literacy Assessment Tools Among Beijing School-Aged Children. *Children (Basel, Switzerland)*, 9(8), 1128. https://doi.org/10.3390/children9081128.

Güler, R. (2022). *Okul Çağı Çocuklarında Sağlık Okuryazarlığı ve Okul Sağlığı Hemşireliği* [Health Literacy in School-Aged Children and School Health Nursing]. *Genel Sağlık Bilimleri Dergisi*, 4(3), 330-338.

Güner, A. E., Şahin, E., Peksu, S., Şengül, K. S., & Güngör, M. (2020). A Study to Determine the Health Literacy Levels of Classroom Teachers, Knowledge, Attitude, Behavior Change, and Educational Needs. *Turkey Health Literacy Journal*, 1(1), 58-76.

Health Literacy in Schools. (2020). *School for Health in Europe Factsheet No:6.* https://www.schoolsforhealth.org/sites/default/files/editor/fact-sheets/factsheet-2020-english.pdf.

Hoffman, S., Marsiglia, F. F., Nevarez, L., & Porta, M. (2017). Health Literacy Among Youth in Guatemala City. *Social Work in Public Health*, 32(1), 30–37. https://doi.org/10.1080/19371918.2016.1188741.

Kickbusch, I., Pelikan, J. M., Apfel, F., & Tsouros, A. D. (2013). *Health Literacy: The Solid Facts.* Copenhagen: World Health Organization Regional Office for Europe. https://www.euro.who.int/__data/assets/pdf_file/0008/190655/e96854.pdf?ua=1.

Kocataş, S., Güler, N., Yağmur, S., Kuzucu, C., & Akkaya, K. (2023). The Relationship Between Hygiene Behaviors and Health Literacy Levels of Secondary School Students. *Cumhuriyet Nursing Journal* 7(2), 39-50.

Liu, C., Wang, D., Liu, C., Jiang, J., Wang, X., & Chen, H. (2020). What is the Meaning of Health Literacy? A Systematic Review and Qualitative Synthesis. *Family Medicine and Community Health*, 8(2), e000351. https://doi.org/10.1136/fmch-2020-000351.

Muslu, L., & Kolutek, R. (2018). Childhood Cancers and Health Literacy. *Current Pediatrics*, 16(3), 117-132. https://doi.org/10.32941/pediatri.485585.

Nutbeam, D. (2000). Health Literacy as a Public Health Goal: A Challenge for Contemporary Health Education and Communication Strategies into the 21st Century. *Health Promotion International*, 15(3), 259-267. https://doi.org/10.1093/heapro/15.3.259.

Paakkari, L., Kokko, S., Villberg, J., Paakkari, O., & Tynjälä, J. (2017). Health Literacy and Participation in Sports Club Activities Among Adolescents. *Scandinavian Journal of Public Health*, 45(8), 854–860. https://doi.org/10.1177/1403494817714189.

Paakkari, L., Torppa, M., Mazur, J., Boberova, Z., Sudeck, G., Kalman, M., & Paakkari, O. (2020). A Comparative Study on Adolescents' Health Literacy in Europe: Findings from the HBSC Study. *International Journal of Environmental Research and Public Health*, 17(10), 3543. https://doi.org/10.3390/ijerph17103543.

Paakkari, O., Torppa, M., Kannas, L., & Paakkari, L. (2016). Subjective Health Literacy: Development of a Brief Instrument for School-Aged Children. *Scandinavian Journal of Public Health*, 44(8), 751–757. https://doi.org/10.1177/1403494816669639.

Qiao, H., Wang, X., Qin, Z., Wang, N., Zhang, N., & Xu, F. (2021). The Relationship Between Health Literacy and Health-Related Quality of Life Among School-Aged Children in Regional China. *Health and Quality of Life Outcomes*, 19(1), 262. https://doi.org/10.1186/s12955-021-01895-6.

Ran, M., Peng, L., Liu, Q., Pender, M., He, F., & Wang, H. (2018). The Association Between Quality of Life (QOL) and Health Literacy Among Junior Middle School Students: A Cross-Sectional Study. *BMC Public Health*, 18(1), 1183. https://doi.org/10.1186/s12889-018-6082-5.

Sørensen, K., Van den Broucke, S., Fullam, J., Doyle, G., Pelikan, J., Slonska, Z., Brand, H., & (HLS-EU) Consortium Health Literacy Project European. (2012). Health Literacy and Public Health: A Systematic Review and Integration of Definitions and Models. *BMC Public Health*, 12, 80. https://doi.org/10.1186/1471-2458-12-80.

Şenyurt, Ö. (2021). The Place of Health Literacy in Curricula: Increasing Importance of Libraries and Librarians. *Information Management,* 4(2), 264-282. https://doi.org/10.33721/by.933441.

Türkoğlu, N., & Kılıç, D. (2021). Adaptation of the Health Literacy Scale to Turkish: A Validity and Reliability Study. *Anatolian Journal of Nursing and Health Sciences*, 24(1), 25-33. https://doi.org/10.17049/ataunihem.662054.

Üstündağ, A. (2020). Examining School-Aged Children's Health Literacy Knowledge Levels. *Journal of Human and Social Sciences*, 3(2), 567-577. https://dergipark.org.tr/tr/download/article-file/1247561

Vamos, S., Okan, O., Sentell, T., & Rootman, I. (2020). Making a Case for "Education for Health Literacy": An International Perspective. *International Journal of Environmental Research and Public Health*, 17(4), 1436. https://doi.org/10.3390/ijerph17041436.

Yilmazel, G., & Cetinkaya, F. (2015). Health Literacy Among Schoolteachers in Çorum, Turkey. *Eastern Mediterranean Health Journal La Revue de Santé de la Méditerranée Orientale*, 21(8), 598–605. https://doi.org/10.26719/2015.21.8.598.

Chapter 17

The Assessment of Health in School-Age Children

Asiye Kartal*, **PhD**
and Edanur Özkaya Bozkurt, MSc
Department of Public Health Nursing, Faculty of Health Science, Pamukkale University, Denizli, Türkiye

Abstract

School is an important environment where children come together apart from their family life. Health assessment in school-age children is crucial for development of a healthy life. Through the assessment process, school nurses can identify children's growth, developmental needs, and potential problems. Assessment of health contributes to early identification of problems, and health prevention and promotion. The primary method for assessment of school-age children's health history is through regular and long-term follow-up. Therefore, assessing the health of school-age children is a process that requires significant dedication and effort. When working with children, school nurses should conduct health assessments by considering developmental patterns appropriate for each age group to plan timely health interventions. In this chapter, health assessment is discussed under the headings of health history, physical examination, developmental characteristics, general examination, system evaluation, and mental health evaluation.

Keywords: assessment of health, health history, examination

Introduction

The health assessment process involves collecting both objective and subjective data, encompassing health problems, health-related practices, lifestyle choices, experiences, and perceived needs (Berman et al., 2022a, 2022b). Schools are the most appropriate settings to collect data and create preventive interventions and assessments for health promotion (Vaivada et al., 2022). Health assessment in school-age children contributes to the early detection of health problems and health promotion (Riley et al., 2019). Nursing interventions can be implemented by identifying risks, needs, and priorities based on the data obtained from health

* Corresponding Author's Email: akartal@pau.edu.tr

In: Health Promotion and Prevention
Editor: Eda Kılınç İşleyen
ISBN: 979-8-89530-758-8

assessment (Berman et al., 2022a, 2022b). The school-age period is an important time for conducting health assessments and fostering the development of a healthy lifestyle. Through this process, school nurses can identify the growth patterns, developmental needs, and potential health problems of school-age children (Berman et al., 2022c).

The school-age period covers from 6 to 12 years (Berman et al., 2022c; Chiocca, 2020a). As children transition from childhood to adolescence, they require healthy physical, sexual, psychological, and neurocognitive development (WHO, 2021). Globally, children and adolescents experience similar problems, including unintentional injury, sexual and reproductive health problems, interpersonal violence, infectious diseases, mental health conditions, and non-communicable diseases. Furthermore, risky behaviors such as alcohol and tobacco use, physical inactivity, and unhealthy dietary habits are frequently observed in these age groups (WHO, 2021). Studies have shown that the majority of the approximately 1 million global deaths among children aged 5-14 years in 2016 were preventable (Hill et al., 2015; Masquelier et al., 2018).

Patton and Azzopardi (2018) highlighted the lack of comprehensive data on school-age children aged 5-14 years in the literature (Patton and Azzopardi, 2018). The most effective way to obtain health-related data in school-age children is through regular and long-term monitoring and evaluation (Vaivada et al., 2022). Consequently, the health assessment of school-age children is a process that requires much dedication and effort. When working with this age-group, school nurses should assess health status while taking into account age-appropriate developmental patterns and plan timely, suitable health interventions (Sawyer et al., 2021). For these reasons, this section focuses on the health assessment of school-age children.

Assessment of Health in School-Age Children

Reviewing a Health History

The first step in a health assessment of school-age children involves reviewing their health history, which provides essential insights into their past and present health status. Reviewing the health history involves gathering information from the individual and other sources about the their health status, as well as their social, physical, emotional, developmental, cultural, and spiritual conditions (Estes et al., 2020a). Therefore, the health history should be taken accurately and completely (Chiocca, 2020b). Since the data collected in the health history is subjective, reflecting what the individual communicates—such as attitudes, beliefs, and concerns—it can be verified through physical examination. Analyzing this information serves as the foundation for planning the necessary health education and highlights areas requiring attention during the physical examination (Estes et al., 2020a).

While reviewing the health history of school-age children, both family history and past and present health status are evaluated. If there is a current health history, complaints, signs, symptoms are identified. The type, location, severity, frequency, and factors affecting symptoms are assessed. Additionally, the status of chronic disease, previous illnesses, injuries, and surgical operations are assessed. Furthermore, allergy status, medications, immune status, growth and development are also evaluated (Foote, 2019; Jarvis and Eckhardt, 2020a).

A family history reveals diseases and conditions to which the child may be at high risk. The health of family members is important as it highlights the child's prolonged exposure to infectious diseases or environmental hazards such as tobacco smoke. A family history can lead to early screening and periodic medical follow-up when there are risk factors for a specific disease.

In conclusion, the assessment of health in school-age children is a critical process that involves reviewing both their health history and physical condition. By considering factors such as family history, past illnesses, and current health status, healthcare providers can ensure early detection of potential health issues and promote the overall well-being of children. Regular health assessments also contribute to the creation of individualized care plans, fostering better health outcomes and supporting a healthy school environment (Foote, 2019; Jarvis and Eckhardt, 2020a).

Considerations When Reviewing a Health History

Firstly, it is essential to provide an appropriate physical environment. The room should have enough seating for everyone, be clean, well-lit, maintained at a comfortable temperature, free from noise, and arranged to ensure the safety of school-age children (Chiocca, 2020b). The school nurse responsible for reviewing the health history of school-age children should possess well-developed communication skills. Effective communication forms the basis for a trusting relationship and makes both the parent and the child feel valued. During interviews with the child and parents, questions should be posed in a non-judgmental, and unhurried manner, while minimizing interruptions to promote open and honest communication. The school nurse should remain seated when reviewing the child's health history, demonstrating that sufficient time allocated for the child and parent, and emphasizing a genuine interest in their perspectives. Safeguarding confidentiality and privacy throughout the interview is important for increasing trust. Furthermore, it is essential that the questions posed are fully comprehended; therefore, the use of medical terminology should be minimized to ensure clarity (Balog et al., 2014; Chiocca, 2020b).

When developmentally appropriate, school-age children should be included in the interview process. This provides the school nurse to assess the language, social, and health-related comprehension of the school-age children (Balog et al., 2014). Moreover, this inclusive approach provides insights into the child's overall behavior, temperament, cognitive and intellectual abilities. It also prepares the child to be an active, lifelong participant in their own healthcare. Initially, it is important to start the interview with the parent present to ensure the child feels comfortable and safe. School-age children have an increased need for privacy as they approach adolescence. Therefore, when discussing sensitive topics such as their sexual activity, drug or alcohol use, or risk-taking behaviors, the parent should be requested to leave the room. Without a parent there, adolescents are more likely to provide honest and accurate responses. However, before delving into these sensitive areas, the school nurse should first engage the school-age children with general questions about such as school, friends, activities, hobbies, and interests to build rapport (Balog et al., 2014; Chiocca, 2020b).

Physical Examination

A physical examination is a crucial component in the assessment of child health. During the physical examination phase, objective data gathered using a variety of testing procedures. An accurate and comprehensive health history is essential for guiding the physical examination (Chiocca, 2020c; Estes et al., 2020c).

To reduce gaps in the assessments of body system, it is recommended that a comprehensive physical examination be conducted systematically from head to toe. However, this sequence should be adapted according to the child's age, health status, and developmental stage. School-age children can easily adapt to a head-to-toe physical examination (Chiocca, 2020a, 2020c).

Considerations When Performing a Physical Examination

The physical examination area should be well lit, maintained at an appropriate temperature, and decorated in an age-appropriate manner. Additionally, the examination area should be child-proofed, and all medical equipment should be kept out of the school-age children's direct line of sight until it is required for use. Age-appropriate reading materials and toys should be readily accessible within the examination area to support developmental assessment and provide distraction as needed. Furthermore, the preservation of each child's privacy must be rigorously maintained throughout all stages of the clinical encounter to promote a sense of safety and trust (Chiocca, 2020c; Estes et al., 2020c).

Advanced physical examination skills, combined with a thorough understanding of school-age children's developmental stages, are essential competencies for school nurse. Core assessment techniques include inspection, palpation, percussion, and auscultation, each of which plays a critical role in obtaining accurate health data (Chiocca, 2020c). Before the assessment begins, school-age children should be given the opportunity to handle the equipment to ensure they will not experience any pain. For example, allowing the child to listen to the heartbeat of the school nurse or a parent often helps to alleviate anxiety. During the physical assessment, the nurse should clearly explain each step to the child. It is important to maintain honesty and inform the child in advance if any part of the physical assessment may cause discomfort. The least distressing part of the physical examination should be performed first, while the most upsetting or potentially painful components should be conducted at the end (Chiocca, 2020c; Estes et al., 2020b).

General Examination

The child's mobility, posture, facial expressions, behavior, level of consciousness, attitude, nutritional status, hygiene, and interpersonal interactions with school nurses and parents are assessed. Additionally, the child's developmental stage, speech, and motor skills should be evaluated and compared with age-appropriate norms. An evaluation of the child's general appearance also includes a brief assessment of their respiratory status and skin color. The child should exhibit no signs of respiratory distress and should have a healthy pink coloration. If the school-age children appear to be in discomfort, this should be noted, along with any visible injuries. The child's current mental and physical health status can often be inferred from their facial expression. Facial expressions can convey a range of emotions, including respiratory distress, pain, fear, worry, sadness, or despair. As a child's emotion changes, their facial features typically reflect these shifts in expression (Chiocca, 2020b, 2020c; Estes et al., 2020b).

The child's posture should be upright and balanced, with the back straight. They should also walk proper posture and maintain normal balance. During the general examination, any changes in limb mobility or limitations should be assessed. A quick inspection of the child's nails, hair, skin, and teeth is also necessary. Ideal conditions include skin and hair that are clean and well-groomed, smooth nails, and teeth that are free from cavities. Overall, the child should appear healthy, with appropriate height, weight, muscle tone, and mass (Chiocca, 2020b, 2020c).

Developmental Characteristics of School-Age Children

Physical Development

The school-age children experience rapid weight gain, with individual variations becoming more apparent due to environmental and genetic factors (Berman et al., 2022c). During this period, significant development occurs in gross motor skills (such as running, jumping, climbing, cycling, and general coordination), fine motor skills (such as tying shoelaces, using scissors, writing letters and numbers, and drawing pictures), and language skills (including vocabulary expansion, verbal ability, telling time, and reading proficiency) (Foote, 2019; Jarvis and Eckhardt, 2020a).

Anthropometric Measurements

Measuring physical growth of school-age children is crucial for assessing their current health status. Common physical growth parameters include arm circumference, height, and weight. Plotting these measurements on percentile charts enables comparison of the child's growth patterns with those of the general population. Body Mass Index (BMI) is used to assess the risk of overweight and obesity in school-age cgildren aged (Chiocca, 2020c; Foote, 2019).

The Centers for Disease Control and Prevention (CDC) has developed specialized growth charts to monitor very high BMI values in children and adolescents by adding extended reference curves. These modified growth charts also include percentile curves up to 20 years of age (CDC, 2022b, 2022c). School-age children at risk of obesity or growth retardation should have their growth closely monitored. Growth retardation should be evaluated periodically, as it may indicate an underlying illness or nutritional deficiency. Additionally, obesity can lead to significant physical and mental health problems (Chiocca, 2020c; Foote, 2019). problems (Chiocca, 2020c; Foote, 2019).

Weight

The weight of a child is a critical indicator of their general health. Boys weigh around 21 kg at the age of six, approximately 1 kg more than girls. School-age children, between six and twelve years of age, typically gain approximately 3.2 kg of weight per year. The most significant weight gains occur between the ages of 10-12 for boys and 9-12 for girls. By the age of 12, the average weight for both boys and girls are approximately 40-42 kg, with girls generally being heavier at this stage. If the child has developed regular physical activity and a healthy diet during earlier growth periods, overweight and obesity are less likely to occur at this age (Berman et al., 2022c; Foote, 2019). The CDC recommends using BMI as a guideline to monitor weight after two years of age (CDC, 2022c).

Height

At the age of six, both boys and girls are approximately 115 cm tall. By the age of twelve, their height typically reaches around 150 cm. A growth spurt occurs before puberty, between the ages of 10 and 12 in girls and between 12 and 14 in boys. As a result,, girls may be taller than boys around the age of twelve. Generally, the extremities grow more rapidly than the trunk during this period, causing the bodies of school-age children to appear somewhat disproportionate (Berman et al., 2022c; Foote, 2019).

Body Mass Index

Measuring a child's BMI is considered a routine practice for the early identification of overweight and obesity. BMI provides a guideline to determine a healthy weight based on the child's height. It is calculated by dividing the child's weight in kilograms by the square of their height in meters. Table 1 shows the standardized BMI values for children. For those older than two years, BMI should be plotted on the CDC's current age- and sex-specific growth charts. A BMI above the 85th percentile indicates the need for further assessment (CDC, 2022a, 2022c; Chiocca, 2020c).

Table 1. Standard values of BMI for children aged 2-20 years (CDC, 2022a)

Category	Percentile
Underweight	Less than the 5
Healthy Weight	Between 5-85
Overweight	Between 85-95
Obesity	Equal or greater than the 95

Cognitive Development

According to Piaget, the school-age period is characterized as the stage of concrete operations, during which abstract ideas are not yet fully understood. School-age children at this stage develop an understanding cause-and-effect relationships and are able to consider the perspectives of others. They become more objective and realistic, displaying a strong curiosity about how things work and why actions are taken. School-age children begin to recognize that their behaviors can influence others. They are capable of processing significant amounts of information by using symbols to represent objects and events. Thinking during this period becomes more stable and logical. School-age children can evaluate multiple aspects of a situation to reach a conclusion, although their reasoning abilities remain still limited (Berman et al., 2022c; Jarvis and Eckhardt, 2020b).

Psychosocial Development

According to Erikson, the psychosocial developmental stage of school-age children is characterized by industry versus inferiority. During this stage, children strive to achieve success through effort and perseverance but are at risk of developing feelings of inadequacy if they experience repeated failure. Children who have experienced success in earlier developmental stages are more likely to work diligently and collaborate effectively with others to shared goals. Freud defines the period between the ages of 6 and 12 as the latency stage, during which academic and physical pursuits are prioritized. Although sexual impulses are largely repressed during this time, children may still show curiosity about sexual topics. It is important to recognize children's knowledge and emotions related to these subjects and provide appropriate guidance to help them cope and develop healthily (Berman et al., 2022c; Rodgers, 2019).

As school-age children grow older, they develop the ability to play cooperatively with others. Throughout the process of socialization, they learn to work more effectively in groups. During this period, their self-concept continues to develop as they increasingly compare themselves to their peers. Bullying can have a profoundly negative impact on psychological development (Ali et al., 2016; Berman et al., 2022c; Rodgers, 2019).

Spiritual Development

As school-age children grow older, they enter the mythic-literal stage of psychological development. During this stage, school-age children learn to distinguish between fiction and reality, with fiction referring to the thoughts and images formed in their minds. Fiction is the thoughts and images that form in the child's mind. Parents help their children separate fact from fiction. School-age children may also have many questions about God and religion. Parents should support their child's spiritual development by answering their questions. When provided with religious education, most children at this stage are ready to apply reasoning rather than relying solely on blind faith (Berman et al., 2022c; Papaleontiou-Louca, 2016).

Physiological Measurements

Vital signs, or physiological measurements, are essential indicators of a child's physical health. These include blood pressure, heart rate, body temperature, and respiration rate. It is recommended that the child's vital signs be compared both with standard age-specific values and with the child's previous baseline measurements (Chiocca, 2020c; Foote, 2019).

Temperature

Fever is a common symptom in children and often indicates an underlying medical condition. Infections are the most frequent cause of fever in otherwise healtly children. Body temperature can be measured orally, tympanically, axillary, temporally, or rectally. If the measurement exceeds 101°F (38.3°C), it is recommended that the temperature be checked for accuracy (Chiocca, 2020c).

Pulse

Assessing peripheral pulses is important for identifying circulatory abnormalities. Key peripheral pulses include the popliteal, pedal, radial, and femoral pulses. In school-age children, the pulse rate typically ranges from 75 to 120 beats per m,nute between the ages of 5 and 8 years, and from 50 to 90 beats per minute after the age of 10, approaching adult valuee (Berman et al., 2022d; Chiocca, 2020c).

Respiration

Respiratory assessment includes observation of the rate, rhythm, depth, and effort of breathing. Respirations should be regular in rhythm, normal in depth, and symmetrical in chest expansion. Breathing should appear unlabored and fluid. The normal respiratory rate ranges from 20 to 24 breaths per minute at age 6, and decreases to 16 to 22 breaths per minute by age 12 (Chiocca, 2020c; Jarvis and Eckhardt, 2020d).

Blood Pressure (BP)

Primary hypertension in adolescents and children is on the rise due to the significantly higher prevalence of overweight and obesity in childhood (Flynn et al., 2017). Updated BP charts include sex, age, height, and 50th, 90th, 95th, and 99th percentiles (NHLBI, 2012). CDC growth charts are used to determine the child's height percentile (CDC, 2022b). Based on the child's age and height percentile, the measured systolic and diastolic blood pressure values are compared to the CDC reference tables. Blood pressure below the 90th percentile is considered normotensive. If the BP is at or above the 90th percentile, the measurement should be repeated elevated BP. Measurements between the 90th and 95th percentile indicate prehypertension and require further assessment and consideration of additional risk factors. Additionally, if an adolescent's BP exceeds 120/80 mm Hg, it may be classified as prehypertension, even if it falls below the 90th percentile. Blood pressure at or above the 95th percentile suggests hypertension, and at least two additional measurements are necessary to confirm the diagnosis (Foote, 2019; NHLBI, 2012).

Pain

Self-reporting remains the most reliable indicator of pain in school-age children. Between the ages of 7 and 10, children develop cognitive abilities such as measuring, classifying, and sorting, which enables them to use a numerical rating scale for pain assessment. Therefore, most school-age children have the cognitive ability to use a numerical rating scale. Many self-report pain rating scales are available (Manworren and Stinson, 2016). There are many different "face" scales for measuring pain intensity. Children of all ages can point to the face representing pain intensity to report their pain (Quinn et al., 2014). For children aged 8 years and older, several numerical rating scales are appropriate. The 0 to 10 numerical scale is widely used in clinical practice due to its simplicity (Bailey et al., 2010). Alternatively, the visual analog scale which is typically a continuous scale ranging from 0 to 10 or 0 to 100. Additionally, word graph scales, such as "no pain" and "very much pain," are arranged along a line, provide a subjective assessment of pain intensity (Martin et al., 2019).

Assessment of Systems

Skin

The skin should be assessed for texture, color, temperature, turgor, moisture, rashes, and lesions. Typically, children's skin is smooth, slightly dry, and not oily or sticky. Tissue turgor or skin elasticity, is evaluated by gently grasping the abdominal skin between the thumb and forefinger, stretching it, and then quickly. In healthy children, the elastic tissue immediately returns to its original position, preventing the formation of wrinkles or blemishes. In contrast, in children with reduced skin turgor, the skin remains elevated for a few seconds before gradually returning to the abdominal surface. Skin turgor is considered one of the most reliable indicators of adequate nutrition and hydration (Chiocca, 2020c; Foote, 2019).

Head and Neck

The head is assessed for trauma, macrocephaly, microcephaly, and abnormalities in size and shape. Symptoms such as headache, dizziness, and limitation in movement are also evaluated. In the neck, the examination focuses on signs of pain, stiffness, torticollis, thyroid enlargement, or lymphadenopathy (Chiocca, 2020b; Foote, 2019).

Eyes

In school-age children, both eyes are able to focus simultaneously on a single object due to the coordination and maturation of ocular muscles. As a result of structural changes during development, preschoolers typically achieve 20/20 vision by school age, with full visual acuity usually established between the ages of 9 and 11 (Berman et al., 2022a). The eyes should be evaluated for issues such as sitting too close to the television or computer screen, blurred vision, bumping into objects, double vision, squinting, holding a book too close to the face, difficulty seeing the blackboard, frequent eye rubbing, photophobia, and the use of glasses or contact lenses. Additionally, assessments should be made for signs of strabismus, dizziness, excessive tearing, eyelid edema, ocular discharge, or infections (Chiocca, 2020b).

Ears

Auditory perception is fully developed in school-age children, allowing them to detect subtle differences in sounds. These children should be assessed for a history of ear infections, ear pain, ear drainage, surgical interventions, delayed speech, hearing loss, the date and results of the their most recent hearing examination, and symptoms of tinnitus (Berman et al., 2022b; Chiocca, 2020b).

Mouth, Nose, Throat, and Sinuses

The frontal sinuses become a common site of infection between the age of 6 and 10 years. School-age children should be assessed for frequent runny noses, obstructive sleep apnea, sinusitis, upper respiratory tract infections, nasal congestion, allergic rhinitis, mouth breathing, nosebleeds, snoring, and changes in the sense of smell (Chiocca, 2020a).

Regarding oral health, evaluations should include dental care practices, fluoride use, dental caries, age at the first dental check-ups, the date of the most recent dental visit, history of dental trauma, frequency of examinations, reports of toothache, oral candidiasis, sores in the mouth or on the tongue, mouth breathing, and bleeding gums. In terms of throat health, it is important to assess the history of tonsillectomy, presence of enlarged tonsils or infections, nasal discharge, sore throat, cleft lip or palate, difficulty chewing or swallowing, streptococcal infections, and hoarseness (Chiocca, 2020a, 2020b).

Thorax and Lungs

In school-age children, respiration becomes thoracic, similar to that of adults, and the respiratory rate aligns with adult values (Chiocca, 2020c). Assessment of the respiratory system should include evaluation for apnea, dyspnea, croup, stridor, pneumonia, chest pain, frequent respiratory infections, chronic cough, asthma, sputum production, wheezing, cystic fibrosis, cyanosis, or tuberculosis. Additionally, it is important to assess for dyspnea at rest or during exercise, skin reaction to tuberculosis skin tests, the date of the last chest radiograph, exposure to secondhand smoke, and decreased exercise tolerance (Chiocca, 2020a, 2020b).

Cardiovascular

Cardiac health in school-age children should be assessed for congenital heart defects, murmurs, chest pain, dyspnea on exertion, sweating, slow or decreased weight gain, fatigue, hypertension, tachycardia, tachypnea, palpitations, fainting spells, cyanosis, dizziness, cold extremities, edema, exercise intolerance. Additionally, conditions such as anemia, rheumatic fever, bleeding disorders, petechiae, pallor, bruising, lymphadenopathy, recent blood transfusion, and gums should also be evaluated (Chiocca, 2020b, 2020c).

Abdominal

Gastrointestinal health in school-age children should be assessed by monitoring symptoms such as dietary history, loss of appetite, nausea, belching, bloating, vomiting, abdominal pain, food intolerances, ulcers, and reflux. In addition, recent changes in bowel regularity, stool type and frequency, gastrointestinal infections, constipation, diarrhea, blood in stool, jaundice, use of laxatives, presence of fissures or pinworms, and anal itching should be carefully evaluated (Chiocca, 2020b, 2020c).

Liver

In children, the liver occupies a larger portion of the abdominal cavity compared to adults and may be palpated 1-2 cm below the right costae margin (Hockenberry et al., 2019). The liver typically reaches adult size and functions during puberty. In school-age children, the liver is usually not palpable. An enlarged liver may indicate right-sided heart failure and should be further evaluated (Chiocca, 2020a).

Lymph and the Immune System

Lymph tissue reaches adult size by around 6 years of age. It continues to grow and typically reaches its maximum size—about twice the adult size—between 10 and 12 years. Following puberty, lymphatic tissue rapidly decreases to normal adult size (Chiocca, 2020a). Signs such as pain, frequent infections, chills, tenderness or swelling in any lymph node, fever, night sweats, pallor, and hepatosplenomegaly may indicate problems with the immune system and should be carefully assessed (Chiocca, 2020b).

Kidney and Urinary System

Symptoms such as dysuria, frequency of urination, changes in urination patterns, urinary tract infections, enuresis, pyuria, discharge, hematuria, flank pain, oliguria, and polyuria may signal urinary system issues in children. If any of these symptoms are detected, the child should be referred for further evaluation (Chiocca, 2020b, 2020c).

Genital

In boys, a history of cryptorchidism, epispadias or hypospadias, scrotal swelling during crying, inguinal hernia, surgery, hydrocele, and sexually transmitted infections should be assessed. Additionally, testicular self-examination in adolescent boys is important. If the testicles enlarge before the age of 9.5 years, it could indicate early puberty (Chiocca, 2020b). In girls, it is important to evaluate for genital anomalies, vaginal discharge, abnormal vaginal bleeding, and genital infection. For those with signs of precocious puberty, the age at menarche, last menstrual period, menstrual duration, frequency, dysmenorrhea, and history of severe menstrual bleeding should be assessed (Chiocca, 2020b, 2020c).

Musculoskeletal

The school-age children should be assessed for their usual activity level, coordination, history of cramps or inflammation, fatigue, unusual movements, clumsiness, joint or muscle pain, ataxia, mobility problems, swelling, sprains, abnormal gait, back or joint stiffness, limping, spinal curvatures, and fractures (Chiocca, 2020a, 2020b).

Neurological System

By the age of 6, the brain reaches 90% of its adult size and reaches full adult size by the age of 12 (Chiocca, 2020a; Hockenberry et al., 2019). In assessing the neurological system, it is important to observe for general affect, paresthesias, ataxia, mood changes, tics, dizziness, tremors, unusual movements, memory loss, syncope, tingling, headaches, seizures, aphasia, or other speech problems, loss of consciousness, nightmares, unusual habits, and fears (Chiocca, 2020b).

Assessment of Mental Health

Behavioral Assessment

A child's behavior can often be the earliest indicator of a health issue, making behavioral assessment a crucial part of evaluation. This assessment includes observing the child's affect, mood, activity level, personality, response to parents, and any parental comfort measures. School-age children should be able to engage with the nurse, comply during the examination, and maintain eye contact. Separation fear or the lack of eye contact could signal signs of child abuse or neglect. However, in some cultural contexts, avoiding eye contact is considered polite and natural. Attention span is another important factor, as children at this age can usually collaborate, concentrate for brief periods, and follow basic directions (Berman et al., 2022c; Chiocca, 2020a; Foote, 2019). Behavioral and emotional issues can also arise during this stage, so school-age children should be evaluated for signs of breath-holding, sleep disorders, school failure, bedwetting, substance abuse, irritability, and social withdrawal. Additionally, they should be assessed for potential depression, eating disorders, or psychiatric problems that may manifest during this period (Chiocca, 2020b; Jarvis and Eckhardt, 2020c).

Conclusion

Health assessment in school-age children is a comprehensive process that requires regular evaluation to ensure the child's well-being and development. The health assessment process begins with gathering a thorough health history, which is then supplemented by physical examination. The school nurse should know the developmental characteristics of this age group to determine whether the findings obtained are normal or not. A developmental assessment that covers various processes provides a comprehensive view of the child's growth and well-being. Physiological measurements and an evaluation of all systems should be conducted to detect any signs of illness or abnormalities. Psychological assessment is equally vital, as behavioral and emotional health are central to overall well-being. Each stage of the assessment process requires considerable effort and professional knowledge. School nurses have important roles and responsibilities for regular and comprehensive health assessment in schools.

Disclaimer

None.

References

Ali, M. M., Virani, S. F., & Alamans, A. (2016). Bullying: It's impact on child's personality. *i-Manager's Journal on Nursing, 6*(4), 1.

Bailey, B., Daoust, R., Doyon-Trottier, E., Dauphin-Pierre, S., & Gravel, J. (2010). Validation and properties of the verbal numeric scale in children with acute pain. *PAIN®, 149*(2), 216-221.

Balog, E. K., Hanson, J. L., & Blaschke, G. S. (2014). Teaching the essentials of "well-child care": inspiring proficiency and passion. *Pediatrics, 134*(2), 206-209.

Berman, A., Snyder, S., & Frandsen, G. (2022a). Assessing. In A. Berman, S. Snyder, & G. Frandsen (Eds.), *Kozier & Erb's Fundamentals of Nursing Concepts, Process, and Practice* (pp. 190-211). Pearson Education Limited.

Berman, A., Snyder, S., & Frandsen, G. (2022b). Health Assessment. In A. Berman, S. Snyder, & G. Frandsen (Eds.), *Kozier & Erb's Fundamentals of Nursing Concepts, Process, and Practice* (pp. 570-650). Pearson Education Limited.

Berman, A., Snyder, S., & Frandsen, G. (2022c). Promoting Health from Conception Through Adolescence. In A. Berman, S. Snyder, & G. Frandsen (Eds.), *Kozier & Erb's Fundamentals of Nursing Concepts, Process, and Practice* (pp. 454-480). Pearson Education Limited.

Berman, A., Snyder, S., & Frandsen, G. (2022d). Vital Signs. In A. Berman, S. Snyder, & G. Frandsen (Eds.), *Kozier & Erb's Fundamentals of Nursing Concepts, Process, and Practice* (pp. 532-569). Pearson Education Limited.

CDC. (2022a). About Child & Teen BMI. Retrieved January from https://www.cdc.gov/healthyweight/assessing/bmi/childrens_bmi/about_childrens_bmi.html.

CDC. (2022b). CDC Extended BMI-for-age Growth Charts. Retrieved January from https://www.cdc.gov/growthcharts/extended-bmi.htm.

CDC. (2022c). Vital and Health Statistics. Retrieved January from https://www.cdc.gov/nchs/data/series/sr_02/sr02-197.pdf.

Chiocca, E. (2020a). Child Health Assessment: An Overview. In E. Chiocca (Ed.), *Advanced Pediatric Assessment* (3rd ed., pp. 3-20). Springer Publishing Company, LLC.

Chiocca, E. (2020b). Obtaining the Pediatric Health History. In E. Chiocca (Ed.), *Advanced Pediatric Assessment* (3rd ed., pp. 101-122). Springer Publishing Company, LLC.

Chiocca, E. (2020c). The Pediatric Physical Examination. In E. Chiocca (Ed.), *Advanced Pediatric Assessment* (3rd ed., pp. 153-176). Springer Publishing Company, LLC.

Estes, M. E. Z., Calleja, P., Theobald, K., & Harvey, T. (2020a). The complete health history including documentation. In M. E. Z. Estes, P. Calleja, K. Theobald, & T. Harvey (Eds.), *Health Assessment and Physical Examination* (3rd ed., pp. 51-83). Cengage AU.

Estes, M. E. Z., Calleja, P., Theobald, K., & Harvey, T. (2020b). The pediatric patient. In M. E. Z. Estes, P. Calleja, K. Theobald, & T. Harvey (Eds.), *Health Assessment and Physical Examination* (3rd ed., pp. 737-801). Cengage AU.

Estes, M. E. Z., Calleja, P., Theobald, K., & Harvey, T. (2020c). Physical Examination. In M. E. Z. Estes, P. Calleja, K. Theobald, & T. Harvey (Eds.), *Health Assessment and Physical Examination* (3rd ed., pp. 103-120). Cengage AU.

Flynn, J. T., Kaelber, D. C., Baker-Smith, C. M., Blowey, D., Carroll, A. E., Daniels, S. R., de Ferranti, S. D., Dionne, J. M., Falkner, B., & Flinn, S. K. (2017). Clinical practice guideline for screening and management of high blood pressure in children and adolescents. *Pediatrics, 140*(3).

Foote, J. (2019). Communication, Physical, and Developmental Assessment of the Child and Family. In M. Hockenberry, D. Wilson, & C. Rodgers (Eds.), *WONG'S Nursing Care of Infants and Children* (11th ed., pp. 80-132). Elsevier Inc.

Hill, K., Zimmerman, L., & Jamison, D. T. (2015). Mortality risks in children aged 5–14 years in low-income and middle-income countries: a systematic empirical analysis. *The Lancet Global Health, 3*(10), e609-e616.

Hockenberry, M., Wilson, D., & Rodgers, C. (2019). *Wong's Nursing Care of Infants and Children* (11th ed.). Elsevier.

Jarvis, C., & Eckhardt, W. A. (2020a). The Complete Health History. In C. Jarvis & W. A. Eckhardt (Eds.), *Physical Examination & Health Assessment* (8th ed., pp. 106-137). Elsevier Inc.

Jarvis, C., & Eckhardt, W. A. (2020b). The Interview. In C. Jarvis & W. A. Eckhardt (Eds.), *Physical Examination & Health Assessment* (8th ed., pp. 72-105). Elsevier Inc.

Jarvis, C., & Eckhardt, W. A. (2020c). Mental Status Assessment. In C. Jarvis & W. A. Eckhardt (Eds.), *Physical Examination & Health Assessment* (8th ed., pp. 139-162). Elsevier Inc.

Jarvis, C., & Eckhardt, W. A. (2020d). Vital Signs. In C. Jarvis & W. A. Eckhardt (Eds.), *Physical Examination & Health Assessment* (8th ed., pp. 241-261). Elsevier Inc.

Manworren, R. C., & Stinson, J. (2016). Pediatric pain measurement, assessment, and evaluation. In *Seminars in Pediatric Neurology* (Vol. 23, No. 3, pp. 189-200). WB Saunders.

Martin, S., Maxtin, M., Smalling, K., & Park, S. (2019). Pain Assessment and Management in Children. In M. Hockenberry, D. Wilson, & C. Rodgers (Eds.), *WONG'S Nursing Care of Infants and Children* (11th ed., pp. 137-169). Elsevier Inc.

Masquelier, B., Hug, L., Sharrow, D., You, D., Hogan, D., Hill, K., Liu, J., Pedersen, J., & Alkema, L. (2018). Global, regional, and national mortality trends in older children and young adolescents (5-14 years) from 1990 to 2016: an analysis of empirical data. *Lancet Global Health, 6*(10), e1087-e1099. https://doi.org/10.1016/s2214-109x(18)30353-x.

National Heart, Blood and Lung Institute. (2012). Integrated guide lines for cardiovascular health and risk reduction in children and adolescents. Retrieved from https://www.nhlbi.nih.gov/files/docs/guidelines/peds_guidelines_full.pdf.

Papaleontiou-Louca, E. (2016). Spiritual development in children and adolescents. *Weber Psychiatry and Psychology, 2*(2), 1-3.

Patton, G. C., & Azzopardi, P. (2018). Missing in the middle: measuring a million deaths annually in children aged 5–14 years. *The Lancet Global Health, 6*(10), e1048-e1049.

Quinn, B. L., Sheldon, L. K., & Cooley, M. E. (2014). Pediatric pain assessment by drawn faces scales: a review. *Pain Management Nursing, 15*(4), 909-918.

Riley, M., Morrison, L., & McEvoy, A. (2019). Health maintenance in school-aged children: part I. History, physical examination, screening, and immunizations. *American Family Physician, 100*(4), 213-218.

Rodgers, C. (2019). Health Promotion of the School-Age Child and Family. In M. Hockenberry, D. Wilson, & C. Rodgers (Eds.), *WONG'S Nursing Care of Infants and Children* (11th ed., pp. 460-494). Elsevier Inc.

Sawyer, S. M., Raniti, M., & Aston, R. (2021). Making every school a health-promoting school. *Lancet Child & Adolescent Health, 5*(8), 539-540. https://doi.org/10.1016/s2352-4642(21)00190-5.

Vaivada, T., Sharma, N., Das, J. K., Salam, R. A., Lassi, Z. S., & Bhutta, Z. A. (2022). Interventions for health and well-being in school-aged children and adolescents: a way forward. *Pediatrics, 149*(Supplement 6).

WHO. (2021). *WHO guideline on school health services.* Retrieved December from https://iris.who.int/bitstream/handle/10665/341910/9789240029392-eng.pdf?sequence=1.

Chapter 18

School Health Screenings

Eda Kılınç İşleyen[1,*], PhD
and Edanur Özkaya Bozkurt[2], MSc
[1]Uşak University, Faculty of Health Sciences, Department of Public Health Nursing, Uşak, Türkiye
[2]Pamukkale University, Faculty of Health Sciences, Department of Public Health Nursing, Denizli, Türkiye

Abstract

School age represents a critical period in a child's physical, cognitive, and social development. Timely health screenings during this stage are essential for preventing potential health problems and mitigating negative long-term consequences. Health screenings for school-age children are considered a fundamental strategy in preventive healthcare. According to the United States National Association of School Nursing (NASN), the core responsibilities of school nurses include conducting screenings, making appropriate referrals, and monitoring students' health outcomes. Screenings carried out by school nurses may target general well-being or specific conditions. Routine screenings commonly include measurement of vital signs, assessment of oral and dental health, height, weight, body mass index, vision, and hearing evaluations, posture assessments for conditions such as scoliosis, and screening for head lice. To ensure effectiveness, screening tests must meet essential criteria: they should be simple, acceptable to students and families, accurate, reliable, and valid. These features are simplicity, acceptability, accuracy, reliability, and validity. Screening tests that meet these criteria are selected and implemented in accordance with standardized protocols. School nurses are responsible for accurately performing and documenting screenings, identifying risks, initiating referrals, and ensuring follow-up and monitoring. Risks or problems detected in students are recorded, and then referral and monitoring are carried out. As a result, for the school-age child to have a healthy development period, risk factors should be identified and controlled at an early stage.

Keywords: school health, health screening, school nurses

* Corresponding Author's Email: eda.isleyen@usak.edu.tr

In: Health Promotion and Prevention
Editor: Eda Kılınç İşleyen
ISBN: 979-8-89530-758-8

Introduction

School screenings are crucial for supporting healt promotion of school-age children, identifying potential health problems, and providing early intervention (Bobo et al., 2012). Therefore, health screenings within the framework of school health programs have an important place. Health screening is defined as the evaluation of a group or population at higher risk for health problems, using disease-specific tests to provide treatment before complications and disability arise. School health screening is recognized as one of the seven core roles of school nurses (caregiver, health educator, counselor, case manager, advocate, investigator, screener for health conditions, and referrer) established by the National Association of School Nurses (NASN). (Akgül and Ergün, 2021; Bobo et al., 2012; Erol, 2016). Screenings, referrals, and follow-up activities are secondary prevention strategies to detect and treat health problems in their early stages, often before signs and symptoms appear. School health screenings are a key component of the Community/Public Health principle, one of the five core principles outlined by the NASN (Maughan et al., 2016).

The school nurse conducts health screenings to assess vital signs, height, weight, body mass index, vision, hearing, posture disorders (such as scoliosis, lordosis, kyphosis etc.), psychosocial development, hypertension, hyperlipidemia, anemia, oral and dental health, diabetes mellitus, head lice, and lead. Health screenings may also include evaluations for school-age children neglect and abuse, pervasive developmental disorders such as autism, attention deficit and hyperactivity, developmental characteristics (motor skills, speech, and social relations), and emotional development (Erol, 2016). For each of these areas, the school nurse should maintain detailed records of all screening results for each student (Pedersen Turner, 2016).

Essential Features of Health Screening Tests

For screening programs to be successful, the test or examination methods must be accurate, reliable, and easily applicable. A good screening test should effectively identify individuals with a condition and distinguish them from those who are healthy. According to Erol (2016), a suitable screening test should have the following features:

- Simplicity: The test should be straightforward, easily understood, and applicable by both healthcare providers and participants.
- Acceptability: The test should be well-tolerated, causing no physical or psychological trauma, and should be engaging enough to encourage participation.
- Accuracy: The test must be capable of correctly detecting the targeted disease or condition.
- Cost-effectiveness: Since screenings are typically applied to large populations, the test should be affordable and economically viable.
- Consistency (reliability): The test should produce consistent results when repeated under the same conditions, on the same individuals, and by the same observers.
- Sensitivity and specificity (validity): Sensitivity refers to the test's ability to correctly identify those with the disease, while specificity refers to its ability to correctly identify

those without the disease. An appropriate balance between sensitivity and specificity is essential.

Health Screenings in School-Age Children

Monitoring and supporting children's health and development during childhood increases their quality of life and reduces morbidity. Screenings conducted during this period represent the most fundamental preventive health services. By identifying and addressing health problems at an early stage, these screenings enable children to live healthy lives under conditions equal to those of their peers. Screenings for school-age children may vary depending on the child's age, health history, and individual needs (Aktürk, 2023; NASN, 2024). However, in general, common screenings include measurement of Body Mass Index (BMI), vision and hearing screening, oral and dental health screening, scoliosis screening, blood pressure screening, and screening for scalp lice. These screenings are important to monitor the child's health and detect potential health issues at an early stage. However, the exact content and frequency of screenings may differ based on the child's age, gender, health history, and local health policies (Nelson and Rajan, 2018).

Body Mass Index (BMI) Screening

To assess and monitor growth in school-age children, both height (see Table 1) and body weight (see Table 2) should be measured annually and evaluated using standardized references. Evaluations should be performed more frequently in children who have a disease or have a problem with height growth. Health issues typically manifest first in a child's growth, with deviations in growth curves often serving as early indicators. Deviations in the normal growth process can stem from various causes, including systemic diseases (e.g., malnutrition), gastrointestinal vdiseases, psychosocial issues (e.g., eating disorders), congenital disorders (e.g., Turner syndrome, intrauterine growth restriction), and endocrine system disorders (e.g., hypothyroidism, growth hormone deficiency) (CDC, 2022a; 2022b; Chiocca, 2020a; Erol, 2016).

To determine BMI percentile, the child's height and weight are assessed relative to age and gender using standardized growth charts. The body mass index on standardized growth charts is 85.-94. Children with BMI values between the 85th and 94th percentiles are classified as overweight, and those above the 95th percentile are classified as obese (see Table 3). Following these measurements, children identified as overweight or obese should receive counseling on lifestyle changes and balanced nutrition. When appropriate, a referral to a pediatrician or dietitian should be made. These children should be re-evaluated every 3 to 6 months to monitor progress (CDC, 2022a; Erol, 2016) (see Chapter 17).

Table 1. Height screening implementation steps (Erol, 2016)

Preparation
• Ensure that all necessary equipment is available and calibrated before beginning the procedure. • Preferably use a stadiometer; if unavailable, a fixed paper or wooden tape measure attached to a wall may be used. • A stadiometer provides the most accurate results and should be used when possible. • The device must have a flat, vertical surface with an attached measurement scale and a movable headpiece. • If the device includes its own platform, the student should stand on it; if wall-mounted, the student should stand on a flat floor surface. • Measurements should be taken with 0.1 cm (1 mm) precision. • Select an appropriate room or area that ensures privacy during measurement. • Ensure that students being measured cannot see or hear one another during the process.
Implementation
• Students should be brought into the room individually. • Shoes must be removed before measurement. • Ensure the student's head, shoulders, back, calves, and heels are aligned with the measuring surface, and the student stands comfortably upright. • Support the student's chin with the index finger and thumb to keep the head level, and instruct the student to look straight ahead. • Mark the height accurately on the measurement scale.
Evaluation
• Evaluate the measured height by calculating the percentile value according to the child's age.
Registration and Referral
• Record the child's height on the appropriate registration form. • Refer children who grow less than 5 cm annually. • Refer children whose height falls above the 95th percentile or below the 3rd percentile. • Monitor all referred cases regularly.

Table 2. Weight screening implementation steps (Erol, 2016)

Preparation
• Ensure all necessary materials are available and properly calibrated before starting the process. • Required equipment: A scale with 100-gram sensitivity. • Verify that the scale is properly set before each measurement. • Place the scale on a hard, flat surface. • Choose an appropriate environment or room for the measurements. • Students should be prevented from seeing or hearing each other's measurements to maintain privacy. • Select a time when children are not immediately post-meal for the most accurate results.
Implementation
• Students should enter the room one at a time. • Ask students to remove their shoes and any excess clothing before measurement. • Have the student stand with both feet evenly distributed on the scale platform. • Instruct the student to stand still and upright; incorrect posture may lead to inaccurate measurements. • Record the student's body weight from the scale.
Evaluation
• Assess the child's weight by calculating the percentile value according to age and gender.
Registration and Referral
• Record the child's weight on the designated registration form. • Children identified with weight concerns should receive increased attention. • Any child whose weight or BMI is below the 5th percentile or above the 95th percentile should be referred immediately for further evaluation. • Referred cases must be followed up and monitored regularly.

Table 3. Standard values of body weight for children aged 2-20 (CDC, 2022a)

Weight Status Category	Percentile Range
Underweight	Less than the 5
Healthy Weight	Between 5-85
Overweight	Between 85-95
Obesity	Equal or greater than the 95

Table 4. Vision screening implementation steps (Erol, 2016)

Preparation
• Various eye charts to assess visual acuity: *Snellen E chart* for children aged 3–6 years and *Snellen chart* for children aged 7 years and older. • Nails or adhesive materials to hang the chart. • Plastic or paper eye covers to occlude one eye. • Chair for the child and the practitioner. • Pointer or stick to indicate letters or symbols. • Measuring tape or meter stick to mark the distance. • Prepared record forms to document screening results.
Implementation
• Inform the student about the procedure in age-appropriate language. • Select a quiet room with natural lighting and no distractions. • Hang the Snellen chart on a non-reflective, plain wall at the child's eye level while seated. • Mark a distance of 6 meters (20 feet) from the chart. • Confirm that the lighting, chart height, and visibility are appropriate from the marked position. • Invite the students into the room one at a time. • Briefly inspect the eyes for visible issues (e.g., redness, discharge, strabismus). • Begin the test with both eyes open, starting at the 6th line on the Snellen chart. • Seat the child and ask them to read at least four letters or symbols from the line. • If the child cannot correctly identify at least 3 out of 4 symbols, move to the next larger line. • Start by covering the left eye gently (without pressure). Begin at the 20/80 line using the pointer to guide. • For older children, you may start at the 20/60 line. • Ask for one symbol from each subsequent line until reaching the 20/30 line. • Ask questions rhythmically and at a steady pace that the child can comfortably follow. • Praise the child for correct responses to maintain cooperation. • Mark and record the last line where at least 3 out of 4 symbols were read correctly. • Repeat the same steps with the right eye covered. • If the child wears glasses or contact lenses: • Perform the test both with and without corrective lenses. • A child is considered to have correctly read a line if they identify 3 out of 4 symbols accurately.
Evaluation
• 20/20 vision is considered normal for children of all ages. • 20/30 vision is acceptable for 5-year-old children; by age 6, full **20/20** vision is expected. • Visual acuity is defined by the last line in which the child correctly identifies at least 3 out of 4 symbols.
Registration and Referral
• Record the results for each eye and both eyes together on the vision screening form. • Children who do not meet the age-appropriate visual acuity standard should be referred for further evaluation. • In addition to visual acuity results, note any signs of eye abnormalities or complaints related to vision. • Monitor and follow up on all referred cases.

Vision Screening

Good vision is crucial for a child's academic success and overall well-being. Without clear vision, a child may struggle to read books, use digital devices, or see instructional materials posted in the classroom. Since the majority of learning is visually based, undetected vision problems can significantly hinder educational development. The school nurse plays a key role in secondary prevention by conducting vision screenings to identify children who may need corrective measures. Often, vision changes are subtle and go unnoticed until academic performance begins to decline. Therefore, early screening and intervention are critical. Vision typically matures by the age of 8, underscoring the importance of timely evaluations (Loschiavo, 2021). Research by Rodriguez et al., (2018) demonstrated that a school nurse-led, follow-up-focused intervention improved the effectiveness of vision screenings, allowing for earlier detection of visual impairments.

The most common test to measure visual acuity is the Snellen chart, which displays rows of letters in decreasing size (Table 4). During the screening: The child stands with heels aligned on a line 20 feet away from the chart. The nurse begins by testing the right eye, while the left is covered. Both eyes should remain open. Children who wear glasses should be screened while wearing them. If the child cannot read a particular line, the nurse moves up to the next larger line and continues until the child can read. Then, the nurse returns to smaller lines until the child cannot read a line. To pass a line, the child must correctly identify at least 4 out of 6 symbols. The same procedure is repeated for the left eye (Erol, 2016; Foote, 2019).

Hearing Screening

Hearing loss is the most common developmental disorder seen at birth. Because the auditory system is almost fully developed at birth, most states now require newborn hearing screenings to enable early detection. Despite this, the number of children identified with hearing deficits tends to increase throughout the school years. This highlights the critical role of the school nurse in the early identification, referral, and support of affected children. The primary goal is to detect and address hearing issues before they lead to academic, social, language or emotional difficulties (Loschiavo, 2021).

Hearing screening typically conducted using with an audiometer, especially for students in the first grade of primary school (Table 5). When necessary, it may also be performed during the preschool years or for children identified as being in high-risk groups. The American Academy of Pediatrics recommends annual hearing screenings from kindergarten through third grade, and then once again during middle and high school. If there is no response of 20 dB signal at any tested frequency or in either ear during the screening, the child should be referred to an ear, nose, and throat (ENT) specialist for further evaluation. In addition, children with known risk factors should be referred for specialist assessment regardless of their screening result (Bower et al., 2023; Loschiavo, 2021).

Table 5. Hearing screening implementation steps (Erol, 2016)

Preparation
• Prior to the screening, the student is informed about the procedure in an age-appropriate manner. • All required materials are prepared in advance. • A suitable room is selected and prepared for the screening process. • Visual and auditory distractions are minimized to ensure an optimal testing environment. • The screening area is arranged to prevent students from seeing or hearing one another during testing. • Ambient noise levels are reduced to ensure a quiet environment conducive to accurate hearing assessment.
Implementation
• The examiner positions themselves 30–60 cm away from the student, ensuring they are not in the student's line of sight. • The student is instructed to plug one ear with their finger. • Using a soft whisper, the examiner pronounces numbers with non-consecutive syllables and equal stress (e.g., "fourteen"). • The student is then asked to repeat the number heard. • The same procedure is repeated for the other ear.
Evaluation
• If the student correctly repeats the whispered number, their hearing acuity is considered within normal limits.
Registration and Referral
• The results of the hearing screening are documented on the student's health record form. • Students who are unable to accurately identify the whispered numbers are referred for further evaluation.

Mouth and Dental Health Screening

Schools and school nurses play an important role in promoting the oral health of students and their families. School nurses are responsible for coordinating oral health education for students, parents, and school staff. They serve as valuable resource for teachers implementing oral health curricula and actively conduct or facilitate oral health screenings and dental caries prevention programs. In addition, school nurses conduct or facilitate oral health screenings and dental caries prevention programs (NASN Oral Health Connections, 2021). Dental caries are largely preventable, and providing preventive oral health services in schools is critical to helping students remain healthy and academically successful (CDC, 2023). In a study conducted on school-age children (12-15 years), a four-month school health education program was implemented significantly reduced both gum issues and plaque accumulation (Bhardwaj, 2013). Oral and dental health screenings are conducted by school nurses in accordance with standardized procedures (Table 6). The outcomes are recorded and evaluated, and appropriate referrals are made based on the results (Erol, 2016).

Scoliosis Screening

Scoliosis is a musculoskeletal condition characterized by an abnormal lateral curvature of the spine. Depending on the angle and direction of the curvature, it may present as lordosis (inward curvature) or kyphosis (outward curvature) (Chiocca, 2020b). The primary goal scoliosis screening is to detect spinal deviations at the earliest possible stage, allowing for early intervention that may prevent progression and reduce the need for surgical treatment. Scoliosis screening is mandatory in many educational institutions and is usually carried out in students between the ages of 10 and 18. However, considering individual differences in physical development, earlier screening may be appropriate for some children (Loschiavo, 2021). In a large-scale study conducted by Zou et al., (2022), scoliosis screenings were performed on 45,547 school-aged children, and the prevalence of scoliosis was found to be 3.9%. These findings underscore the importance of early detection through school-based screening in reducing long-term health burdens for individuals and the broader community (Zou et al., 2022). School nurses play a critical role in this process by conducting routine screenings and ensuring appropriate referrals and follow-ups. Scoliosis screening is performed in accordance with established procedural steps, as outlined in Table 7 (Chiocca, 2020b; Erol, 2016).

Table 6. Mouth and dental health screening implementation steps (Erol, 2016)

Implementation Steps
Preparation
• In case of infection, it is useful, if possible, to assign a staff member to each scanner to record the results.
• Try to avoid screening immediately after a meal. If necessary, distribute sugar-free chewing gum to students before the screening.
Prepare the necessary materials: • A good light source (a suitable lantern or a lamp with a tilting neck) • Glove • Disposable wooden tongue spoon • Garbage bin and bag • Alcohol-based disinfectant • Charts, pens, a writing platform for each staff member, or an alternative method for recording. • A good light source is essential. LED lighting should be preferred. • The tongue spoon is used during the scanning to pull the inside of the tongue and cheeks so that the scanner can see the teeth; it is discarded after each use. • The student is informed and explained about the procedure.
Implementation and Evaluation
• The students take turns in the room.
• The student's oral mucosa and gums are checked with the help of an abeslang and a light source (redness, swelling, bleeding, etc.).
• The student's teeth are checked for internal-external and chewing surfaces.
• The learner moves the tongue so that the scanner can see the desired parts of the tooth, and if necessary, the scanner can gently push the tongue and the inside of the cheek with the tongue spoon. • With the help of the light source, dental defects are observed (tooth wear or an unexpected shape, abnormal tooth color, severe tooth dislocation).
Registration and Referral
• Problems with the students' oral mucosa and gums are recorded.
• Missing teeth, caries, and structural defects in the jaw are recorded. Record the students according to the following categories: 0- No obvious problems with teeth 1-There are observable dental defects in one or two areas. Their parents should be informed that dental treatment is needed. 2-There are observable dental defects in three or more areas. Their families should be informed that dental treatment is needed. • Indicate the areas where there are defects in the teeth by marking them on the quad chart (according to the student - upper right, lower right, upper left, lower left). • Any problems with the oral mucosa or gums that the screener sees should be noted and reported to parents.
• The notes should include the date and the name of the nurse who performed the screening.
• Parents and teachers of students with identified problems are informed.
• Students with identified problems are referred.
• Students are trained in oral and dental health.

Table 7. Scoliosis screening implementation steps (Erol, 2016)

Implementation Steps	
Preparation	
• The student is informed, and an explanation is given about the process.	
• Permission is obtained from the student to scan.	
• The environment is prepared to protect privacy (a section surrounded by a screen should be prepared, the area should be well-lit and ventilated, the temperature of the room should be 22-24 degrees, and male and female students should be screened separately).	
• The student is prepared for screening, leaving only underwear on. Shoes must be removed.	
Implementation and Evaluation	
Back view	The student should stand with his/her back to the person who will perform the scan. The student should stand upright, straight without bending the knees, and with the weight of the body equally distributed on both feet. Arms on their side and relaxed.
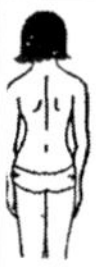	*Normal*
	The head should be in the center of the midline
	Shoulder level should be equal
	The shoulder blades should be at the same level
	Equal distance between arm and body
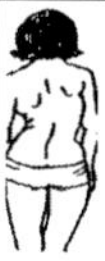	*Suspected scoliosis*
	The head is located on one side of the midline.
	One shoulder is higher.
	One shoulder blade is more protruding and higher.
	One hip is more prominent and protruding than the other hip.
	The pleats (folds) are deeper on one side of the waist than on the other.
	The distance between the arm and body is not equal.
Adam's Test	The student should stand away from the screener. The student should lean forward so that the waist is 90 degrees. Feet apart, knees straight, arms hanging comfortably on the sides with palms facing each other. The head is down.
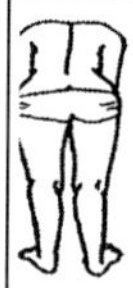	*Normal*
	The upper and lower parts of the back are symmetrical on both sides.
	Hips are flat and symmetrical.
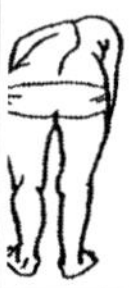	*Suspected scoliosis*
	The lower back and rib cage are not symmetrical.
	Spinal processes are irregular.
Front View	The student faces the screener and repeats the Adam's test.
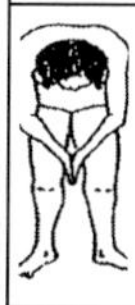	*Normal*
	Both sides are balanced and symmetrical in the upper and lower back.
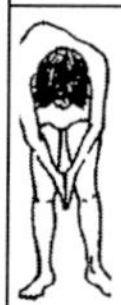	*Suspected scoliosis*
	The lower and upper parts of the back or both parts are not symmetrical.
Registration and Referral	
	The scan and findings are recorded on the recording form (such as the left shoulder higher than the right). Suspicious cases are referred. Referred cases are monitored.

Head Lice Screening

Head lice infestation (*Pediculus humanus capitis*) is a prevalent condition among school-age children globally, carrying both social and medical implications. Screening for head lice involves careful examination of the scalp and hair to detect the presence of live lice, nits (lice eggs), or scalp irritation. A key component of the screening process is distinguishing between lice, nits, and dandruff—misidentification is common, and the use of a magnifying glass and a fine-toothed comb may be necessary to ensure accuracy (NASN, 2020). Transmission of head lice occurs primarily through direct head-to-head contact. Because lice live their entire life cycle on the scalp, educating families about prevention is essential. Children with head lice may experience sensations of movement in their hair, and allergic reactions to lice bites can lead to itching and subsequent scratching. This can cause open sores, which may become secondarily infected. Additionally, head lice are more active in the dark, which can contribute to irritability and sleep disturbances (CDC, 2020).

Table 8. Head lice screening implementation steps (Erol, 2016)

Preparation
• The student is informed and explained about the process. • Prepare the materials to be used (abeslang, wooden applicator stick, disposable gloves, frequent tooth comb). • The screening environment is prepared. • Determine the appropriate environment (well-lit) or room for measurement. • The students to be screened are taken to the room one by one.
Implementation and Evaluation
• Wearing disposable gloves. • If the student's hair is tied/tangled, it can be untied with permission. • One or two tongue depressors are used to check the hair behind the ears, on the nape, and on the crown of the head for lice and nits. • To distinguish vinegar from dandruff, it is tried to be removed from the hair, if it is easily removed, it is understood that it is dandruff, and if it does not leave the hair and is bright in color, it is understood that it is vinegar. • Lice are concentrated in warm areas of the head. More attention is paid to the skin folds, behind the ears, on the nape, and under the crown. • Students who have only nits in their hair during combing can return to class. Contact the parents of these students and talk about how to treat lice and nits.
Registration and Referral
• Record if the student has lice or nits. • Students with live lice should stay with the nurse in the health office until they are picked up by their parents. If the students' siblings are in different classes at school, they will also be screened. Discuss with the parents the process of treating the lice. • The student is readmitted to school after being treated for head lice. Hair may be checked again before being admitted to class. • The student is followed up with the parent for 8-10 days. If the treatment is not positive, a second and different treatment is recommended. • 8-10 days after the second treatment, the family is contacted to see if there are still live lice or nits. If a live louse is still seen, it is referred. • Parents and teachers are informed if lice or nits are detected in the student. • Family members are educated on the prevention and treatment of lice/nits.

Head lice infestation is best diagnosed by finding a live nymph or adult louse on a person's scalp or hair (Table 8). However, due to their small size, quick movement, and aversion to light, live lice can be difficult to detect. The presence of viable nits attached within ¼ inch of the scalp may strongly suggest active infestation, though it is not definitive. In contrast, nits found farther than ¼ inch from the scalp are typically nonviable and do not require treatment. Nymphs may be misidentified as dandruff, hairspray residue, or dirt particles, further complicating diagnosis (CDC, 2020; NASN, 2020).

Screening should be conducted before hair washing, using a fine-toothed comb. Nits appear gray-white, about the size of a thread knot, and are difficult to remove. Adult lice are red-black and approximately the size of a sesame seed (Eisenhower and Farrington, 2012). When lice infestation is suspected, treatment orders for pediculicides and vinegar combing should be obtained. The nurse conducting the examination should wear appropriate personal protective equipment (PPE), such as gloves, an apron, and head covering (Anderson and Herring, 2019).

In addition to treating the affected child, it is important to assess other household members and provide family education on the use of personal hair care items and general prevention strategies. School nurses have a critical role in debunking myths about lice transmission and promoting non-stigmatizing, evidence-based management approaches. Such strategies aim to reduce unnecessary school absenteeism while supporting student engagement and academic success (NASN, 2020).

Conclusion

School health screenings are essential components of health promotion and disease prevention during school-age childhood. These screenings are carried out by school nurses to identify and address preventable health problems at an early stage. They are implemented regularly and systematically, following standardized procedures established by national and local health authorities. Common school health screenings include height and weight measurement, BMI calculation, vision abd hearing assessments, oral and dental health evaluations, scoliosis screening, and head lice screening. All these screenings are nurse-led, underscoring the pivotal role school nurses play in prevention and promotion of school-age children's health. It should be ensured that at least one school nurse is employed in every school all over the world to ensure that screening processes are not disrupted and are sustainable.

Disclaimer

None.

References

Akgül, E., & Ergün, A. (2021). School health nursing in the development of community health. *Journal of Public Health Nursing, 3*(2), 141-153.

Aktürk, Ü. (2023). School Health Nursing. In R. Aylaz & R. Hacıhasanoğlu-Aşılar (Eds.), *Public Health Nursing and Practices* (Ch. 13, pp. 293-310). Akademi Basın Publishing.

Anderson, C. E., & Herring, R. A. (2019). Pediatric Nursing Interventions and Skills. In M. Hockenberry, D. Wilson, & C. Rodgers (Eds.), *WONG'S Nursing Care of Infants and Children* (11th ed., pp. 678-735). Elsevier Inc.

Bhardwaj, V. K., Sharma, K. R., Luthra, R. P., Jhingta, P., Sharma, D., & Justa, A. (2013). Impact of school-based oral health education program on oral health of 12- and 15-year-old school children. *Journal of Education and Health Promotion, 2*(1), 33.

Bobo, N., Kımel, L., & Bleza, S. (2012). Promoting Health at School. In J. Selekman (Ed.), *School Nursing: A Comprehensive Text* (pp. 440-472). FA Davis Company. Ebook.

Bower, C., Reilly, B. K., Richerson, J., Hecht, J. L., Hackell, J. M., Almendarez, Y. M., ... & Spooner, S. A. (2023). Hearing assessment in infants, children, and adolescents: Recommendations beyond neonatal screening. *Pediatrics, 152*(3).

CDC. (2020). Head Lice General Information. https://www.cdc.gov/parasites/lice/head/gen_info/faqs.html.

CDC. (2022a). *About Child & Teen BMI.* Retrieved January from https://www.cdc.gov/healthyweight/assessing/bmi/childrens_bmi/about_childrens_bmi.html.

CDC. (2022b). *Vital and Health Statistics*. Retrieved January from https://www.cdc.gov/nchs/data/series/sr_02/sr02-197.pdf.

CDC. (2023). Oral Health. Retrieved January from https://www.cdc.gov/healthyschools/npao/oralhealth.htm.

Chiocca, E. (2020a). Assessment of the Musculoskeletal System. In E. Chiocca (Ed.), *Advanced Pediatric Assessment* (3rd ed., pp. 457-480). Springer Publishing Company, LLC.

Chiocca, E. (2020b). The Pediatric Physical Examination. In E. Chiocca (Ed.), *Advanced Pediatric Assessment* (3rd ed., pp. 153-176). Springer Publishing Company, LLC.

Eisenhower, C., & Farrington, E. A. (2012). Advancements in the treatment of head lice in pediatrics. *Journal of Pediatric Health Care, 26*(6), 451–461.

Erol, S. (2016). School Health Screenings. In S. Gözüm (Ed.), *Improving the Health of School Children* (pp. 146-149). Vize Publishing.

Foote, J. (2019). Communication, Physical, and Developmental Assessment of the Child and Family. In M. Hockenberry, D. Wilson, & C. Rodgers (Eds.), *WONG'S Nursing Care of Infants and Children* (11th ed., pp. 80-132). Elsevier Inc.

Maughan, E. D., Bobo, N., Butler, S., & Schantz, S. (2016). Framework for 21st Century School Nursing Practice. *NASN School Nurse, 31*(1), 45-53. https://doi.org/10.1177/1942602X15618644.

NASN Oral Health Connections. (2021). *Linking School Nurses to Health and Wellness Resources.* https://www.oralhealthconnections.org/home.

NASN. (2020). *Head Lice Management in Schools*. https://www.nasn.org/nasn-resources/professional-practice-documents/position-statements/ps-head-lice.

NASN. (2024). *Health Screenings and Immunizations*. https://schoolnursenet.nasn.org/covid19ref/screenings-immunizations.

Nelson, H., & Rajan, S. (2018). Barriers and Facilitators to Successful School-based Health Screenings. *Health Behavior and Policy Review, 5*(4), 57-71.

Pedersen Turner, L. (2016). The Nurse in School. In M. Stanhope & J. Lancaster (Eds.), *Public Health Nursing: Population-Centered Health Care in the Community* (pp. 914-936). Elsevier.

Rodriguez, E., Srivastava, A., & Landau, M. (2018). Increasing Screening Follow-Up for Vulnerable Children: A Partnership with School Nurses. *International Journal of Environmental Research and Public Health, 15*(8), 1572. https://doi.org/10.3390/ijerph15081572.

Zou, Y., Lin, Y., Meng, J., Li, J., Gu, F., & Zhang, R. (2022). The Prevalence of Scoliosis Screening Positive and Its Influencing Factors: A School-Based Cross-Sectional Study in Zhejiang Province, China. *Frontiers in Public Health, 10*, 773594. https://doi.org/10.3389/fpubh.2022.773594.

Chapter 19

The Management of Chronic Diseases in Schools

Leyla Muslu*, **PhD**
Department of Public Health Nursing, Akdeniz University Faculty of Nursing, Antalya, Türkiye

Abstract

The prevalence of chronic diseases in school-age children is increasing worldwide. A large proportion of children with chronic diseases are school-age children. Precautions should be taken to prevent the stigmatization of students with chronic diseases at school and to maintain their optimum level of health. Prevention of chronic diseases should focus specifically on the self-management abilities of these students, proactive strategies, and interventions for lifestyle change to prevent disease recurrence, progression, and long-term complications. These interventions can promote students' self-care capacities and health literacy and support the health and well-being of students and their families. Effective management of chronic diseases within the school setting requires collaboration with the school nurse, students, parents, school administrators, teachers, other school staff, healthcare providers, and the community.

Keywords: chronic diseases, tertiary prevention, school health, school nurses

Introduction

Chronic diseases are the leading cause of death worldwide (Alexander et al., 2022; World Health Organization (WHO), 2024a). The prevalence of children and adolescents with chronic diseases has increased in many countries in the last two decades (United Nations Children's Fund (UNICEF), 2024). Globally, more than 2.1 billion children and adolescents under the age of 20 are affected by chronic diseases. Approximately 1 million people under the age of 20 die each year from treatable chronic diseases, accounting for more than 15.85% of deaths in this age group (UNICEF, 2024a).

Chronic disease is defined as a condition that affects or is likely to affect a person's daily functioning for at least three months of the year, or that requires hospitalization for more than

* Corresponding Author's Email: leylamuslu@akdeniz.edu.tr

In: Health Promotion and Prevention
Editor: Eda Kılınç İşleyen
ISBN: 979-8-89530-758-8

one month per year (Pless and Pinkerton, 1975). Chronic diseases such as asthma, type 1 diabetes, epilepsy, obesity, cancers, and mental health problems, which are common in children, negatively affect children and adolescents' potential to attend school and participate in school activities and their growth and development. Risk factors for chronic diseases are lifestyle behaviors during childhood and adolescence. Today, 81% of adolescents do not get enough physical activity, 41 million children over the age of 5 are overweight or obese, and more than 90% of those under 15 breathe toxic air every day (UNICEF, 2024a). At the same time, these children and adolescents may also have chronic diseases as a result of various risk factors, including the socio-economic and environmental conditions in which their families live and work, poor dietary habits, and exposure to unhealthy products such as tobacco, alcohol, and foods high in fat, sugar, and salt. Many children and adolescents also grow up in environments that offer limited opportunities for physical activity that do not promote healthy behaviors, such as urban areas, unsafe roads, and high levels of air pollution (Center for Chronic Disease Prevention (CDC), 2022a; Peltzer and Pengpid, 2020; UNICEF, 2024a).

Children and adolescents with chronic diseases spend most of their day at school, as well as other children. Therefore, these students with chronic health conditions may face various challenges related to managing their illness in school (CDC, 2021; Thongseiratch and Chandeying, 2020). The school life and academic achievement of students diagnosed with chronic diseases are often hindered by factors such as hospitalizations, check-ups, treatment, and side effects of medications. It is reported that these students experience problems such as absenteeism or dropping out of school, negative school experiences, and low life satisfaction (American Academy of Pediatrics (AAP), 2021; Sentenac et al., 2023; Thongseiratch and Chandeying, 2020; Yetiş and Aylaz, 2021).

The health needs of students diagnosed with chronic disease can be complex, requiring both daily management and preparedness for potential emergencies (CDC, 2021). Effective management necessitates collaboration among school nurses, parents, students, school staff, and health institutions to ensure that students with chronic diseases receive equitable educational opportunities in a safe and supportive environment (McClanahan and Weismuller, 2015). It is important that students have access to the health services they need at school to manage their chronic conditions and to help them stay healthy and ready to learn. Improved chronic disease management is associated with increased school attendance, enhanced physical resilience, reduced symptoms burden, fewer limitations in participating in special activities. Therefore, it is essential to improve the delivery of health services in the school setting for students of all ages. School nursing plays a key role in addressing these challenges by providing critical support for students with chronic diseases (Davis et al., 2021; National Association of School Nurses (NASN), 2020). This chapter examines the most common chronic diseases in school-age children and their management strategies within the school context are described below.

Asthma

Asthma is the most common chronic respiratory disease in children (WHO, 2023). Asthma is often described as a heterogeneous disease that makes breathing difficult due to chronic airway inflammation and muscle tension. Symptoms can include coughing, wheezing, shortness of breath, and chest tightness (Global Initiative for Asthma (GINA), 2023). The majority of asthma-related deaths occur in low- and lower middle-income countries, where challenges in diagnosis and treatment persist (WHO, 2023). According to the latest Global Asthma Study (GAN), the global prevalence of asthma was 11% in children aged 6-7 years and 9.1% in those aged 13-14 years (García-Marcos et al., 2022).

Predisposing factors for asthma include low birth weight, prematurity, frequent early childhood infections, family history of asthma or allergy, obesity, physical inactivity, exposure to tobacco smoke, air pollution, house dust mites, and molds. Students with asthma are more prone to physical and emotional challenges, which may negatively impact academic performance and cognitive development. In addition, asthma-related complications often cause increased school absenteeism (Holst et al., 2020; WHO, 2023).

Asthma Management in School Settings

School nurses, school administrators, teachers, school staff, and parents working together to address risk factors for students with asthma and to prepare an appropriate school environment can improve asthma management. The following are the steps to be taken for asthma management at school.

- A healthy school environment should be created to reduce asthma symptoms by eliminating asthma triggers (e.g., tobacco smoke, chemical cleaning products, etc.) and indoor and outdoor pollutants.
- Daily management of asthma and emergency protocol should be established.
- Establish procedures that allow students with asthma to carry and use quick-relief medications (e.g., bronchodilators). Additionally, the school should have backups of these medications to ensure quick and reliable access.
- Teachers, students with asthma, and their families should be educated about recognizing asthma symptoms, appropriate asthma treatment strategies, common triggers to avoid, and effective management of asthma-related emergencies both at home and in the school setting.
- Individualized health plans (e.g., Emergency Care Plan, Individualized Education Plan) or intensive case management should be established for students with uncontrolled asthma.
- Measures should be taken to avoid stigmatization of children with asthma (e.g., education of other students about asthma, help in emergencies, etc.) (American Lung Association (ALA), 2024; Al Kindi et al., 2021; Szefler et al., 2020; WHO, 2023).

Diabetes

Diabetes is a chronic metabolic disease that occurs when the pancreas does not produce enough insulin, or the body cannot effectively use the insulin it produces. The most common is type 2 diabetes, which usually occurs in adults. Type 1 diabetes is more common in children. Around 1.1 million children and adolescents worldwide have Type 1 diabetes, and many do not have access to life-saving care and treatment (International Diabetes Federation (IDF), 2021; UNICEF, 2024a). In Turkey, there are around 30.000 children under the age of 18 with Type 1 diabetes, and at least 23.000 of them are school-age children (Diabetes in School Platform, 2022).

In Type 1 Diabetes, no single clinical feature is sufficient alone to confirm the diagnosis. The most distinguishing feature is younger age at diagnosis (<35 years), low BMI (<25 kg/m 2), involuntary weight loss, ketoacidosis, and glucose >20 mmol/L (>360 mg/dL) at presentation. Autoimmune β-cell destruction is present in 90% of patients, and non-autoimmune (idiopathic) β-cell destruction in 10% (Diabetes Mellitus Study and Education Group, 2022). In Type 1 diabetes, the pancreas produces little or no insulin on its own, and daily insulin therapy is required. Currently, blood glucose measurement 6-10 times a day, continuous glucose monitoring with a sensor, insulin injection 4 times a day, or insulin pump therapy based on this information is used in the treatment of patients with Type 1 diabetes. In addition, pancreas and islet transplantation, immunotherapy, antibody therapy, and stem cell therapy are promising new treatment approaches (Holt et al., 2021).

Diabetes Management in School Settings

Students with diabetes spend almost half of their time at school, making the school environment a critical setting for effective diabetes management. These students require consistent support from school nurses, administrators, teachers, and staff to manage their condition effectively during school hours (Diabetes in School Platform, 2022). When provided with adequate support, the risk of both short- and long-term complications from diabetes can be reduced. Additionally, this support helps ensure that students can maintain optimal academic performance, normal growth, and development (American Diabetes Association (ADA), 2024; An et al., 2022; Lindholm Olinder, 2022). The following items are essential in diabetes management at school:

- A policy and cultural environment that supports self-care for students, respects privacy, and prevents discrimination should be created in school.
- Students with diabetes should be supported in field trips, extracurricular activities, and all activities.
- It is important to educate and support students with diabetes to achieve diabetes self-management. Mostly, cognitive behavioral therapy techniques related to problem-solving, goal setting, communication skills, motivational interviewing, family conflict resolution, coping skills, and stress management should be used.
- The use of technologies such as insulin pumps and continuous glucose monitoring systems should be supported in diabetes management.
- To keep children with diabetes safe, they should have easy access to a measuring device, insulin, food (e.g., carbohydrate-containing food, fruit juice), water, and a toilet in case of emergency (e.g., hypoglycemia and hyperglycemia, etc.). Spare medicines and supplies should be available at school and should be easily accessible when needed (ADA), 2024; Diabetes in School Platform, 2022; Lindholm Olinder., 2022).

Epilepsy

Epilepsy is a chronic, non-communicable brain disease that affects people of all ages. Epilepsy, one of the most common neurological diseases in the world, affects approximately 50 million people (WHO, 2024a). It is reported that the prevalence in the age group under the age of 20 is 8.96% (Olusanya et al., 2020).

Epileptic seizures are the result of excessive and abnormal cortical cell electrical activity in the brain. Such discharges can occur in different parts of the brain. Seizures can range from the briefest loss of attention or muscle tremors to severe and prolonged convulsions. About 40 different types of seizures have been identified (Berg, 2010; Fleeman et al., 2022; WHO, 2024b). The cause is unknown in approximately half of the cases. It is stated that genetic predisposition and some environmental risk factors are effective in the occurrence of seizures (Beghi, 2020). Epilepsies of unknown etiology are more common in poor communities. This is probably a reflection of the increased multifactorial risk in these communities (Joseph D Symonds, Katherine S Elliott, 2021).

The diagnosis of the disease is usually based on the identification of persistent or recurrent seizures, and an Electroencephalogram (EEG) assessment can be useful (Minardi et al., 2019). Epilepsy is treated with antiepileptic drugs (AEDs), diet therapy, and surgery. In almost all patients with multiple seizures, medications are the first treatment option. They are highly effective and completely control seizures in the majority of patients (about 70%). Antiepileptic drugs can prevent the onset of seizures by reducing the tendency of brain cells to send excessive and mixed electrical signals (American Association of Neurological Surgeons (AANS), 2024).

Students diagnosed with epilepsy may experience physical problems (such as a slightly increased risk of fractures, bruising, and sudden death) as well as social problems due to stigma. At school, these students may experience absenteeism problems, restrictions, and limitations on their activities at school, which can negatively affect their academic progress and social and emotional development. These students and their families may experience social isolation, shame, fear, and discrimination (Fleeman et al., 2022; Johnson et al., 2021). Special approaches are needed for students with recurrent seizures, such as epilepsy, and their parents. The components of these approaches are the core issues and education, including self-management, medication adherence, and effective stress management (Leviton et al., 2023).

Epilepsy Management in School Settings

It is important to manage the disease and seizures of students with epilepsy at school and provide academic and social support (AAP, 2024; Minardi et al., 2019). What needs to be done for the management of epilepsy at school is listed below.

- Students with epilepsy, their parents, teachers, other school staff, and other students should be educated about the nature and treatment of epilepsy and first aid for seizures. These children need to have open airways during seizures and be protected from injuries caused by uncontrolled movements.
- Students with seizure disorders should be identified (e.g., spreadsheet, logbook), and their treatment compliance and self-management should be monitored.

- Students should be helped to avoid seizure triggers such as flashing lights and other triggers identified in seizure intervention plans.
- Students with epilepsy and their families should be informed about disability, medical conditions, and relevant laws.
- To prevent bullying against students with epilepsy, their peers must be educated about this disease, the fear of this condition must be minimized, and student behavior must be monitored. Students with epilepsy should be evaluated for comorbid cognitive and behavioral difficulties and provided with appropriate support (AAP, 2024; CDC, 2024a; Johnson et al., 2021; Fleeman et al., 2022; Leviton et al., 2023; Minardi et al., 2019).

Obesity

Childhood obesity is a global public health problem with significant impacts on children's health and well-being (Balasundaram and Krishna, 2023; WHO, 2024c). Childhood obesity is associated with increased morbidity and premature mortality, and its prevention is a high priority (Smith and Kobayashi, 2020; Balasundaram and Krishna, 2023). The word obesity means excessive accumulation of fat in the body. Body mass index (BMI) is used to indirectly assess body fat. BMI is measured using the formula [BMI= weight (kg)/height $(m)^2$]. As growth in children varies by age and gender, BMI norms also vary. The following definitions are used to classify the weight status according to the BMI of children aged 5 to 19 years. WHO recommends using BMI Z-score cut-offs of >1, >2, and >3 to define overweight, overweight, and obesity risk, respectively. The Z-score is measured in standard deviations from the mean. A child is considered obese if their BMI is higher than the 95th percentile (Table 1) (WHO, 2024d) (see Chapter 17).

Tablo 1. BMI-for-age (5-19 years) (WHO, 2024d)

Obesity	>+2SD (BMI equivalent to 30 kg/m^2 at age 19)
Overweight	>+1SD (equivalent to BMI 25 kg/m^2 at age 19)
Weakness	<-2SD>
Severe weakness	< >

The prevalence of childhood obesity is increasing rapidly worldwide. In 2022, more than 390 million children and adolescents aged 5-19 years are overweight; 160 million of them are obese. This has increased from 8% in 1990 to 20% in 2022 (WHO, 2024c). In the USA, 1 in every five children and adolescents are obese (CDC, 2022b). In a study conducted in Turkey, the prevalence of childhood obesity was determined at 15.7% (Alkan et al., 2022).

Chronic diseases such as obesity in children and adolescents are directly related to genetic and lifestyle behaviors such as taking certain medications, participation in physical activity and dietary preferences (e.g., consumption of sugary drinks, eating out), screen time, and sleep duration. Social determinants such as access to healthy, affordable food and beverages, lack of safe and appropriate places for physical activity and a supportive school environment, and cultural, socioeconomic, and environmental factors also contribute (Alexander et al., 2022; Mazur et al., 2022; Zavala et al., 2024). The consequences of childhood obesity can extend into later life and have a lasting impact on a child's life throughout adolescence and adulthood. These children tend to remain obese into adulthood and may develop diseases such as type II diabetes, high blood pressure, heart disease, sleep apnea, orthopedic problems, and asthma at a younger age. Obesity can also affect reproduction and increase the risk of certain cancers (Balasundaram and Krishna, 2023; WHO, 2024c). Obese students may be prone to develop psychological problems. Students who are obese often face stigmatization, low self-esteem, depression, and an increased risk of eating disorders (Sahoo et al., 2015).

Obesity Management in School Settings

Physical activity and healthy eating approaches carried out jointly with society, families, and schools, as well as students choosing the right and healthy foods at home, school, and in restaurants, and being active by exercising can be effective in protecting against obesity or overweight. What should be done to prevent overweight and obesity in students by promoting healthy behaviors in schools is explained below (Klein et al., 2023; Mazur et al., 2022; Sahoo et al., 2015).

- Physical education classes should be part of the school curriculum, and family activities such as physical activity, walking, or cycling should be planned. Active breaks should be encouraged at school with dance, music, competitions, and games, and adequate infrastructure and materials (e.g., balls, ropes, hoops, etc.) should be provided for physical activity.
- Increasing the availability of fresh foods such as fruits and vegetables in school canteens by developing guidelines that include a list of healthy foods (for example, breakfasts containing fruits and vegetables, no sugar-sweetened beverages, and eliminating the sale of unhealthy foods) (including ultra-processed products containing high amounts of sodium, sugar, fat, and calories) should be provided. Advertising and sponsorship of the unhealthy food and beverage industries should also be banned.
- It is recommended that the Ministries of Health and Education prepare and implement legal procedures (e.g., policies, laws, regulations, government agreements, or decrees focusing on school meals and health promotion in schools) for health promotion in the school environment (Nury et al., 2022; Pallan and Adap, 2023; UNICEF, 2020).

Cancers

Cancer is the leading cause of death in children. An estimated 400.000 children develop cancer each year. The most common types of childhood cancers include leukemias, brain cancers, lymphomas, and solid tumors such as neuroblastoma and Wilms' tumors (WHO, 2024e). In high-income countries, more than 80% of children with cancer are cured, but in low- and middle-income countries, only 30% of children with cancer are cured (Figure 1).

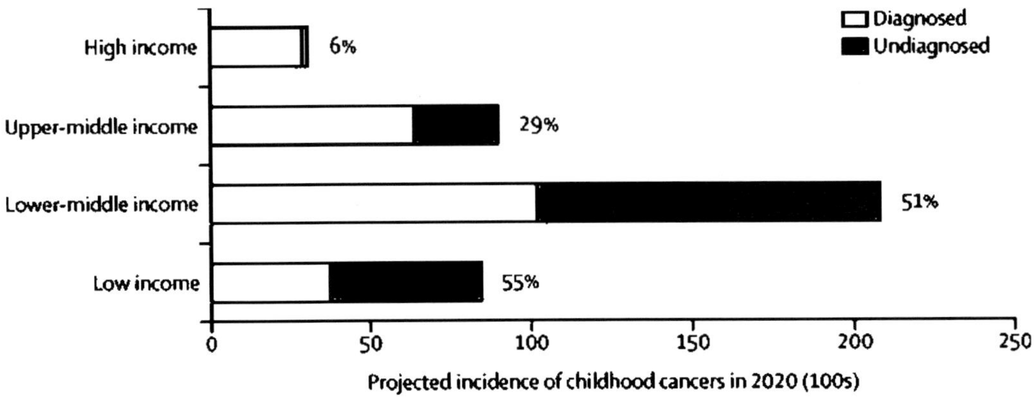

Figure 1. Predicted childhood cancer incidence in 2020 by country income group. (Altın et al., 2020).

Hereditary changes and environmental exposures such as smoking, asbestos, and ultraviolet radiation from the sun are known to be risk factors for cancer in these children (National Cancer Institute (NCI), 2023). Childhood cancer survivors are at risk of various serious physical, mental, and psychological health problems related to cancer and its treatment, as well as adverse socioeconomic conditions (Atun et al., 2020; Erdmann et al., 2021). This leads to academic difficulties and limited interaction with classmates. When these students return to school after cancer treatment, 50% of them experience social, psychological, or school-related problems, requiring 20% of them to repeat a grade (Bryan, 2021).

Cancer Management in School Settings

Collaborative efforts are needed for the care and long-term follow-up of students diagnosed with cancer. What needs to be done for cancer management at school is described below.

- Clinicians, teachers, and policymakers should be made aware of the diversity of students diagnosed with cancer, and early educational support should be provided for survivors.
- It should be developed effective interventions and policies to mitigate the harmful bio-psychosocial effects experienced by students diagnosed with cancer.
- Robot/digital technologies with the potential to help students diagnosed with cancer stay socially and academically connected with their classrooms during cancer treatment should be utilized. These interventions can improve children's daily hospital life and the organization of their care and treatment (Bryan et al., 2021; Weibel et al., 2020).

Mental Disorders

Childhood and adolescence are critical periods with a higher propensity for mental illness (McGorry et al., 2022). Mental disorders in children and adolescents are common but often overlooked around the world. These illnesses can significantly hinder their health, education, and ability to reach their full potential (Friedmann et al., 2022; UNICEF, 2021a). It is estimated that more than 13% of adolescents aged 10-19 have a mental disorder (WHO, 2024f). Anxiety and depression are among the most common mental health conditions in children and adolescents, accounting for around 40% of diagnosed mental disorders. Other mental health conditions in this population include attention-deficit/hyperactivity disorder (ADHD), conduct disorder, intellectual disability, bipolar disorder, eating disorders, autism spectrum disorder, schizophrenia, and various personality disorders. These diseases can have a profound impact on a child's social, academic, and emotional development. Proper diagnosis, treatment, and support are essential for helping these students manage their diseases and thrive in both academic and social environments (UNICEF, 2021b).

Mental health risks in students stem from adverse childhood experiences such as physical and emotional abuse, chronic neglect and violence, harsh parenting, severe socioeconomic problems, pressure to fit in with peers and explore identity, media influence, and gender norms, and disparities between their lived reality and their perceptions or aspirations for the future (Friedmann et al., 2022; WHO, 2024f;). It has been determined that the school attendance rates for students with mental disorders are lower than for their peers without disorders. Untreated mental health disorders in these students can have negative consequences ranging from poor educational attainment, unemployment and poverty, deterioration in physical health throughout life, substance abuse, juvenile delinquency and unemployment, and even early death (e.g., suicide) (Friedmann et al., 2022).

Management of Mental Disorders in School Settings

Mental health should be recognized as an important part of general health. Ensure that schools are kinder, safer places for students' mental health and are able to meet their social and emotional needs. Students and their families should be empowered to recognize, manage, and learn from difficult emotions. At the same time, solutions to the social determinants (economic and social barriers) of these students and families that contribute to poor mental health should be addressed (National Healthcare Quality and Disparities Report, 2022; UNICEF, 2021b). In order to develop an integrated, comprehensive support and service program for mental health at school, the following actions should be taken in collaboration with schools, families, and community mental health institutions (Figure 2).

- Programs should be developed to encourage students to cope with bullying and conflicts, solve their problems, develop healthy peer relationships, and engage in activities to prevent suicide and substance use by providing a positive school climate.
- Early intervention services should be developed for students who need additional support to cope with grief, anger, anxiety, sadness, etc.
- It should establish a school culture that promotes mental health literacy where teachers, other students, and school staff are trained to prevent stigmatization of students with mental health disorders and to recognize early warning signs of mental health problems in students.
- Treatment programs that meet the various mental health needs of students and social support resources for these students and their families should be provided.

- In digital media, health, or social care settings, schools should develop approaches that include a variety of strategies to reach students who are particularly vulnerable (CDC, 2024b; Öncel et al., 2016; Richter et al., 2022; WHO, 2024f).

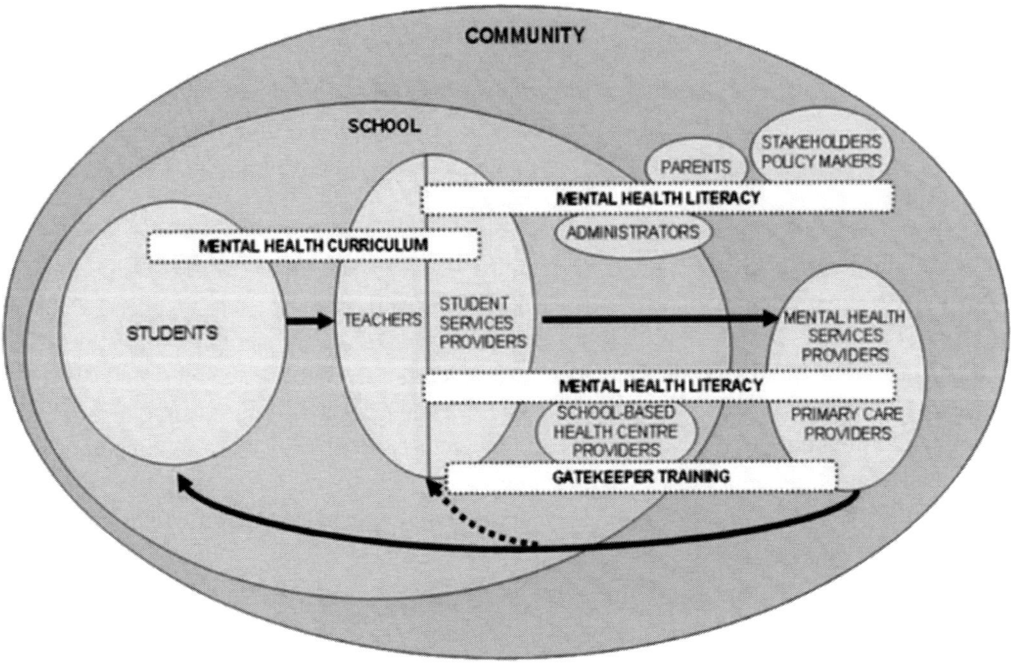

Figure 2. School-based pathway to care model (Wei et al., 2011).

Conclusion

The increasing prevalence of chronic diseases in school-age children presents significant challenges to health care systems worldwide. The changes of the 21st century in health care include a shift from hospital-based acute care to community-based prevention and chronic disease care. School nursing play key role in addressing these challenges by providing critical support for students with chronic diseases. They can make effective interventions to promote school attendance and academic success by meeting the health needs of students in chronic disease management.

School nurses should provide care coordination in the management of chronic diseases. Care coordination includes student-centered, purposeful, and intentional activities in the delivery of health services. Chronic disease management includes effective collaborative communication, direct care, student-centered interventions to meet acute, urgent, or chronic health needs, and tertiary prevention. Student-centered care can contribute to the school nurse working in collaboration with students, parents, and the school, meeting the needs of students and increasing the caregiving abilities of families and students. It is important to evaluate the student with a chronic disease holistically with a biopsychosocial approach, implement the necessary interventions, and monitor the results. Thus, these students can reach their optimal health level and look toward their future with more hope.

Disclaimer

None.

References

Al Kindi, Z., McCabe, C., & McCann, M. (2021). School nurses' available education to manage children with asthma at schools: A scoping review. *Journal of Pediatric Nursing, 60*, 46–57. https://doi.org/10.1016/j.pedn.2021.01.027.

Alexander, J., Gilreath, T., Grant, M., & Curran, L. (2022). Racial/ethnic differences in chronic disease predictors among American high school students. *Journal of School Health, 92*(12), 1177–1185. https://doi.org/10.1111/josh.13218.

Alkan, H., Enç, N., Yeni, K., Yıldız Ayvaz, M., Kayıkcı, E. E., & Kalkan Uğurlu, Y. (2022). Evaluation of childhood obesity, prevalence, and related factors in Istanbul. *Florence Nightingale Journal of Nursing, 30*(3), 267–273. https://doi.org/10.5152/FNJN.2022.20106.

American Association of Neurological Surgeons. (2024). *Epilepsy*. Retrieved from https://www.aans.org/en/Patients/Neurosurgical-Conditions-and-Treatments/Epilepsy.

American Diabetes Association. (2024). *Safe at School*. Retrieved from https://diabetes.org/advocacy/safe-at-school-state-laws.

American Lung Association. (2024). *Improve Asthma Management in Schools*. Retrieved from https://www.lung.org/lung-health-diseases/lung-disease-lookup/asthma/health-professionals-educators/asthma-in-schools.

An, R., Li, D., Cole, M., Park, K., Lyon, A. R., & White, N. H. (2022). Implementation of school diabetes care in the United States: A scoping review. *The Journal of School Nursing, 38*(1), 61–73. https://doi.org/10.1177/10598405211026328.

Atun, R., Bhakta, N., Denburg, A., Frazier, A. L., Friedrich, P., Gupta, S., … Rodriguez-Galindo, C. (2020). Sustainable care for children with cancer: A Lancet Oncology Commission. *The Lancet Oncology, 21*(4), e185–e224. https://doi.org/10.1016/S1470-2045(20)30022-X.

Balasundaram, P., & Krishna, S. (2023). *Obesity effects on child health*. In NCBI Bookshelf. Retrieved from https://www.ncbi.nlm.nih.gov/books/NBK570613/.

Berg, A. T., Berkovic, S. F., Brodie, M. J., Buchhalter, J., Cross, J. H., van Emde Boas, W., … Scheffer, I. E. (2010). Revised terminology and concepts for organization of seizures and epilepsies: Report of the ILAE Commission on Classification and Terminology, 2005–2009. *Epilepsia, 51*(4), 676–685. https://doi.org/10.1111/j.1528-1167.2010.02522.x.

Bryan, G., Kelly, P., Chesters, H., Franklin, J., Griffiths, H., Langton, L., Wakefield, C. E., & Gibson, F. (2021). Access to and experience of education for children and adolescents with cancer: A scoping review protocol. *Systematic Reviews, 10*(1), 167. https://doi.org/10.1186/s13643-021-01723-4.

Centers for Disease Control and Prevention. (2021). *Managing chronic health conditions*. Retrieved from https://www.cdc.gov/healthyschools/chronicconditions.htm.

Centers for Disease Control and Prevention. (2022a). *Healthy Schools*. Retrieved from https://www.cdc.gov/healthyschools/chronicconditions.htm.

Centers for Disease Control and Prevention. (2022b). *Obesity*. Retrieved from https://www.cdc.gov/healthyschools/obesity/index.htm.

Centers for Disease Control and Prevention. (2024a). *Epilepsy in schools*. Retrieved from https://www.cdc.gov/epilepsy/groups/schools.htm.

Centers for Disease Control and Prevention. (2024b). *Promoting mental health and well-being in schools*. Retrieved from https://www.cdc.gov/healthyyouth/mental-health-action-guide/index.html.

Davis, D., Maughan, E. D., White, K. A., & Slota, M. (2021). School nursing for the 21st century: Assessing scope of practice in the current workforce. *The Journal of School Nursing, 37*(5), 374–386. https://doi.org/10.1177/1059840519880605.

Diabetes in School Platform. (2022). *Having diabetes at school*. Retrieved from https://okuldadiyabet.meb.gov.tr/anasayfa.

Diabetes Mellitus Study and Education Group. (2022). *Diabetes mellitus and complications diagnosis, treatment and monitoring guide*. Ankara: Scientific Research Publications.

Erdmann, F., Frederiksen, L. E., Bonaventure, A., Mader, L., Hasle, H., Robison, L. L., & Winther, J. F. (2021). Childhood cancer: Survival, treatment modalities, late effects and improvements over time. *Cancer Epidemiology, 71*(Pt B), 101733. https://doi.org/10.1016/j.canep.2020.101733.

Friedmann, J. A., DelPozo-Banos, M., Frizzati, A., Ford, T., & Thapar, A. (2022). Association of school absence and exclusion with recorded neurodevelopmental disorders, mental disorders, or self-harm: A nationwide, retrospective, electronic cohort study of children and young people in Wales, UK. *The Lancet Psychiatry, 9*(1), 23–34. https://doi.org/10.1016/S2215-0366(21)00367-9.

García-Marcos, L., Asher, M. I., Pearce, N., Ellwood, E., Bissell, K., Chiang, C. Y., El Sony, A., Ellwood, P., Marks, G. B., Mortimer, K., Martínez-Torres, A. E., Morales, E., Perez-Fernandez, V., Robertson, S., Rutter, C. E., Silverwood, R. J., Strachan, D. P., & Global Asthma Network Phase I Study Group. (2022). The burden of asthma, hay fever and eczema in children in 25 countries: GAN Phase I study. *The European Respiratory Journal, 60*(3), 2102866. https://doi.org/10.1183/13993003.02866-2021.

Global Initiative for Asthma. (2023). *Report: Global strategy for asthma management and prevention*. Retrieved from www.ginasthma.org/2023-gina-main-report.

Holst, G. J., Pedersen, C. B., Thygesen, M., Brandt, J., Geels, C., Bønløkke, J. H., & Sigsgaard, T. (2020). Air pollution and family related determinants of asthma onset and persistent wheezing in children: Nationwide case-control study. *BMJ (Clinical Research Ed.), 370*, m2791. https://doi.org/10.1136/bmj.m2791.

Holt, R. I., DeVries, J. H., Hess-Fischl, A., Hirsch, I. B., Kirkman, M. S., Klupa, T., ... & Peters, A. L. (2021). The management of type 1 diabetes in adults: A consensus report by the American Diabetes Association (ADA) and the European Association for the Study of Diabetes (EASD). *Diabetes Care, 44*(11), 2589–2625. https://doi.org/10.2337/dci21-0043.

International Diabetes Federation. (2021). *Diabetes Atlas* (9th ed.). Retrieved from https://www.diabetesatlas.org/en/resources/.

Johnson, E., Atkinson, P., Muggeridge, A., Cross, J. H., & Reilly, C. (2021). Inclusion and participation of children with epilepsy in schools: Views of young people, school staff and parents. *Seizure, 93*, 34–43. https://doi.org/10.1016/j.seizure.2021.10.007.

Klein, D. H., Mohamoud, I., Olanisa, O. O., Parab, P., Chaudhary, P., Mukhtar, S., Moradi, A., Kodali, A., Okoye, C., & Arcia Franchini, A. P. (2023). Impact of school-based interventions on pediatric obesity: A systematic review. *Cureus, 15*(8), e43153. https://doi.org/10.7759/cureus.43153.

Leviton, A., Patel, A. D., & Loddenkemper, T. (2023). Self-management education for children with epilepsy and their caregivers: A scoping review. *Epilepsy & Behavior, 144*, 109232. https://doi.org/10.1016/j.yebeh.2023.109232.

Lindholm Olinder, A., DeAbreu, M., Greene, S., Haugstvedt, A., Lange, K., Majaliwa, E. S., Pais, V., Pelicand, J., Town, M., & Mahmud, F. H. (2022). ISPAD Clinical Practice Consensus Guidelines 2022: Diabetes education in children and adolescents. *Pediatric Diabetes, 23*(8), 1229–1242. https://doi.org/10.1111/pedi.13418.

Mazur, A., Zachurzok, A., Baran, J., Dereń, K., Łuszczki, E., Weres, A., Wyszyńska, J., Dylczyk, J., Szczudlik, E., Drożdż, D., et al., (2022). Childhood obesity: Position statement of Polish Society of Pediatrics, Polish Society for Pediatric Obesity, Polish Society of Pediatric Endocrinology and Diabetes, the College of Family Physicians in Poland and Polish Association for Study on Obesity. *Nutrients, 14*(18), 3806. https://doi.org/10.3390/nu14183806.

McClanahan, R., & Weismuller, P. C. (2015). School nurses and care coordination for children with complex needs: An integrative review. *The Journal of School Nursing, 31*(1), 34–43. https://doi.org/10.1177/1059840514550484.

McGorry, P. D., Mei, C., Chanen, A., Hodges, C., Alvarez-Jimenez, M., & Killackey, E. (2022). Designing and scaling up integrated youth mental health care. *World Psychiatry, 21*(1), 61–76. https://doi.org/10.1002/wps.20938.

Minardi, C., Minacapelli, R., Valastro, P., Vasile, F., Pitino, S., Pavone, P., Astuto, M., & Murabito, P. (2019). Epilepsy in children: From diagnosis to treatment with focus on emergency. *Journal of Clinical Medicine, 8*(1), 39. https://doi.org/10.3390/jcm8010039.

National Association of School Nurses. (2020). Framework for 21st century school nursing practice™: Clarifications and updated definitions. *NASN School Nurse, 35*(4), 225–233. https://doi.org/10.1177/1942602X20928372.

National Cancer Institute. (2023). *Cancer in children and adolescents*. Retrieved from https://www.cancer.gov/types/childhood-cancers/child-adolescent-cancers-fact-sheet.

National Healthcare Quality and Disparities Report. (2022). *Child and adolescent mental health*. Rockville (MD): Agency for Healthcare Research and Quality (US). Retrieved from https://www.ncbi.nlm.nih.gov/books/NBK587182/.

Olusanya, B. O., Wright, S. M., Nair, M. K. C., Boo, N. Y., Halpern, R., Kuper, H., Abubakar, A. A., Almasri, N. A., Arabloo, J., Arora, N. K., ... Global Research on Developmental Disabilities Collaborators (GRDDC). (2020). Global burden of childhood epilepsy, intellectual disability, and sensory impairments. *Pediatrics, 146*(1), e20192623. https://doi.org/10.1542/peds.2019-2623.

Öncel, S., Akcan, A., & Meydanlıoğlu, A. (2016). Health promotion and disease prevention. In A. B. Temel, Z. Bahar, A. Ergün, H. Kadıoğlu, S. Erol, & S. Öncel (Eds.), *Improving the health of school children* (p. 215). Ankara: Vize Press.

Pallan, M., & Adab, P. (2023). Preventing obesity through school-based approaches to improve nutrition. *BMJ Medicine, 2*, e000463. https://doi.org/10.1136/bmjmed-2022-000463.

Peltzer, K., & Pengpid, S. (2020). Chronic disease behavioural risk factors among in-school adolescents in Mozambique. In *Adolescence: Behavioural risk factors of non-communicable diseases* (pp. 27–39). Nova Science Publishers, Inc.

Pless, I. B., & Pinkerton, P. (1975). *Chronic childhood disorder: Promoting patterns of adjustment*. YearBook Medical.

Richter, A., Sjunnestrand, M., Romare Strandh, M., & Hasson, H. (2022). Implementing school-based mental health services: A scoping review of the literature summarizing the factors that affect implementation. *International Journal of Environmental Research and Public Health, 19*(6), 3489. https://doi.org/10.3390/ijerph19063489.

Sahoo, K., Sahoo, B., Choudhury, A. K., Sofi, N. Y., Kumar, R., & Bhadoria, A. S. (2015). Childhood obesity: Causes and consequences. *Journal of Family Medicine and Primary Care, 4*(2), 187–192. https://doi.org/10.4103/2249-4863.154628.

Smith, J. D., Fu, E., & Kobayashi, M. A. (2020). Prevention and management of childhood obesity and its psychological and health comorbidities. *Annual Review of Clinical Psychology, 16*, 351–378. https://doi.org/10.1146/annurev-clinpsy-100219-060201.

Szefler, S. J., Fitzgerald, D. A., Adachi, Y., Doull, I. J., Fischer, G. B., Fletcher, M., ... & Lenney, W. (2020). A worldwide charter for all children with asthma. *Pediatric Pulmonology, 55*(5), 1282–1292. https://doi.org/10.1002/ppul.24713.

Thongseiratch, T., & Chandeying, N. (2020). Chronic illnesses and student academic performance. *Journal of Health Science and Medical Research, 38*(3), 245–253. https://doi.org/10.31584/jhsmr.2020738.

United Nations Children's Fund. (2021b). *The State of the World's Children 2021: On my mind – Promoting, protecting and caring for children's mental health*. UNICEF.

United Nations Children's Fund. (2020). *Prevention of overweight and obesity in children and adolescents*. Retrieved from https://www.unicef.org/documents/prevention-overweight-and-obesity-children-and-adolescents.

United Nations Children's Fund. (2021a). *UNICEF stresses mental health in State of the World's Children report*. Retrieved from https://www.unicefusa.org/stories/unicef-stresses-mental-health-state-worlds-children-report.

United Nations Children's Fund. (2024). *Non-communicable diseases: Behaviors that lead to disease often emerge during childhood and adolescence*. Retrieved from https://www.unicef.org/health/non-communicable-diseases.

Weibel, M., Hallström, I. K., Skoubo, S., Bertel, L. B., Schmiegelow, K., & Larsen, H. B. (2023). Telepresence robotic technology support for social connectedness during treatment of children with cancer. *Children & Society, 37*(5), 1392–1417. https://doi.org/10.1111/chso.12776.

World Health Organization. (2023). *Asthma*. Retrieved from https://www.who.int/news-room/fact-sheets/detail/asthma.

World Health Organization. (2024a). *The top 10 causes of death*. Retrieved from https://www.who.int/news-room/fact-sheets/detail/the-top-10-causes-of-death.

World Health Organization. (2024b). *Epilepsy*. Retrieved from https://www.who.int/news-room/fact-sheets/detail/epilepsy.

World Health Organization. (2024c). *Obesity and overweight*. Retrieved from https://www.who.int/news-room/fact-sheets/detail/obesity-and-overweight.

World Health Organization. (2024d). *BMI-for-age (5–19 years)*. Retrieved from https://www.who.int/tools/growth-reference-data-for-5to19-years/indicators/bmi-for-age.

World Health Organization. (2024e). *Childhood cancer*. Retrieved from https://www.who.int/news-room/fact-sheets/detail/cancer-in-children.

World Health Organization. (2024f). *Mental health of adolescents*. Retrieved from https://www.who.int/news-room/fact-sheets/detail/adolescent-mental-health.

Yetiş, G., & Aylaz, R. (2021). Effect of the perceived social support on school success of children with chronic disease. *Journal of Inonu University Health Services Vocational School, 9*(3), 808–819. https://doi.org/10.33715/inonusaglik.941220.

Zavala, G. A., García, O. P., Ronquillo, D., Doak, C. M., Caamaño, M. D. C., Camacho, M., & Rosado, J. L. (2024). Dietary energy density is associated with biomarkers of chronic diseases—A cross-sectional study of school-aged children in rural Mexico. *Current Developments in Nutrition, 8*(3), 102096. https://doi.org/10.1016/j.cdnut.2024.102096.

Chapter 20

The Management of Children with Special Needs in Schools

Kamer Gür[1,*], PhD
and Bahar Doğan[2], MSc
[1]Department of Public Health Nursing, Marmara University, Faculty of Health Science, Istanbul, Türkiye
[2]Department of Public Health Nursing, Marmara University, Health Science Institute, Istanbul, Türkiye

Abstract

According to the World Disability Report (2011), more than one billion people worldwide are estimated to be living with disabilities. This includes approximately 93 million children aged 0-14 years with "moderate or severe disability" (5.1%), of whom 13 million (0.7%) experience severe functional difficulties. The majority of these children with special needs reside in low- and middle-income countries. Children with special needs are less likely to start school, continue their education, or transition to higher levels of education. To ensure educational participation, efforts must focus on strengthening the capacity of educational systems to respond to diverse needs, while also providing specialized services and support. School nurses play a critical role in health promotion and academic success of children with special needs. This chapter aims to explore approaches to supporting school-age children with special needs, emphasizing tertiary prevention strategies and the multifaceted roles of school nurses.

Keywords: children with special needs, nursing interventions, prevention levels

Introduction

Schools are important institutions where children begin to socialize within groups. During this period, children undergo many critical developmental stages, and the behaviors and habits they acquire often carry into adulthood. Therefore, the school environment plays a vital role in shaping healthy, conscious individuals and integrating them into society (Tunçeli and Zembat, 2017). This role becomes even more significant for children with special needs. Today, the

* Corresponding Author's Email: kamergur@gmail.com

In: Health Promotion and Prevention
Editor: Eda Kılınç İşleyen
ISBN: 979-8-89530-758-8

educational system is changing in order to support students with different needs equally and fairly and emerges as a dynamic structure. Identifying and addressing the difficulties faced by children with special needs is among the core objectives of school health services (Gözüm, 2016).

When discussing special needs, physical disabilities—such as wheelchair dependency—may be the first conditions that come to mind. However, many challenges these children face are not immediately visible (Loschiavo, 2019). Children with special needs may struggle with emotional, educational, behavioral, and health-related issues, as well as difficulties in communication and access to social resources. Reducing disparities and enhancing their social skills is a long and delicate process, especially as their needs may be either temporary or lifelong (Hazar, 2023).

According to United Nations Children's Fund (UNICEF) report, children with special needs are often at a disadvantage compared to their peers across numerous indicators of child well-being (UNICEF, 2021). In this context, school nurses play a vital role in working with and advocating for disadvantaged students. Their responsibilities encompass providing care through all levels of prevention. Primary prevention involves proactive efforts to reduce the risk of disease before symptoms appear, while secondary prevention focuses on early diagnosis, intervention, and monitoring. Tertiary prevention aims to manage chronic conditions, slow progression, and improve quality of life (Selekman, 2019). These strategies are designed to support children's resilience, address their health needs, and ensure a safe and inclusive learning environment. Ultimately, school nurses are indispensable in creating inclusive, supportive, and health-promoting school environments for children with special needs.

Concepts Related to Special Needs

The concept of *special needs* is multifaceted, complex, and often controversial, and dynamic phenomenon. It encompasses a wide range of physical, mental, emotional, behavioral, and developmental conditions that may affect an individual's ability to function effectively in daily life. Understanding who qualifies as having special needs—and what that means in educational and health contexts—requires examining key concepts that underlie this term.

Impairment

Impairment, in the context of health, refers to the loss or abnormality of psychological, physiological, or anatomical structure or function. It may result from congenital conditions, disease, trauma, or other health-related factors and can be either temporary or permanent in nature. Impairments manifest as measurable signs or symptoms that affect the individual's functioning at the organ or system level. As such, impairment primarily reflects the individual and physical dimension of a health problem (Loschiavo, 2019).

Handicap

Handicap refers to the disadvantage or limitation in an individual's ability to perform tasks or fulfill roles that are considered typical for their age, gender, or sociocultural context. It results from the interaction between a person's impairments or disabilities and the environmental and societal barriers that hinder participation. As defined by the World Health Organization, a handicap reflects a restriction in performing activities of daily living and engaging in social life within the scope of what is considered normal, due to physical or mental limitations (WHO, 2022a).

Handicaps may arise from hereditary, congenital, acquired, or unknown causes and may involve a loss of physical and/or mental capabilities. This situation may affect a student's ability to learn, communicate, or behave in the same way as their peers (Loschiavo, 2019; Güloğlu, 2022).

Disability

The concept of disability is very comprehensive, and the definitions show diversity and complexity. This conceptual ambiguity can affect not only which terms are used but also how these terms are interpreted. Barton (1998) stated that the way disability is defined shapes societal attitudes, interactions, and expectations. It is crucial to recognize that individuals with disabilities have unique service needs that differ from the general population, and these needs are shaped by both individual characteristics and the definitions applied to their condition (WHO, 2011).

Disability arises from the interaction of health conditions—such as dementia, blindness, or spinal cord injury—with various contextual factors, including personal characteristics and environmental barriers such as societal attitudes, infrastructure inaccessibility, and discriminatory policies (Güloğlu, 2022). For instance, a blind child may be unable to attend school not because of the impairment itself, but due to a lack of appropriate assistive technologies and educational resources. Importantly, individuals with disabilities can lead healthy, fulfilling lives by actualizing their aspirations, meeting their needs, and transforming their environments (Öztabak, 2017).

The United Nations (UN) Convention on the Rights of Persons with Disabilities (CRPD) defines people with disabilities as those "with long-term physical, mental, intellectual or sensory impairments which in interaction with various barriers may hinder their full and effective participation in society on an equal basis with others" (UN, 2009). As a result, the concept of disability itself is an umbrella concept that points to the individual and social aspects of disability (Güloğlu, 2022).

Special Needs

Individuals with special needs are those who differ from their peers in emotional, physical, social, or mental characteristics and therefore require different types of support or interventions (Kılıçkaya and Zelyurt, 2015).

The Declaration of the Rights of Persons with Disabilities, adopted by the United Nations General Assembly, describes individuals with special needs as those who, due to a congenital or acquired deficiency in their mental or physical capabilities, are unable to carry out necessary daily tasks independently in social life (UN, 2009). Similarly, the American Medical Association defines a child with special needs as one who is unable to perform the same activities as their peers and may have difficulties in play, learning, or general development. It further notes that these children may experience one or more cognitive, physical, emotional, or developmental impairments.

Therefore, the term *special needs child* encompasses children with behavioral and learning difficulties, sensory or physical impairments, and those who are intellectually gifted (Ersan and Kartal, 2020). Special needs are commonly classified under six primary categories: physical/orthopedic, vision, hearing, language and speech, intellectual, and chronic diseases (Gür et al., 2019; Demirarslan, 2022).

Characteristics of Children with Special Needs

Physical and Psychomotor Development Characteristics

- Children with special needs acquire developmental skills such as sitting, crawling, and walking later than their peers,
- They may experience challenges in using both gross and fine motor skills including tasks requiring hand-eye coordination.
- Issues such as limited mobility and physical weakness are common.

Mental Development Characteristics

- These children often have a very short attention span and struggle with concentration.
- Academic concepts are learned more slowly and with difficulty.
- They may forget previously learned material within a short time.
- Difficulties in generalizing learned knowledge to new situations are frequent.
- Concepts related to time are especially challenging, and confusion is common.
- Cognitive differences such as intellectual disability or autism may be present.

Language Development Characteristics

- The stages of language development are typically slower in children with special needs with variability in the duration required for language acquisition.
- They may struggle to express their emotions and thoughts, which can sometimes lead to aggressive behavior.
- Common issues include phonological disorders (e.g., problems with voice pitch and loudness); echolalia and stereotypical speech patterns; articulation disorders (e.g., difficulty producing certain sounds); fluency disorders, such as stuttering, affecting speech rate and smoothness.

These characteristics can vary significantly among children. Therefore, children should be supported in accordance with their specific needs (Parent Consciousness Raising Studies, 2019).

According to data from a report published by UNICEF, compared to children without disabilities, children with disabilities:

- They are 24% less likely to benefit from early stimulation and responsive care.
- 42% less likely to acquire basic reading and arithmetic skills.
- 25% more likely to be underweight and 34% more likely to be stunted.
- 53% more likely to exhibit symptoms of acute respiratory infection.
- 49% more likely to have never attended school.
- They are 47% more likely to drop out of primary schooll, 33% more likely to drop out of secondary school, and 27% more likely to drop out of high school.
- They are 51% more likely of feeling unhappy.
- 41% more likely to experience discrimination.
- 32% more likely to be subjected to severe corporal punishment (UNICEF, 2021).

At the same time, children with disabilities also face substantial health inequalities. For example;

- Compared to individuals without disabilities, they are likely to die up to 20 years earlier.
- They have more than twice the risk of developing chronic conditions such as diabetes, stroke, or depression.
- They encounter up to six times more barriers when trying to access healthcare services (WHO, 2022a).
- Among hearing-impaired adolescents, 70.5% have inadequate health literacy; 43.2% do not understand the instructions provided by nurses, and 56.8% struggle to comprehend health education materials (Gür et al., 2020).

Prevalence of Individuals with Special Needs

The first multinational *World Health Survey* was conducted in 2002 to determine the global prevalence of individuals with special needs. In this survey, participants were interviewed face-to-face about their living conditions and health status (Karcı, 2021). The World Health Organization (WHO) has since utilized data from the Global Burden of Disease (GBD) study to estimate current prevalence of disability. Over the past two decades, the GBD study has served as the most comprehensive source of global, regional, and national epidemiological evidence on all health conditions and injuries (WHO, 2022a).

According to WHO data, an estimated 1.3 billion people worldwide — approximately 16% of the global population—live with a significant disability. In the European Region, the prevalence of disability ranges from 6% to 10% among member states (16% of the global population) (WHO, 2022b). These statistics indicate that one in every six individuals experiences a disability. The number of people with disabilities has risen markedly in the past decade, largely due to population growth and demographic and epidemiological transitions—such as increased longevity among people with non-communicable diseases and aging populations living with functional limitations.

Notably, approximately 80% of the 1.3 billion individuals with disabilities reside in low- and middle-income countries, where access to essential health services remains particularly limited (Karatana and Gür, 2019; WHO, 2022a).

According to Table 1, the most significant increase in health problems contributing to moderate and severe disability between 2010 and 2021 is observed in musculoskeletal system and mental health conditions. These are followed by respiratory infections and tuberculosis, as well as neurological and cardiovascular diseases (WHO, 2022a).

Table 1. Change in the prevalence of health conditions associated with moderate and severe disability globally, 2010 and 2021

Health Condition	2010 (In Millions)	2021 (In Millions)
Musculoskeletal conditions	298.5	370
Mental health conditions	180	252
Neurological conditions	159.7	191.4
Sense organ conditions	81.2	100
Cardiovascular diseases	62.5	84.3
Respiratory infections and tuberculosis	14	60
Injuries	47.9	56
Other non-communicable diseases	46.5	52
Chronic respiratory diseases	41	51
Maternal and neonatal conditions	38.2	44
Skin and subcutaneous diseases	38	43
Substance use disorders	27	31.5
Diabetes and kidney diseases	14.6	20.5
Neglected tropical diseases and malaria	14	16.5
Neoplasms	9	11.5
Digestive diseases	9	10.2
HIV/AIDS and sexually transmitted infections	9.7	5.5
Nutritional deficiencies	2.8	2.4
Other infectious diseases	0.3	2.3
Enteric infections	0.01	0.02

According to health board reports received from public institutions and organizations affiliated with the Ministry of Family, Labor and Social Services of Turkey (MoFLSS), the number of individuals with disabilities who are registered in the National Disability Data System and currently living is 2,511,950. Of these, 1,414,643 are men and 1,097,307 are women (Figure 1). The number of individuals with severe disabilities is reported to be 775,012 (MoFLSS, 2022).

According to Table 2, among the disability conditions of registered and living individuals, chronic diseases rank first as the leading cause of disability, followed by mental and orthopedic disorders (MoFLSS, 2022). The reports on children and adolescents with special needs, published by UNICEF in 2021, and based on internationally comparable data from 42 countries, estimates that approximately 240 million children with special needs are living worldwide (UNICEF, 2021).

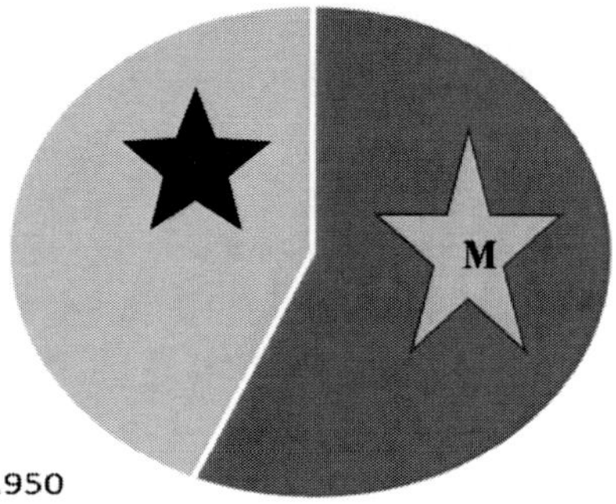

Figure 1. Distribution of individuals with disabilities, who are registered in the data system and currently alive, according to gender.

Table 2. Distribution of individuals with disabilities, who are registered in the data system and currently alive, according to disability groups

Disability Group	Number of People	Rate (%)
Chronic Disease	917.259	40.63
Mental	385.313	17.07
Orthopedic	311.131	13.78
Visual	215.076	9.53
Hearing	179.867	7.97
Spiritual and Emotional	170.927	7.57
Other	44.248	1.96
Language and Speech	33.686	1.49

According to data obtained from the 2022 National Disability Data System in Turkey, the number of individuals with disabilities aged 0-24 and their distribution by gender are presented in Table 3 (MoFLSS, 2022).

Table 3. Distribution of individuals with disabilities, who are registered in the database and currently alive, according to age group and gender

Age Groups	Male	Female	Total
0-4	19.304	13.881	33.185
5-9	56.267	34.792	91.059
10-14	74.525	48.282	122.807
15-19	79.897	54.181	134.078
20-24	87.544	59.814	147.358

Prevention Levels

Primary Prevention

Primary prevention strategies in schools aim not only to reduce the risk of health problems in individuals or society but also aim to combat harmful effects and enhance individuals' resilience to these effects (Murray et al., 2009). The primary goal is to identify and address potential health threats before any symptoms or signs of illness emerge.

Primary Prevention Strategies for Children with Special Needs

- Health education
- Forward guidance
- Promoting healthy lifestyles
- Staying up to date immunization

For example, these can include walking programs that include all students in the school, planning pre-lunch hand washing times, and coordinating anti-bullying programs.

Secondary Prevention

The goal of secondary prevention is to detect diseases as early as possible, before symptoms appear, reduce the duration and severity of consequences, prevent disability or complications, and help the person to return to optimal health function.

Secondary Prevention Strategies for Children with Special Needs

- Early diagnosis
- Screenings
- Focus on early treatment.

Early diagnosis and referral to when necessary are crucial for ensuring students' learning and academic success (Loschiavo, 2021; Selekman, 2019). For example, school nurses can use physical examinations for preliminary diagnosis and early identification of potential health issues before implementing primary prevention strategies. During these examinations, nurses can detect problems such as hypertension, obesity, or missed vaccinations.

Tertiary Prevention

Tertiary prevention strategies aim to improve the health and quality of life of individuals living with chronic health issues. These strategies focus on minimizing the effects of existing health problems, slowing down or halting the disease's progression, and helping individuals maintain optimal functionality through long-term treatment and rehabilitation. Tertiary prevention seeks to reduce complications with early diagnosis and treatment, prevent existing complications from worsening, and avoid recurrence or exacerbation of the condition (Loschiavo, 2021; Selekman, 2019).

For children with special needs, the goal is to ensure their participation integration into educational experiences similar to those of their peer in line with their abilities (CDC, 2025). In addition to typical childhood needs, these children often have special requirements, such as medication use, disease management, and rehabilitation (Çakır and Altay, 2021). Tertiary prevention aims to enhance self-care skills, prevent secondary complications, and help individuals with chronic diseases and disabilities maximize their life skills (Bobo et al., 2012).

As awareness grows, school health and education professionals have taken steps to improve their roles in supporting children with special needs and eliminate barriers to their success. A comprehensive and integrated approach is needed for these children (Adelman and Taylor, 2018). Techniques such as individualized training programs, visual supports, social-emotional learning, special communication methods, positive reinforcement, and collaborative learning should be tailored to each child's specific needs. It is essential to develop an individualized approach for each student. These methods should be presented by integrating appropriate nursing skills.

School nursing practice includes providing professional care to meet the child's physical, psychosocial, and academic needs. The goal is to enhance academic success, improve quality of life, treat current and potential health problems, and provide a safe environment (Çakır and Altay, 2021).

Tertiary Prevention Strategies for Children with Special Needs

Some of the tertiary prevention activities provided by school nurses for students with chronic health problems include:

- Ensuring medication is taken at the correct time, dose, and route
- Educating about the importance of completing antibiotic treatments
- Planning and implementing health training tailored to the individual's needs, including empowering students to manage disease symptoms (Bobo et al., 2012).

Asthma:

- Educating children on correct medication use
- Teaching ways to avoid allergens
- Preventing asthma attacks by educating classmates and teachers about proper classroom ventilation

Diabetes:

- Teaching blood sugar control
- Promoting diabetes management through education on nutrition and exercise education.

Children with autism and behavioral disorders:

- Ensuring correct medications use
- Providing behavioral interventions and teaching appropriate behavioral methods (Stanhope and Lancaster, 2008).

These interventions make it easier to manage students' health problems and monitor their progress effectively.

The Role of School Nurses for Children with Special Needs

School nurses play a critical role in supporting children with special needs through interventions at all levels of prevention—primary, secondary, and tertiary. While they are actively involved across the spectrum of care, a particular emphasis is placed on tertiary prevention to help these children achieve a better state of health and an improved quality of life.

Health Assessment

School nurses analyze and assess the situations of students by gathering information from teachers, administrators, parents, and other individuals in the child's environment. During this data collection process, methods such as observation, home visits, and screenings may be employed. If there is no existing registration system for children with special needs that can be accessed and evaluated by professionals, school nurses are responsible for creating appropriate records (Adelman and Taylor, 2018).

Care and Monitoring

Care and monitoring are among the most commonly performed practices by school nurses for children with special needs. The school nurse identifies each child's care needs and develops individualized care plans, which are crucial (Leroy et al., 2017). For children with severe disabilities, assistance should be provided in areas where they struggle or cannot independently perform tasks such as personal hygiene, toileting, feeding, and dressing. Holistic care should also involve education and counseling, resource management, communication, and collaboration (Adelman and Taylor, 2018).

Health Promotion

Promoting and maintaining the health of the school community is one of the main responsibilities of school nurses (Allender et al., 2013). Their goal is to raise awareness and foster a sense of responsibility among individuals to improve their own health levels (Bruzzese et al., 2010). To enhance the well-being of children with special needs, school nurses may implement interventions such as nutrition regulation, planning physical activities, offering education and counseling, and providing psychosocial support.

Nutrition Regulation and Monitoring

The school nurse monitors the dietary needs of children with special requirements and adjusts their diets as necessary. They work with families and teachers to help children maintain healthy eating habits and follow appropriate nutrition plans (Yabancı, 2011). For example, in collaboration with a dietician, a child with diabetes may receive support in carbohydrate counting, blood glucose monitoring, and appropriate interventions. The nurse ensures consistent snack routines and informs parents. For children with sodium restrictions or food allergies, the nurse checks school meal nutritional values and provides guidance to cafeteria staff to ensure safe and adequate meals (Leroy et al., 2017; Staudt et al., 2015).

Physical Activity Planning

School nurse encourage children with special needs to participate in extracurricular and physical activities, offering support to students, teachers, and parents. They develop management plans to address misconceptions about physical activity and to emphasize its safety and importance. For example, they may adapt activities: a longer warm-up for a child with asthma, rhythmic joint exercises for cerebral palsy, or swimming and cycling for those with rheumatoid arthritis. They also create emergency action plans and collaborate with families and teachers (MoH, 2018; Yüzer and Polat, 2014). Gür et al., (2020) found that visually impaired adolescents desire more physical activity, but environmental and familial factors act as barriers.

Education and Counseling

Nurses identify educational needs among students, parents, teachers, and school staff, providing health-related education and consultancy services to the child's family and teachers. Depending on the level of disability, children should receive structured education and be supported in developing daily life and social skills. Children should be encouraged to become as independent as possible. For example, those with mild impairments can learn to use the phone, pay bills, shop, and use public transportation (Yabancı, 2011; Adelman and Taylor, 2018; Bektaş and Aydın, 2018).

Evaluation, Monitoring, and Management

Nurses continuously evaluate the health status of children with special needs, ensuring ongoing monitoring throughout all phases of the nursing process. These evaluations guide necessary plan revisions and include environmental assessments within the school. For instance, in managing chronic diseases like asthma, adjustments are made to ensure physical activity can occur in non-humid, temperature-regulated spaces (Mülayim, 2019; MoH, 2018).

In addition, children with disadvantages are more vulnerable to violence. School nurses must monitor signs of abuse and, when needed, initiate medical and legal actions and ensure access to professional support. For example, Gür and Albayrak (2017) found that many visually impaired children had experienced violence. Risk factors included being male, visually impaired, and residing in boarding schools.

Conclusion

School nurses who work with children with special needs play a vital role in promoting and protecting their health and well-being within the school environment. Their responsibilities include:

- Having a thorough understanding of special education laws and regulations.
- Establishing supportive and collaborative relationships with parents.
- Identifying children with special needs as early as possible.
- Facilitating the integration of children with special needs into the school community.
- Acting as advocates for these children, ensuring their voices are heard and their needs met.
- Developing individualized, health-related goals that support each child's well-being.
- Serving as a coordinator among students, teachers, parents, and healthcare providers.
- Ensuring the confidentiality of sensitive health and personal information.
- Providing education and supervision to non-professional staff involved in the care of children with special needs.
- Leading efforts to create inclusive environments where children with special needs are accepted and supported by their peers.
- Identifying and utilizing appropriate community resources (Loschiavo, 2019).

In summary, school nurses deliver comprehensive healthcare services at the primary, secondary, and tertiary prevention levels, making them essential contributors to the health, inclusion, and educational success of children with special needs.

Disclaimer

None.

References

Adelman, H. S., & Taylor, L. L. (2018). Addressing barriers to learning: *In the classroom and schoolwide.* https://smhp.psych.ucla.edu/pdfdocs/barriersbook.pdf Access Date: 21.03.2024.

Allender, J., Rector, C., Rector, C., & Warner, K. (2013). Community & public health nursing: Promoting the public's health. lippincott williams & wilkins.

Barton, L. (1998). Sociology, disability studies and education: Some observations. *The disability reader: Social science perspectives*, 53-64.

Bektaş, M., & Aydin, B. (2018). The role and functions of the school nurse. *Türkiye Clinics Pediatric Nursing-Special Topics* 2018;4(1):52-64.

Bobo, N., Kımel, L., & Bleza, S. (2012). Promoting Health at School (ed) Selekman, J. in *School Nursing: A comprehensive text* (s. 440-472). FA Davis Company. Ebook.

Bruzzese, J. M., Unikel, L. H., Evans, D., Bornstein, L., Surrence, K., & Mellins, R.B. (2010). Asthma knowledge and asthma management behavior in urban elementary school teachers. Journal of Asthma, 47(2), 185-191.

Centers for Disease Control and Prevention. (2025). *Disability Inclusion.* https://www.cdc.gov/disability-inclusion/about/index.html Access Date: 20.03.2024.

Parent Consciousness Raising Studies. (2019). Characteristics of Individuals with Special Education Needs. Guidance and Psychological Counseling Services Service. Number of Publications: 2019-01 https://manisaisuygulamamerkezi.meb.k12.tr/meb_iys_dosyalar/45/01/747618/dosyalar/2019_03/20093540_Yzellikler.pdf Access Date: 10.03.2024.

Çakır, G., Altay, N. (2021). Duties and responsibilities of the school nurse in the care of children with chronic diseases. *Dokuz Eylül University Faculty of Nursing Electronic Journal*, 14(1), 55-61.

Demirarslan, S. (2022). Spatial need awareness for children with disabilities. *TURAN-SAM*, 14(55), 127-130.

Ersan, V. D. K., & Kartal, M. S. (2020). Determining the opinions of preschool teachers who have children with special needs in their classrooms about adaptations. *Eskişehir Osmangazi University Turkish World Application and Research Center Education Journal,* 5(2), 74-100.

Gözüm, S. (2016). *Improving the health of school children.* Ankara: Vize Publishing.

Güloğlu, F. (2022). Reasons for conceptual confusion about disability and the situation in Turkey. *Society and Social Work*, 33(1), 291-315. doi: 10.33417/tsh.989123.

Gür, K., & Albayrak, S. (2017). Exposure to violence of secondary school children with visual impairment. *Journal of interpersonal violence*, 32(15), 2257-2274.

Gür, K., Beyhan, A., Aktan, C., Akbulut, E., Sezer, M., Çelik, Ş., & Çakıcı, T. (2020). Physical activity levels, enjoyment, and perceptions of barriers to physical activity of adolescents with visual impairments in Turkey. J*ournal of Visual Impairment & Blindness,* 114(6), 502-515.

Gür, K., Dolaner, G., & Turan, S. R. (2020). Health literacy of hearing-impaired adolescents, barriers and misunderstandings they encounter, and their expectations. *Disability and Health Journal,* 13(4), 100929.

Gür, K., Sezer, A. B., Şentürk, M. K., Sağlam, E. & Top, K. (2019). The effectiveness of a self-care development program in visually impaired students. *Acıbadem University Journal of Health Sciences,* (2), 282-287.

Hazar, Z. (2023). *Examination of the Relationship Between Watchdog Behaviors of Mothers with Children with Special Needs and Father Involvement* (Master's thesis, Ankara University).

Karatana, Ö., & Gür, K. (2019). Access to health services and barriers for disabled individuals. *Journal of Public Health Nursing,* 1(1), 43-53.

Karcı, E. (2021). Mothers' views on the placement of their children with special needs in pre-school education institutions (Master's thesis, Hasan Kalyoncu University).

Kılıçkaya, A., & Zelyurt, H. (2015). Examining the inclusion of individuals with special needs in preschool programs (1989-2013). *International Turkish Journal of Educational Sciences,* 2015(4), 200-212.

Leroy, Z. C., Wallin, R., & Lee, S. (2017). The role of school health services in addressing the needs of students with chronic health conditions: A systematic review. *The Journal of School Nursing,* 33(1), 64-72.

Loschiavo, J. (2019). *Fast Facts for the School Nurse: What You Need to Know.* Springer Publishing Company.

Ministry of Family, Labor and Social Services (2022). *Disabled and Elderly Statistics Bulletin*, August 2022. https://www.aile.gov.tr/media/117257/eyhgm_istatistik_bulteni_agustos2022.pdf Access Date: 21.03.2024.

Ministry of Health (MoH). (2018). General Directorate of Public Health, Physical Activity Guide for Children and Adolescents in Chronic Diseases. https://krtknadmn.karatekin.edu.tr/files/sbf/Cocuk_ve_

Ergen_Rehberi__________________%C3%87OCUK%20GEL%C4%B0%C5%9E%C4%B0M%C4%B0_BESLENME____.pdf Publication No: 1089. 1st Edition. Ankara; 2018. Access Date: 20.03.2024.

Murray, R., Zentner, J., & Yakimo, R. (2009). *Health promotion strategies through the life span.* Upper Saddle River, NJ: Pearson/ Prentice Hall.

Mülayim, A. (2017). Solution suggestions for disabled people in interior design. *Kırklareli University Journal of Engineering and Science,* 3(1), 68-94.

Öztabak, M. Ü. (2017). Examining the life expectations of disabled individuals. *FSM Journal of Scientific Research, Humanities and Social Sciences,* (9), 355-375.

Selekman, J., Shannon, R. A., & Yonkaitis, C. F. (2019). *School nursing: A comprehensive text.* FA Davis.

Stanhope, M., & Lancaster, J. (2008). *Public health nursing: Population-centered health care in the community.* Elsevier Health Sciences.

Staudt, A. M., Alamgir, H., Long, D. L., Inscore, S. C., & Wood, P. R. (2015). Developing and Implementing a Citywide Asthma Action Plan: A Community Collaborative Partnership. *Southern medical journal,* 108(12), 710-714.

Tunçeli, H. İ., & Zembat, R. (2017). Evaluation and importance of development in early childhood. *Journal of Educational Theory and Practice Research,* 3(3), 1-12.

UNICEF. (2021). https://www.unicef.org/turkiye/bas%C4%B1n-b%C3%BCltenleri/unicefin-kapsaml%C4%B1-istatistiksel-analizine-g%C3%B6re-d%C3%BCnya-%C3%A7ap%C4%B1nda-yakla%C5%9F%C4%B1k-240-milyon Access Date: 21.03.2024.

United Nations. (2009). *Convention on the Rights of Persons with Disabilities.* https://www.ohchr.org/sites/default/files/Documents/HRBodies/CRPD/CRPD-C-2-3.pdf Access Date: 21.03.2024.

Yabancı, N. (2011). School health and nutrition programs. TAF Preventive Medicine Bulletin,10(3).

Yüzer, S., & Polat, S. (2014). Asthmatic Children and Sports. TAF Preventive Medicine Bulletin, 13(3).

World Health Organization. (2011). *World Disability Report.* https://www.engellilerkonfederasyonu.org.tr/wp-content/uploads/2020/04/D%C3%BCnya-Engellilik-Raporu-2011.pdf Access Date: 20.03.2024.

World Health Organization. (2022a). *Global report on health equity for persons with disabilities.* https://www.who.int/publications/i/item/9789240063600 Access Date: 20.03.2024.

World Health Organization. (2022b). *Health equity for persons with disabilities.* https://cdn.who.int/media/docs/default-source/ncds/3054-dp-infographic-key-message-291122.pdf?sfvrsn=de68ccfa_1 Access Date: 20.03.2024.

Chapter 21

The Management of Neglect and Abuse in School-Age Children

Aysun Erdal*, **MSc**
and Naile Bilgili, PhD
Gazi University, Faculty of Nursing, Department of Public Health Nursing, Ankara, Turkey

Abstract

Child neglect and abuse, defined as child maltreatment, is a significant public health problem worldwide, affecting millions of children of all ages, races, and socioeconomic levels. Any action or inaction by parents, caregivers, or other individuals that causes, or has the potential to cause, harm to a child is categorized as neglect and abuse. Research shows that approximately one in four children, regardless of age, race, or socio-economic status, are affected at some point in their lives. The management of child neglect and abuse requires a multi-sectoral and multi-stage system. In addition to implementing similar policies in all age groups, school-based prevention and management programs for school-age children are promising in terms of their results. It has been shown that school-based neglect and abuse prevention programs increase children's knowledge about neglect and abuse and provide them with self-protection skills. The programs should be standardized and included in the compulsory curriculum, and their long-term results should be evaluated. Standardized procedures should be established for the management of neglect and abuse cases in schools. In this way, case diagnosis, follow-up, and rehabilitation can be carried out healthily. School nurses are the most competent personnel in preventing and managing neglect and abuse in schools. They actively perform the roles of caregiver, educator, researcher, collaborator, and case manager throughout at-risk school-age children's prevention education, follow-up, diagnosis, and rehabilitation process.

Keywords: neglect, abuse, school-age children, school-based program, school nursing

---

* Corresponding Author's Email: aysun.mutlu@gazi.edu.tr

In: Health Promotion and Prevention
Editor: Eda Kılınç İşleyen
ISBN: 979-8-89530-758-8

Introduction

Child abuse and neglect, defined as child maltreatment, is a significant public health problem worldwide, affecting millions of children of all ages, races, and socioeconomic levels (Gubbels et al., 2021; McCoy and Keen, 2022; Amin et al., 2023). The World Health Organization (WHO) defines child maltreatment as "any form of abuse or neglect that results in actual or potential harm to the child's health, survival, development, or dignity in the context of a relationship of responsibility, trust, or power" (WHO, 1999). Abuse involves active behaviors that harm a child's development, whereas neglect refers to the failure to meet a child's essential needs—a more passive but equally damaging form of maltreatment (Amin et al., 2023). Common types of child maltreatment are detailed in Table 1.

Table 1. Some common forms of child maltreatment

Maltreatment	Definition	Examples
Physical Abuse	The intentional use of physical force that harms or is likely to harm the child's health, survival, development, or dignity (WHO, 2006)	Beating, hitting, kicking, biting, shaking, drowning, burning, poisoning, etc.
Emotional/ Psychological Abuse	Non-accidental verbal or symbolic actions by a child's parent or caregiver that cause or have the potential to cause significant psychological harm to the child (American Psychiatric Association, 2013)	Yelling, scolding, comparing, humiliating, mocking, rejecting, withholding love, threatening, isolating, etc.
Sexual Abuse	Involving a child in sexual activities that he or she does not fully understand, cannot give informed consent, or is not developmentally ready for, or that violates the laws or social taboos of the community (WHO, 2006)	Fondling, penetration, incest, rape, sodomy, indecent exposure, exposure to sexual activities, etc.
Neglect	A child's basic physical or emotional needs are not met and responded to appropriately, or the child is not protected from harm or potential harm (American Psychiatric Association, 2013)	Abandonment, lack of proper supervision, failure to provide the necessary shelter, food, clothing, education, medical care, etc.

Prevalence of Child Neglect and Abuse

Studies on the global prevalence of child abuse and neglect indicates that approximately one in four children experiences some form of maltreatment during their lifetime (Lippard and Nemeroff, 2020; Massullo et al., 2023; Higgins et al., 2023). According to the WHO's global report (2020), there was a marked increase in reported cases of physical, emotional/ psychological, sexual abuse and neglect between 2003 and 2019 (see Figure 1). The report highlights that, in most cases, the perpetrators of abuse are individuals within the child's immediate family. Specifically, biological fathers are most often the perpetrators, followed by biological mothers and stepfathers. In cases of sexual abuse, male perpetrators are primarily responsible, while emotional abuse and neglect are more frequently attributed to biological mothers (WHO, 2020).

According to WHO data, approximately three out of every four children aged 2-4 years are regularly subjected to physical punishment and/or psychological violence by their parents or caregivers. Additionally, one in five women and one in thirteen men report having been sexually abused during childhood (ages 0-17) (WHO, 2022). In the United States, the *Children's Bureau of the U.S. Department of Health and Human Services* (2022) reported more than four million cases of child maltreatment in 2022. Tragically, nearly 1,990 child fatalities due to abuse and neglect occurred that year—an average of five child deaths per day (Children's Bureau of the U.S. Department of Health and Human Services, 2022).

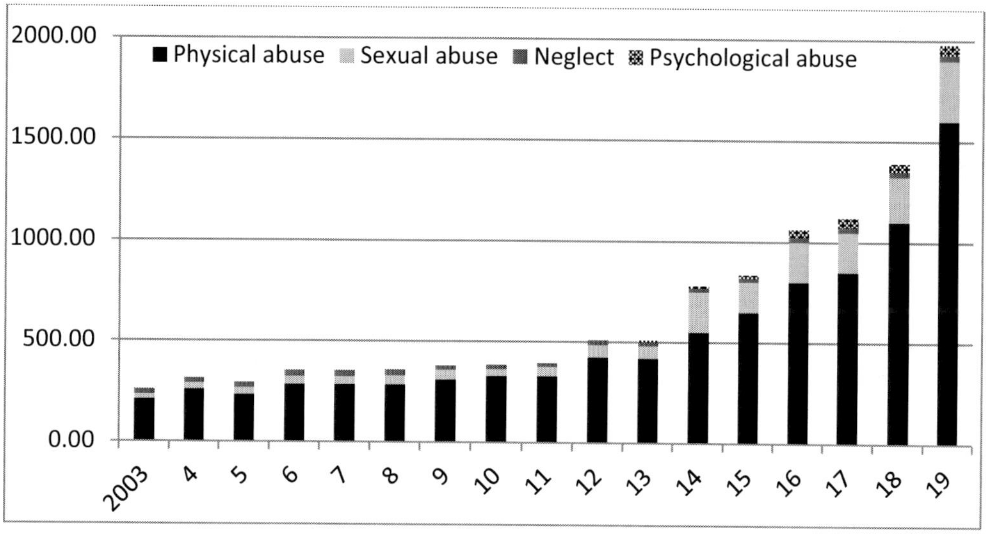

Figure 1. Rates of abuse and neglect (2003-2019) (WHO, 2020).

Although comprehensive national data are lacking in some countries, in Türkiye, statistics from the *Turkish Statistical Institute (TURKSTAT)* indicate that the number of incidents involving children increased by 10.8% in 2021 compared to 2020. Among children who came to or were brought to security units, 57.4% were victims of assault or injury, 13.1% were involved in sexual crimes, 12.4% were exposed to crimes against family integrity, and 4.5% were involved in incidents of threats (TURKSTAT, 2022). Notably, in 2020, 44% of all crimes against sexual immunity in Türkiye consisted of crimes related to child sexual abuse. In the literature, it is emphasized that cases of neglect and abuse are much higher than what is detected, but factors such as the lack of a clear criterion for what is considered maltreatment, different tools used, self-report-based measurements, denial and secrecy of abuse and neglect constitute an obstacle to the accurate estimation of the prevalence of maltreatment against children (Zeanah and Humphreys, 2018; Moody et al., 2018; WHO, 2022). These alarming rates underscore the urgent global need for the development and implementation of effective strategies for the prevention, early detection, and management of child neglect and abuse.

Risk Factors in Child Abuse and Neglect

Understanding the risk factors associated with child abuse and neglect is essential for the development of effective prevention and intervention strategies (Giardino et al., 2018; WHO, 2022). These risk factors can be categorized into four domains: the child, parents, family, and society. Child-related factors include being under the age of four or an adolescent, being the result of an unintended pregnancy, not meeting parental expectations, having special needs or disabilities, possessing physical characteristics that deviate from norms, or identifying with a different sexual orientation (Giardino et al., 2018; McCoy and Keen, 2022; WHO, 2022). Parental risk factors encompass physical or mental health problems, low educational attainment and socioeconomic status, ineffective communication skills, high levels of perceived stress, low self-esteem, poor anger and impulse control, substance and alcohol abuse, a personal history of violence and criminal activity, young age and inexperienced, lack of parenting knowledge and motivation, step-parenting dynamics, and a history of being abused during childhood (Mulder et al., 2018; Giardino et al., 2018; Greene et al., 2020; McCoy and Keen, 2022). Family-related risk factors include a fragmented family structure, single parenthood, extended family structure, the presence of domestic violence, and poorly defined family roles and boundaries (Giardino et al., 2018; WHO, 2022). Societal risk factors involve broader structural and cultural elements such as high unemployment rates, poverty, gender inequality, social marginalization, disability, armed conflict, migration, high crime rates, ease access to substances like alcohol and drugs, cultural acceptance of violence, weak child protection legislation, insufficient reporting procedures, and inadequate access to social services (WHO, 2022; U.S. Department of Health and Human Services, 2022). A comprehensive understanding of these multilayered risk factors is crucial for professionals working in child well-being and health, as it enables targeted and effective prevention, identification, and management of child abuse and neglect cases.

Effects of Neglect and Abuse on Child Health

Child neglect and abuse have profound and lasting effects on children's health, development, and well-being (Fayaz, 2019; Amin et al., 2023). These adverse experiences can result in both immediate and long-term consequences. Physical outcomes may include malnutrition, delayed physical and cognitive development, bruises, fractures, burns, head trauma, permanent disabilities, and even death. In the long term, adults who experienced maltreatment in childhood are at increased risk for a range of chronic health conditions such as sexually transmitted infections, obesity, asthma, cardiovascular disease, diabetes, and certain types of cancer (Giardino et al., 2018; Strathearn et al., 2020; WHO, 2022; McCoy and Keen, 2022).

Children exposed to neglect or abuse are at high risk of developing mental health problems such as depression, anxiety, post-traumatic stress disorder (PTSD), substance and alcohol use disorders, and suicide (Gardner et al., 2019; Humphreys et al., 2020). These children may experience behavioral problems such as aggression, withdrawal, attachment difficulties, and impaired interpersonal relationships. There is a high risk of lifelong negative behaviors such as alcohol, smoking, substance abuse, risky sexual behavior, unintended pregnancy, criminal tendencies, violence, or exposure to violence and harassment. Additionally, studies show that adults who were exposed to neglect and abuse in childhood tend to show similar behaviors to their own children (Jaffee, 2017; Giardino et al., 2018; Strathearn et al., 2020; WHO, 2022; McCoy and Keen, 2022).

It has been found that children exposed to neglect or abuse have interrupted education and show low academic performance. Children exposed to any form of neglect or abuse in childhood are 13% more likely to drop out of school (WHO, 2022). These children may have difficulty establishing healthy relationships with others, leading to social isolation and difficulties establishing healthy relationships in adulthood (Amin et al., 2023). On a societal level, the burden of child maltreatment is reflected in increased healthcare expenditures, treatment needs, lost productivity, and reduced quality of life (WHO, 2022). It is crucial to recognize, however, that not all children exposed to neglect and abuse are affected in the same way. The severity of consequences depends on factors such as the type, frequency, and duration of abuse or neglect, the child's age and developmental level, and the presence of protective factors such as family or community support. Early identification, comprehensive interventions, and sustained support systems play a pivotal role in mitigating adverse outcomes and fostering resilience and recovery (Amin et al., 2023).

Prevention of Neglect and Abuse

Child neglect and abuse are preventable public health problems that require a multifaceted and multisectoral approach involving the individual, family, and society (WHO, 2020; Guastaferro and Shipe, 2023). Early preventive interventions provide greater benefits to both children and society, emphasizing the importance of timely action (Swenson and Schaeffer, 2018). Although existing preventive strategies primarily focus on the early identification of maltreatment and the protection of affected children, these efforts alone are insufficient. Prevention efforts must also address the underlying causes and associated risk factors that contribute to maltreatment. Since neglect and abuse stem from the interaction of numerous risk factors, an effective prevention strategy must be comprehensive and multifactorial. Preventive strategies can be broadly categorized into three levels: individual, relational, and societal/environmental (Fortson et al., 2016; WHO, 2020; McCoy and Keen, 2022; U.S. Department of Health & Human Services, 2023).

Individual strategies: These strategies target changes in individual attitudes, behaviors, and beliefs to prevent child maltreatment.

- Reducing unintended pregnancies
- Educating children to recognize and avoid situations of neglect and abuse
- Raising public awareness on child rights and safety (Fortson et al., 2016; WHO, 2020; U.S. Department of Health & Human Services, 2023).

Relational strategies: These approaches aim to create safe, nurturing environments that promote healthy child development within the family unit:

- Implementing structured home visitation programs
- Strengthening parenting capacities through family-centered services
- Organizing parental education and support programs (Fortson et al., 2016; WHO, 2020; Guastaferro and Shipe, 2023).

Social and environmental strategies: These strategies aim to reduce the risk of maltreatment in environments such as neighborhoods, schools, workplaces, etc., where social relations occur, and aim to influence the formation of the risk: (Fortson et al., 2016; Swenson and Schaeffer, 2018; WHO, 2020; U.S. Department of Health & Human Services, 2023)

- Establishment and enforcing comprehensive child protection laws (e.g., national adaptation of the UN Convention on the Rights of the Child, strengthening legal and security systems),
- Promoting inclusive social and economic policies (e.g., universal access to education, taking measures to reduce unemployment and mitigate its effects, developing and implementing social protection systems)
- Changing harmful cultural and social norms (e.g., disapproval of the culture of violence, creating a culture of reporting suspected abuse and neglect, etc.),
- Reducing economic inequalities (e.g., fighting poverty, reducing income and gender inequalities),
- Reducing environmental risk factors (e.g., limiting the availability of alcohol, monitoring lead levels and cleaning the environment of toxins),
- Establishing shelters and crisis centers for at-risk families,
- Training health and frontline professionals to identify and respond to maltreatment

To ensure successful implementation, it is critical to consider the type, scope, and stakeholders of each strategy. A clearly defined target population enhances the relevance and impact of preventive interventions (Fayaz, 2019; Amin et al., 2023; Guastaferro and Shipe, 2023). In this context, prevention can be categorized into three levels:

Primary prevention targets the general population to reduce the risk of abuse before it occurs.

Secondary prevention focuses on groups identified as at-risk.

Tertiary prevention aims to minimize the negative outcomes of maltreatment and prevent recurrence.

Programs that align their strategies with these levels of prevention tend to show higher efficacy and better adaptability (WHO, 2020; Amin, 2023; Guastaferro and Shipe, 2023).

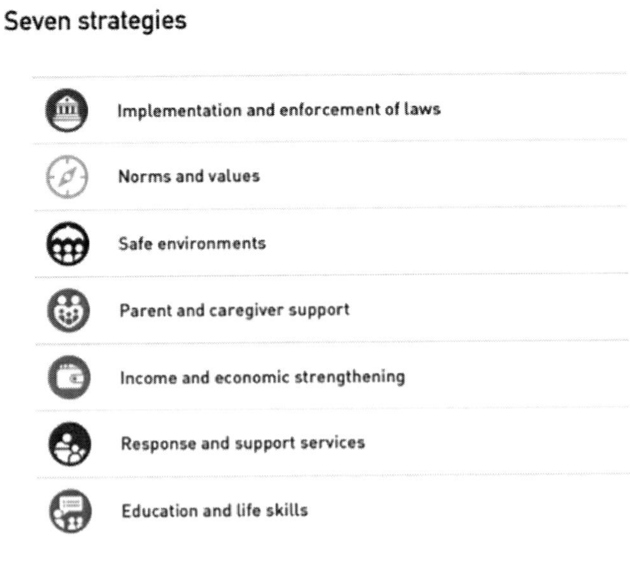

Figure 2. INSPIRE: seven strategies to end violence against children (WHO, 2018).

In addition to these prevention strategies, the World Health Organization, in collaboration with ten global organizations, developed "INSPIRE: Seven Strategies to End Violence Against Children" in 2016 (Figure 2). This evidence-based framework consolidates the most effective interventions and provides a strategic roadmap for governments to address violence against children, including neglect and abuse (WHO, 2018). This resource is a guide for countries to develop their action plans for child neglect and abuse.

Management of Abuse and Neglect

The management of child abuse and neglect involves a systematic and multidisciplinary approach encompassing the identification and reporting of maltreatment, the provision of medical treatment and care, rehabilitation, and long-term follow-up (WHO, 2022). The main stages in the management process are summarized as follows;

1. Identification and Reporting of Neglect and Abuse

Diagnosing child abuse and neglect is complex due to its varied presentations depending on the type and severity of maltreatment. It may include different symptoms and findings depending on the type. It requires a comprehensive assessment of the child's physical and emotional health, as well as the family and social environment (Giardino et al., 2018). When maltreatment is suspected, a physical and mental health assessment of the child should be conducted. According to best practice guidelines, the assessment should include (Swenson and Schaeffer, 2018; WHO, 2022):

- A comprehensive medical history of the child and parents,
- Physical examination of the whole body, including the genital and anal inspection,
- Assessment of mental health,
- Screening for sexually transmitted infections,
- Assessment of pregnancy, if applicable

Procedures, algorithms, workflow charts, or task lists can be used for the early detection of abuse. If the incident is likely to be brought to court, a forensic assessment is also needed. At this point, forensic evidence should be collected and stored appropriately (WHO, 2022; U.S. Department of Health and Human Services, 2023).

2. Provision of Medical Treatment and Care

If physical or mental health problems are identified as a result of abuse or neglect, appropriate treatment must be initiated. In addition to the ongoing medical care, the child is evaluated in terms of mental health, and the necessary psychological support is integrated into the treatment process in the acute stage (WHO, 2022).

3. Rehabilitation of the Child

Rehabilitation aims to reduce the lasting psychological and developmental impacts of maltreatment and should involve both the child and the family. Psychological support should include the child and the family and be coordinated with legal procedures to protect the child (Swenson and Schaeffer, 2018; Humphreys et al., 2020). Therapeutic support may include individual therapy, group sessions, or family counseling. Supporting family members who are suspected of maltreatment of their children can be difficult for service providers, but often, the help provided to the family also means helping the child. Therefore, special support should be provided to the family (Gardner et al., 2019; Humphreys et al., 2020; WHO, 2022). To identify the necessary support interventions (Giardino et al., 2018; WHO, 2022),

- The age and developmental stage of the child,
- The physical and mental health of the child and parents,
- Barriers to family's capacity to raise children,
- Financial and social resources accessible to the child and family should be assessed.

As long as the child's safety is ensured, the least harmful way for the child and the least disturbing way for the family should be preferred (Humphreys et al., 2020; WHO, 2022). Furthermore, considering the health problems that children who have been neglected or abused may experience in adulthood, it is recommended to plan the provision of psychological support and health services in the long term (Lippard and Nemeroff, 2020; Greene et al., 2020).

4. Follow-up

The follow-up phase is critical for monitoring recovery and preventing recurrence. A case manager (typically a primary care health professional or social worker) should be responsible for each child and family who assumes the role of contact person (WHO, 2022). Clearly defined plans and issues to be monitored should be determined for each individual and family affected by abuse or neglect. In this process, it is essential to establish links between service providers from different institutions, to share information quickly and healthily, and to respect confidentiality (WHO, 2022; McCoy and Keen, 2022).

Management of Neglect and Abuse in School-Age Children

Although most child abuse and neglect prevention programs primarily focus on parents—given that they are often the perpetrators—limiting interventions solely to parental education is insufficient (Swenson & Schaeffer, 2018). At this point, schools are seen as appropriate settings to implement universal prevention strategies (Gubbels et al., 2021; Nyberg et al., 2023). School-age children spend most of their days at school, and teachers and school staff are often seen as trusted adults for children (Sharley, 2020; Gubbels et al., 2021). These professionals are in a unique position to detect early signs of abuse and neglect, recognize children at risk, and initiate protective measures when necessary (Walsh et al., 2018). The school environment also facilitates the delivery of structured programs aimed at increasing children's awareness of abuse, improving their ability to recognize unsafe situations, and teaching them how to seek help. Teachers and school staff can be trained to recognize behavioral or physical indicators of maltreatment, respond appropriately, and refer cases to relevant services.

Evidence from existing research underscores the effectiveness of school-based prevention programs. These interventions have been shown to enhance children's knowledge and self-protective skills, increase reporting of abuse, and improve staff confidence in handling suspected cases (Walsh et al., 2018; Gubbels et al., 2021; Nyberg et al., 2023). Thus, integrating abuse prevention strategies into the educational system not only supports at-risk children but also fosters a safer and more informed school community.

School-Based Child Abuse and Neglect Programs

School-based prevention programs are designed to reduce the risk of child abuse and neglect by educating children about maltreatment and teaching them self-protection strategies (Blakey and Thigpen, 2015). These program content generally includes teaching children to recognize signs of neglect and abuse and potential abusers, teaching them how to say "no," how to remove themselves from potentially harmful situations, teaching them that it is not their fault, and encouraging children to report previous or ongoing maltreatment to people they trust (Nickerson et al., 2019; Gubbels et al., 2021; Nyberg et al., 2023). The instructional techniques employed in these programs often include lectures, discussions, storytelling, role-plays, case studies, and video presentations, and the sessions are usually conducted in classrooms or schoolyards. The number of sessions ranges from one to twelve, with individual sessions lasting between 30 minutes and 2 hours. Programs are typically facilitated by trained professionals such as teachers, health personnel, or social workers (Diaz et al., 2021; Wolfersteig et al., 2022; Thompson et al., 2022; Svaljek, 2023).

Empirical studies have demonstrated that these programs significantly improve children's knowledge of abuse and neglect and enhance their protective skills and behaviors (Svaljek, 2023; Nyberg et al., 2023). However, school-based programs vary considerably based on several factors, including the type of abuse addressed, delivery methods, age of participants, qualifications of program facilitators, and program duration. Walsh and colleagues (2018) found that longer programs, programs targeting younger children, and those incorporating hands-on behavioral training yielded more effective outcomes.

When the literature is examined, it is seen that programs are mostly developed to prevent child sexual abuse (Zhang et al., 2021; Che et al., 2022; Guastaferro et al., 2022). The "Play is Safe" program is a good example of school-based prevention programs for physical and sexual abuse. This program teaches children how to recognize abuse, how to respond to potential abuse, and how to report abuse to someone who can help stop it. At the end of the program, children's physical and sexual abuse knowledge scores increased significantly (Blakey and Thigpen, 2015; Thompson et al., 2022). Similarly, a program implemented by Kenny et al., (2022) with minority adolescents, five children directly disclosed that they were sexually or physically abused and were reported. Teachers participating in the program also reported increased satisfaction and competence in identifying abuse (Kenny et al., 2022).

Meta-analyses suggest that various program components and delivery techniques contribute to the effectiveness of school-based neglect and abuse prevention programs (Svaljek, 2023; Nyberg et al., 2023). Programs that emphasize social-emotional learning—such as empathy, emotional regulation, problem-solving, and relationship skills—tend to be more impactful. Teaching children that abuse is never their fault and helping them identify a trusted person to confide in are also associated with better outcomes (Citak Tunc et al., 2018). Additionally, school-based programs using puppets as a presentation technique were found to have a larger effect on knowledge about neglect and abuse. Puppets are generally used in school-based programs as models that children can identify with on emotional and cognitive levels. The use of puppets focuses on increasing children's social-emotional skills or self-esteem. Another technique used in programs that aim to increase knowledge about neglect and abuse is games. Games have a positive impact as they increase students' motivation, confidence, effort, and engagement in learning. Research has shown that school-based prevention programs that encourage children's active participation through games and role-play are more effective than those that use traditional teaching methods (lecture, discussion, video only, use of written materials, etc.). Examining how specific content components of programs relate to overall program effectiveness is important. Identifying effective components is essential for the development or improvement of school-based programs. Future empirical research should examine the effectiveness of programs in more depth (Gubbels et al., 2021).

It is recommended that newly developed school-based programs be expanded to cover all forms of abuse and neglect (Gubbels et al., 2021; Svaljek, 2023; Nyberg et al., 2023). In order to combat the increasing rates of child abuse, these programs should continue to be offered under all circumstances by converting them into a web-based or mobile-based format in addition to face-to-face delivery (Gubbels et al., 2021).

Management of Neglect and Abuse at School

Child neglect and abuse are highly sensitive and traumatic issue for both the affected child and the individual to whom the child discloses the abuse. When a child reports maltreatment to school personnel, the manner in which the disclosure is received and the subsequent actions taken are critical in ensuring the child's safety and well-being (Sharley, 2020; McCoy and Keen, 2022). the following steps should be taken in response to a direct disclosure: (KwaZulu-Natal Department of Education, 2015; Sharley, 2020);

- The child's safety must be ensured.
- Any emergency medical or safety issues must be addressed as a priority.
- A special space should be created for the child to speak freely.
- The child's account should be accepted without judgment, even if it seems implausible.
- The child should not be asked questions that encourage feelings of guilt.
- The child should be reassured that the abuse is not their fault.
- Not make promises that cannot be kept (e.g., "your secret is safe with me").
- The child should be gently informed that the situation may need to be legally reported.
- If the parents are not the alleged offenders, they should be informed with the child's consent.
- A detailed report of the situation should be kept; therefore, interviews should also be recorded.

- All information must be kept strictly confidential. Only the necessary information should be shared with the units.
- A support and rehabilitation plan should be developed for the child.

In cases where child abuse or neglect is suspected based on behavioral or physical signs—rather than explicit disclosure—the following steps are advised (KwaZulu-Natal Department of Education, 2015; Swenson and Schaeffer, 2018; Sharley, 2020),

- The child should be observed in terms of changes in behavior, emotions, physical symptoms, days and periods of absenteeism, and possible signs of abuse should be recorded.
- The child should be given the opportunity to tell without pressure.
- Suspicions of neglect or abuse should be discussed with parents without a judgmental or threatening approach.
- If any physical indicators of neglect and abuse are identified, they must be recorded (location, shape, size, and type, e.g., bruises, burns, belt marks, etc.).
- Even if the child does not express it explicitly, if there are definite physical and behavioral symptoms that indicate that the child has been neglected or abused, they should be reported to the school administration and relevant units.
- A support and rehabilitation plan should be developed for the child.

If child maltreatment is inflicted by teachers or other school staff (the most common form of child maltreatment is corporal punishment) (De Haan et al., 2019; Sharley, 2020).

- The situation should be recorded and reported to school management and relevant units.
- The child who has been maltreated should be protected against threats and similar maltreatment throughout the legal process.
- All information, including the child's identity, must be kept strictly confidential.
- A support and rehabilitation plan should be developed for the child.

In cases of peer-to-peer abuse (i.e., when a student abuses another student), the appropriate response includes (KwaZulu-Natal Department of Education, 2015; Swenson and Schaeffer, 2018; Sharley, 2020)

- The situation should be reported to the school management and the necessary units.
- All records, including the identity of children, must be kept strictly confidential.
- If the action violates the school's code of conduct, the school's disciplinary procedure should be applied.
- If the action is criminal, it should be reported to law enforcement authorities.
- The child victim must be protected against threats and similar ill-treatment.
- Support and rehabilitation plans should be developed for both child victims and perpetrators).

When a case of neglect or abuse is identified, it is essential to implement a support or rehabilitation plan tailored to the needs of the child (KwaZulu-Natal Department of Education, 2015; Swenson and Schaeffer, 2018; Sharley, 2020). Key components include:

- Assessing the severity and impact of the abuse.
- Ensuring the student feels safe and supported during any ongoing legal investigations.
- Initiating support plans regardless of legal outcomes.
- Providing services such as counseling, legal preparation, relocation to a safe environment, and medical care.
- Coordinating with external agencies and ensuring ongoing communication for sustained support.
- Monitoring the child's progress through regular reporting from support institutions.
- Documenting each step of the process in detail.

Research shows that teachers and school staff often experience difficulty in detecting and responding to child maltreatment. Challenges include the emotional complexity of such cases, unclear professional roles, and unsupportive school environments. Teachers' personal beliefs, communication skills, and relationships with families also influence their likelihood of reporting suspected abuse (De Haan et al., 2019; Sharley, 2020).

Role of the School Nurse

The literature underscores the critical role of the school nurse in the prevention, detection, and management of child abuse and neglect. School nurses assess the physical and emotional health needs of at-risk children and support families (Lines et al., 2018; Lucas et al., 2021). At this point, their roles and responsibilities include conducting home visits, following up with the child and family, ensuring that they communicate with different institutions when needed, identifying signs and symptoms of maltreatment, organizing training for children and parents, conducting health screenings, and directing parents to social care or counseling services. Nurses work in collaboration with school staff to manage cases of neglect and abuse, meet the health needs of the child and family, and plan the psycho-social support and rehabilitation process (Lines et al., 2018; Harding et al., 2019; Lucas et al., 2021). However, nurses reported that they had difficulty fulfilling their roles and responsibilities due to a lack of time, workload, and the lack of personnel in matters related to child maltreatment (Lines et al., 2018).

Conclusion

Neglect and abuse are serious and widespread public health problems that can have long-term physical, psychological, and social impacts on school-age children's health. The research results conducted to reveal the importance of the situation are only the tip of the iceberg. Problems related to the identification and reporting of neglect and abuse cause current estimates to be incomplete. Therefore, it is necessary to define the problem correctly, identify the causes and risk factors, and design and implement interventions to minimize risk factors. Prevention efforts should include education and awareness campaigns, policies, and programs that support families and protect children. It is essential to create a society where children can grow up in a safe and supportive environment free of abuse and neglect.

Schools constitute an important part of prevention efforts. School-based neglect and abuse prevention programs have been shown to increase school-age children's knowledge about neglect and abuse and provide them with self-protection skills. However, research on the effectiveness of prevention programs is still quite limited. Therefore, it is recommended that programs be included in standard and compulsory curricula to evaluate their effects in the long term. Standardized procedures need to be established for the management of neglect and abuse cases in schools. In this way, case recording, follow-up, and rehabilitation can be carried out healthily. School nurses are the most competent personnel to prevent and manage neglect and abuse in schools. Time and workload problems should be prevented by employing more nurses in schools, and working environments where they can fulfill their roles and responsibilities better should be created.

Disclaimer

None.

References

American Psychiatric Association. (2013). *Diagnostic and statistical manual of mental disorders: DSM-5* (5th ed., Vol. 21).

Amin, U., Rashid, B., Jan, R., Jan, R., & Malla, A. M. (2023). Child abuse and neglect. *Indian Journal of Continuing Nursing Education, 24*(2), 104–109. https://doi.org/10.4103/ijcn.ijcn_40_22.

Blakey, J. M., & Thigpen, J. W. (2015). Play it safe!®: A school-based childhood physical and sexual abuse prevention program. *Journal of Adolescent and Family Health, 7*(1), 5. https://scholar.utc.edu/jafh/vol7/iss1/5.

Che Yusof, R., Norhayati, M. N., & Mohd Azman, Y. (2022). Effectiveness of school-based child sexual abuse intervention among school children in the new millennium era: Systematic review and meta-analyses. *Frontiers in Public Health, 10*, 909254. https://doi.org/10.3389/fpubh.2022.909254.

Children's Bureau of the U.S. Department of Health and Human Services. (2022). *Child maltreatment 2022*. Retrieved from https://www.acf.hhs.gov/sites/default/files/documents/cb/cm2022.pdf.

Citak Tunc, G., Gorak, G., Ozyazicioglu, N., Ak, B., Isil, O., & Vural, P. (2018). Preventing child sexual abuse: Body safety training for young children in Turkey. *Journal of Child Sexual Abuse, 27*(4), 347–364. https://doi.org/10.1080/10538712.2018.1477001.

De Haan, I., Joy, E., Beddoe, L., & Iam, S. (2019). "The tip of the iceberg": Multiple thresholds in schools' detecting and reporting of child abuse and neglect. *Children and Youth Services Review, 96*, 278–285. https://doi.org/10.1016/j.childyouth.2018.10.034.

Diaz, M. J., Moreland, D., & Wolfersteig, W. (2021). Assessing the effects of Childhelp's Speak Up Be Safe child abuse prevention curriculum for high school students. *Journal of Child & Adolescent Trauma, 14*(3), 425–432. https://doi.org/10.1007/s40653-021-00353-1.

Fayaz, I. (2019). Child abuse: Effects and preventive measures. *The International Journal of Indian Psychology, 7*(2), 871–884. https://doi.org/10.25215/0702.105.

Fortson, B. L., Klevens, J., Merrick, M. T., Gilbert, L. K., & Alexander, S. P. (2016). *Preventing child abuse and neglect: A technical package for policy, norm, and programmatic activities*. Centers for Disease Control and Prevention. http://dx.doi.org/10.15620/cdc.38864.

Gardner, M. J., Thomas, H. J., & Erskine, H. E. (2019). The association between five forms of child maltreatment and depressive and anxiety disorders: A systematic review and meta-analysis. *Child Abuse & Neglect, 96*, 104082. https://doi.org/10.1016/j.chiabu.2019.104082.

Giardino, A. P., Lyn, M. A., & Giardino, E. R. (2018). *A practical guide to the evaluation of child physical abuse and neglect*. Springer.

Greene, C. A., Haisley, L., Wallace, C., & Ford, J. D. (2020). Intergenerational effects of childhood maltreatment: A systematic review of the parenting practices of adult survivors of childhood abuse, neglect, and violence. *Clinical Psychology Review, 80*, 101891. https://doi.org/10.1016/j.cpr.2020.101891

Guastaferro, K., & Shipe, S. L. (2023). Child maltreatment types by age: Implications for prevention. *International Journal of Environmental Research and Public Health, 21*(1), 20. https://doi.org/10.3390/ijerph21010020.

Guastaferro, K., Holloway, J. L., Trudeau, J., Lipson, L. B., Sunshine, S., Noll, J. G., & Pulido, M. L. (2022). Virtual delivery of a school-based child sexual abuse prevention program: A pilot study. *Journal of Child Sexual Abuse, 31*(5), 577–592. https://doi.org/10.1080/10538712.2022.2112347.

Gubbels, J., van der Put, C. E., Stams, G. J. J., & Assink, M. (2021). Effective components of school-based prevention programs for child abuse: A meta-analytic review. *Clinical Child and Family Psychology Review, 24*(3), 553–578. https://doi.org/10.1007/s10567-021-00353-5.

Harding, L., Davison-Fischer, J., Bekaert, S., & Appleton, J. V. (2019). The role of the school nurse in protecting children and young people from maltreatment: An integrative review of the literature. *International Journal of Nursing Studies, 92*, 60–72. https://doi.org/10.1016/j.ijnurstu.2018.12.017.

Higgins, D. J., Mathews, B., Pacella, R., Scott, J. G., Finkelhor, D., Meinck, F., ... Dunne, M. P. (2023). The prevalence and nature of multi-type child maltreatment in Australia. *Medical Journal of Australia, 218*, S19–S25. https://doi.org/10.5694/mja2.51868.

Humphreys, K. L., LeMoult, J., Wear, J. G., Piersiak, H. A., Lee, A., & Gotlib, I. H. (2020). Child maltreatment and depression: A meta-analysis of studies using the Childhood Trauma Questionnaire. *Child Abuse & Neglect, 102*, 104361. https://doi.org/10.1016/j.chiabu.2020.104361.

Jaffee, S. R. (2017). Child maltreatment and risk for psychopathology in childhood and adulthood. *Annual Review of Clinical Psychology, 13*, 525–551. https://doi.org/10.1146/annurev-clinpsy-032816-045005.

KwaZulu-Natal Department of Education. (2015). *Guidelines for the management of child abuse, neglect and exploitation for public schools in KwaZulu-Natal*. Retrieved from https://www.kzneducation.gov.za/images/documents/Resources/SNES/PreventionOfChildAbuse/ChildAbuseProtocols.pdf.

Lines, L., Grant, J., & Hutton, A. (2018). How do nurses keep children safe from abuse and neglect, and does it make a difference? A scoping review. *Journal of Pediatric Nursing, 43*, e75–e84. https://doi.org/10.1016/j.pedn.2018.07.010.

Lippard, E. T., & Nemeroff, C. B. (2020). The devastating clinical consequences of child abuse and neglect: Increased disease vulnerability and poor treatment response in mood disorders. *American Journal of Psychiatry, 177*(1), 20–36. https://doi.org/10.1176/appi.ajp.2019.19010020.

Lucas, C., Crowell, K. R., & Olympia, R. P. (2021). School nurses on the front lines of healthcare: Red flags and red herrings: Improving the recognition of bruises and burns associated with physical abuse in school-age children. *NASN School Nurse, 36*(1), 32–38. https://doi.org/10.1177/1942602X20942922.

Massullo, C., De Rossi, E., Carbone, G. A., Imperatori, C., Ardito, R. B., Adenzato, M., & Farina, B. (2023). Child maltreatment, abuse, and neglect: An umbrella review of their prevalence and definitions. *Clinical Neuropsychiatry, 20*(2), 72. https://doi.org/10.36131/cnfioritieditore20230201.

McCoy, M. L., & Keen, S. M. (2022). *Child abuse and neglect*. Routledge.

Moody, G., Cannings-John, R., Hood, K., Kemp, A., & Robling, M. (2018). Establishing the international prevalence of self-reported child maltreatment: A systematic review by maltreatment type and gender. *BMC Public Health, 18*, 1–15. https://doi.org/10.1186/s12889-018-6044-y.

Mulder, T. M., Kuiper, K. C., van der Put, C. E., Stams, G. J. J., & Assink, M. (2018). Risk factors for child neglect: A meta-analytic review. *Child Abuse & Neglect, 77*, 198–210. https://doi.org/10.1016/j.chiabu.2018.01.006.

Nickerson, A. B., Tulledge, J., Manges, M., Kesselring, S., Parks, T., Livingston, J. A., & Dudley, M. (2019). Randomized controlled trial of the Child Protection Unit: Grade and gender as moderators of CSA prevention concepts in elementary students. *Child Abuse & Neglect, 96*, 104101. https://doi.org/10.1016/j.chiabu.2019.104101.

Nyberg, A., Ferm, U., & Bornman, J. (2023). School-based abuse prevention programs for children: A scoping review. *International Journal of Disability, Development and Education, 70*(2), 137–155. https://doi.org/10.1080/1034912X.2020.1865522.

Sharley, V. (2020). Identifying and responding to child neglect within schools: Differing perspectives and the implications for inter-agency practice. *Child Indicators Research, 13*(2), 551–571. https://doi.org/10.1007/s12187-019-09681-z.

Strathearn, L., Giannotti, M., Mills, R., Kisely, S., Najman, J., & Abajobir, A. (2020). Long-term cognitive, psychological, and health outcomes associated with child abuse and neglect. *Pediatrics, 146*(4). https://doi.org/10.1542/peds.2020-0438.

Svaljek, P. (2023). *Universal school-based programs targeting the prevention of child maltreatment: An effective intervention? Systematic literature review*. Retrieved from https://www.diva-portal.org/smash/get/diva2:1778000/FULLTEXT01.pdf.

Swenson, C. C., & Schaeffer, C. M. (2018). A multisystemic approach to the prevention and treatment of child abuse and neglect. *International Journal on Child Maltreatment: Research, Policy and Practice, 1*(1), 97–120. https://doi.org/10.1007/s42448-018-0002-2.

Thompson, E. L., Zhou, Z., Garg, A., Rohr, D., Ajoku, B., & Spence, E. E. (2022). Evaluation of a school-based child physical and sexual abuse prevention program. *Health Education & Behavior, 49*(4), 584–592. https://doi.org/10.1177/109019812098825.

Turkish Statistical Institute (TURKSTAT). (2022). *Statistics of children coming or brought to the security unit, 2021*. Retrieved from https://data.tuik.gov.tr/Bulten/Index?p=Juvenile-Statistics-Received-Into-Security-Unit-2021-45586.

U.S. Department of Health & Human Services, Administration for Children and Families, Administration on Children, Youth and Families, Children's Bureau. (2023). *Framework for prevention of child maltreatment. Child Welfare Information Gateway*. Retrieved from https://www.childwelfare.gov/topics/preventing/overview/framework/.

Walsh, K., Zwi, K., Woolfenden, S., & Shlonsky, A. (2018). School-based education programs for the prevention of child sexual abuse: A Cochrane systematic review and meta-analysis. *Research on Social Work Practice, 28*(1), 33–55. https://doi.org/10.1177/1049731515619705.

Wolfersteig, W., Diaz, M. J., & Moreland, D. (2022). Empowering elementary and middle school youth to speak up and be safe: Advancing prevention of child maltreatment with a universal school-based curriculum. *International Journal of Environmental Research and Public Health, 19*(19), 11856. https://doi.org/10.3390/ijerph191911856.

World Health Organization (WHO). (1999). *Report of the consultation on child abuse prevention, Geneva, 29–31 March 1999*. Retrieved from https://iris.who.int/handle/10665/65900.

World Health Organization (WHO). (2006). *Preventing child maltreatment: A guide to taking action and generating evidence*. Retrieved from https://iris.who.int/bitstream/handle/10665/43499/9241594365_eng.pdf?sequence=1.

World Health Organization (WHO). (2018). *INSPIRE handbook: Action for implementing the seven strategies for ending violence against children*. Retrieved from https://www.who.int/publications/i/item/inspire-handbook-action-for-implementing-the-seven-strategies-for-ending-violence-against-children.

World Health Organization (WHO). (2020). *Global status report on preventing violence against children 2020*. Geneva. Retrieved from https://iris.who.int/bitstream/handle/10665/332394/9789240004191-eng.pdf?sequence=1.

World Health Organization (WHO). (2022). *Child maltreatment 2022*. Retrieved from https://www.who.int/news-room/fact-sheets/detail/child-maltreatment.

World Health Organization (WHO). (2022). *Responding to child maltreatment: A clinical handbook for health professionals*. Retrieved from https://www.who.int/publications/i/item/9789240048737.

Zeanah, C. H., & Humphreys, K. L. (2018). Child abuse and neglect. *Journal of the American Academy of Child & Adolescent Psychiatry, 57*(9), 637–644. https://doi.org/10.1016/j.jaac.2018.06.007.

Zhang, H., Shi, R., Li, Y., & Wang, Y. (2021). Effectiveness of school-based child sexual abuse prevention programs in China: A meta-analysis. *Research on Social Work Practice, 31*(7), 693–705. https://doi.org/10.1177/10497315211022827.

Chapter 22

The Management of Childhood Infectious Diseases in Schools

Renginar Öztürk Dönmez[1,*], PhD and Gülengül Mermer[2]

[1]Ege University Faculty of Nursing, Public Health Nursing Department, İzmir, Türkiye
[2]Iğdır University Faculty of Health Sciences, Department of Nursing, Iğdır, Türkiye

Abstract

Healthy People 2030 emphasizes the importance of health promotion, safety, and learning in school environments, reducing the incidence of infectious disease and improving outcomes for individuals with chronic infections. Schools are common settings for the spread of infectious diseases such as measles, rubella, chickenpox, mumps, meningococcal infections, enteroviral illnesses (e.g., hand-foot-mouth disease), viral gastroenteritis, hepatitis A, Shigella, Escherichia coli infections, giardiasis, respiratory infections (e.g., influenza, the common cold), streptococcal infections (e.g., scarlet fever, streptococcal pharyngitis, impetigo), and pediculosis capitis (head lice). Key preventive strategies include promoting personal hygiene (e.g., handwashing, respiratory etiquette, nail and oral hygiene), ensuring proper ventilation, educating on safe contact with animals, and maintaining up-to-date immunizations. Supporting informed health decisions and implementing precautions against communicable diseases are vital to safeguarding children's health and preventing outbreaks within school settings.

Keywords: school-age children, infectious diseases, control, school nursing

Introduction

School is an institution that has an important place in public health and is responsible for the social, psychological, physical, and intellectual development of children and adolescents after the family (CDC, 2023). The World Health Organization (WHO) emphasizes this relationship

---

* Corresponding Author's Email: renginarozturk@gmail.com

In: Health Promotion and Prevention
Editor: Eda Kılınç İşleyen
ISBN: 979-8-89530-758-8

between health and education, highlighting that safe and supportive school environments are associated with better health outcomes (WHO, 2021).

School-age children and adolescents (5-19 years old) face a range of preventable health issues, including unintentional injury, interpersonal violence, sexual and reproductive health challenges, communicable and non-communicable diseases, and mental health problems (WHO, 2021). In the United States, the Healthy People 2020 initiative addressed school-based disease management under key themes such as adolescent health, community-based programs, immunization and infectious diseases, injury prevention, nutrition and tobacco use (Healthy People, 2020). The updated Healthy People 2030 goals focus on health promotion, safety, and learning in school environments, reducing infectious disease incidence, and improving the health outcomes in individual with chronic infections (Healthy People, 2030).

Despite global immunization efforts, diseases such as measles, rubella, congenital rubella syndrome, and polio have not yet been fully eliminated. Sustained efforts to improve vaccination coverage are essential to achieving and maintaining disease elimination (Healthy People, 2030). Accordingly, the management of childhood infectious diseases must be revisited using updated guidelines and assessment tools. There is a need for continuous evaluation, classification, and integration of effective treatment strategies into school-based health services (WHO, 2024). According to the WHO, countries also need to critically assess the health needs of children and adolescents, identify the most appropriate evidence-based interventions to address them, and then prioritize them in national health programs (WHO, 2022).

Common infectious diseases in school environment include measles, rubella, chickenpox, mumps, meningococcal infections, enterovirus diseases (e.g., hand-foot-mouth disease), viral gastroenteritis, hepatitis A, Shigella, Escherichia coli, giardiasis, airborne diseases (e.g., influenza, common cold), streptococcal infections (e.g., scarlet fever, streptococcal pharyngitis, impetigo), and infestations such as head lice. Preventing and managing infectious diseases in schools is essential for ensuring children's right to health and education. Schools are not only educational institutions but also critical settings for public health intervention. Coordinated strategies involving school nurses, educators, public health officials, families, and communities are essential to identify, control, and prevent the spread of infectious diseases among school-aged children. Integrating these measures into school health systems can significantly reduce absenteeism, enhancing academic performance.

Common Cold

The common cold is a prevalent upper respiratory tract infection caused by numerous viruses, particularly rhinoviruses, and occasionally by bacteria. Most children experience 8 to 10 colds by the age of two, and the frequency tends to increase in settings with multiple children, such as schools and childcare centers, due to the ease of transmission (Pappas et al., 2008).

Typical symptoms of the common cold include a sore throat, runny nose, coughing, watery eyes, sneezing, restlessness, and a low-grade fever. According to Troullos et al., (2014), children aged 6-11 most frequently report nasal congestion, and sore or itchy throat as the most severe symptoms. The intensity of these symptoms generally peaks within 1-2 days of onset (Jones, 2020). Transmission occurs primarily via respiratory droplets when an infected individual coughs or sneezes, and another person inhales the droplets. The virus may also spread through contact with contaminated surfaces, followed by touching the eyes, nose, or mouth (Troullos et al., 2014). To reduce the spread of the common cold in school, the following preventive measures should be enforced:

- Proper hand hygiene: Regular and effective hand-washing with soap and water by children and staff.
- Surface disinfection: Daily cleaning and disinfection of commonly touched surfaces and toys.
- Ventilation: Ensuring adequate airflow through natural ventilation (e.g., opening windows) or mechanical systems.
- Respiratory etiquette: Teaching children to cough or sneeze into their elbow or a tissue and disposing of tissues properly.

There is no antiviral treatment for the common cold, and antibiotics are ineffective since the condition is viral in nature. Most cases resolve spontaneously with adequate rest, hydration, and supportive care. However, in cases where symptoms persist or worsen, medical evaluation may be necessary to rule out secondary bacterial infections or other complications (Fashner et al., 2012).

Influenza

Influenza is an acute respiratory disease caused by influenza viruses and is highly contagious, affecting individuals of all ages. In school-aged children, the total economic burden of influenza is estimated to be approximately $1.5 billion annually (Molinari et al., 2007). Influenza is different from the common cold, and symptoms usually appear quickly. Symptoms include headache, muscle aches, cough, sore throat, nasal congestion, fatigue, abdominal pain, nausea, and vomiting. A rapid spike in fever is also common in many cases.

The influenza virus is usually transmitted through the respiratory droplets when an infected person coughs or sneezes. It can also spread via contact with contaminated surfaces, followed by touching the eyes, nose, or mouth. While many individuals recover within a few days, influenza can lead to serious complications such as pneumonia, myocarditis, myositis, or even multi-organ failure. Every year, both children and adults die from influenza-related complications (Department of Health and Social Services Delaware, 2020; Principi et al., 2004).

Vaccination is the most effective strategy for preventing influenza. Annual influenza vaccination is recommended for all individuals aged 6 months and older (Coelingh et al., 2015). Randomized controlled trials have demonstrated that the live attenuated influenza vaccine is especially protective for children aged 2-6 years, offering a higher degree of protection than the inactivated vaccine (Wang et al., 2020; Kildegaard et al., 2023). Other general prevention measures align with those recommended for the common cold.

Measles, Mumps, Rubella (MMR)

In recent years, significant outbreaks of mumps and clusters of measles cases in children have underscored the continuing threat posed by these vaccine-preventable diseases. Measles typically begins with symptoms such as a runny nose, sneezing, cough, conjunctivitis (characterized by painful, itchy, watery, red, and sticky eyes), followed by high fever. A hallmark sign is the appearance of small white spots on the inside of the cheeks and behind the lips. By the third day of illness, a red or brown rash generally begins on the face and ears, then spreads throughout the rest of the body. This usually begins on the third day of illness (Lee et al., 2005).

Rubella presents more mildly and includes a low-grade fever, loss of appetite, nausea, fatigue, cough, headache, and conjunctivitis (less pronounced than in measles). A non-itchy or mildly itchy erythematous, maculopapular rash typically starts on the face and spreads to the trunk and limbs (Jaber, 2006).

Mumps is characterized by fever, painful swelling of the salivary glands (usually the parotid), headaches, joint pain, malaise, fatigue, and reduced appetite (Harling et al., 2005).

The infectious periods of these diseases vary:

- Measles is contagious from 4 days before to 4 days after the appearance of the rash (Lee et al., 2005).
- Rubella is infectious 1–2 days before the rash begins and remains contagious for 5–7 days afterward (Jaber, 2006).
- Mumps can spread a few days before symptom onset, and children should stay home for at least 5 days after glandular swelling begins (Harling et al., 2005).

Vaccination is the most effective preventive measure. The MMR vaccine, which protects against measles, mumps, and rubella, should be routinely administered to all children (Defay et al., 2013). A cross-sectional study conducted in England between January and March 2013 identified 28 cases of mumps (24 students and 4 staff). Among these, 21 had received two MMR doses, two had received one dose, and two were unvaccinated. The study recommended administering an additional MMR dose as an acceptable control strategy in outbreak settings, even where vaccination coverage is high (Aasheim et al., 2013).

To prevent transmission within school settings:

- Thorough cleaning of high-touch surfaces—such as light switches, handrails, kitchens, and bathrooms—should be conducted regularly.
- Children should be taught to cover their nose and mouth with a tissue or sleeve when coughing or sneezing, dispose of tissues immediately, and wash their hands afterward.
- Regular hand hygiene with soap and water or alcohol-based hand sanitizer should be emphasized, especially before eating, after using the toilet, and after coughing or sneezing.
- Adequate ventilation must be ensured without compromising thermal comfort.
- Sharing personal items such as cutlery, towels, bedding, clothing, and bathrooms should be discouraged (Kauffmann et al., 2021).

Haemophilus Influenzae

Haemophilus influenzae type b (Hib) is a bacterium that causes a variety of infections in humans, particularly in school-age children. These infections include otitis media (ear infections), bacteremia (bloodstream infections), and more severe conditions such as meningitis, epiglottitis, and pneumonia (Department of Health and Social Services Delaware, 2020). Clinical manifestations of Hib infection vary depending on the site of infection but may include fever, irritability, cough, vomiting, joint swelling, facial swelling or discoloration, neck stiffness, and difficulty breathing. Complications of Hib infections can include meningitis, epiglottitis, pneumonia, and death (Oh et al., 2008). A longitudinal study assessing children infected with Hib found that those who experienced neurological complications during the acute phase were at increased risk for long-term neuropsychological, academic, and behavioral sequelae, particularly those with early, widespread brain damage (Taylor et al., 2000).

The treatment of Hib infections usually includes the use of appropriate antibiotics. In certain cases, prophylactic antibiotics therapy is recommended for unvaccinated or incompletely immunized individuals who have been exposed to Hib. Transmission of Hib occurs through respiratory droplets when an infected person coughs or sneezes. The bacterium can also spread via contact with contaminated objects or surfaces, followed by touching the eyes, nose, or mouth (Bou et al., 2000; Department of Health and Social Services Delaware, 2020).

Immunization is the most effective strategy to prevent Hib infections. Routine Hib vaccination is essential and should be part of all school immunization programs (See *Immunization in School-Age Children and Adolescents*). Preventive measures in schools should include:

- Promoting regular and effective handwashing practices among children and staff, especially after using the toilet or changing diapers.
- Daily cleaning and disinfection of toys and frequently touched surfaces, particularly when visibly soiled.
- Teaching children to cough or sneeze into their elbows or into a tissue, followed by appropriate hand hygiene.
- Ensuring that children diagnosed with Hib infection return to school only after receiving medical clearance from a physician (Ortiz et al., 2017).

Diphtheria

Diphtheria is a serious bacterial infection caused by the Corynebacterium diphtheriae, primarily affecting the mucous membranes of the nose and throat. Diphtheria causes a thick coating in the nose and throat that can make breathing difficult. The hallmark of diphtheria is the formation of a thick, grayish coating in the throat and nose, which can obstruct breathing and swallowing (Adler, 2013). Initial symptoms typically resemble those of a common cold—fever, sore throat, runny nose, and swollen cervical lymph nodes—but the disease can rapidly progress and become life-threatening if untreated.

Transmission occurs through respiratory droplets when an infected person coughs or sneezes, or through direct contact with respiratory secretions. Diphtheria can also spread by touching contaminated objects and surfaces such as toys, books, doorknobs, or desks. Although less common, contact with open skin lesions of an infected individual may also transmit the bacteria (Department of Health and Social Services Delaware, 2020).

Vaccination is the most effective method of prevention. There are four vaccines available that protect against diphtheria: DTaP, Tdap, DT, and Td. These vaccines are typically administered as part of routine childhood immunization schedules (Clarke, 2017). For further information, refer to the section Immunization in School-Age Children and Adolescents. School health protocols should include:

- Reviewing and documenting students' immunization status upon school entry and conducting periodic follow-ups.
- Promptly referring children with incomplete or missing vaccinations to healthcare providers or local health departments for immunization updates.
- Ensuring that children who have been infected with diphtheria receive appropriate medical care and are cleared to return to school only after obtaining negative cultures, confirming that they are no longer contagious (Clarke, 2017; Department of Health and Social Services Delaware, 2020).

Chickenpox

Chickenpox is a highly contagious disease caused by the *varicella-zoster* virus. Although it is generally a mild illness in healthy children, it can result in serious complications or even death, particularly in individuals with weakened immune systems—such as newborns, individuals undergoing chemotherapy, those with AIDS, or individuals taking immunosuppressive medications like corticosteroids (Gould, 2014).

The disease typically begins with that progresses from small red bumps to fluid-filled blisters, initially appearing on the scalp and then spreading to the torso and face. However, the distribution and severity of the rash can vary among individuals (Wan, 2024). Some individuals may exhibit no symptoms at the early stage of the infection or may display mild symptoms that resemble the common cold.

A study conducted in England by Camoerin et al., (2007), reported that the average age of confirmed chickenpox cases was 3 years (range: 0–14 years). Among hospitalized children, serious complications were frequently observed, including bacteremia/septic shock (n = 30), pneumonia (n = 30), encephalitis (n = 26), ataxia (n = 25), toxic shock syndrome or toxin-mediated illness (n = 14), necrotizing fasciitis (n = 7), purpura fulminans/disseminated intravascular coagulation (n = 5), fulminant chickenpox (n = 5), and neonatal varicella (n = 3). Nearly half (46%) of the patients developed secondary bacterial infections. The average hospital stay was 7 days, with durations ranging from 1 to 68 days (Cameron et al., 2007).

Immunization is the most effective preventive measure against chickenpox. The varicella vaccine is recommended for all individuals aged 12 months and older (Ministry of Health, 2025). For additional information, refer to the section *Immunization in School-Age Children and Adolescents.*

Prevention of transmission also involves:

- Maintaining strict hand hygiene,
- Avoiding contact between infected and non-immune individuals,
- Encouraging respiratory etiquette, and
- Disinfecting surfaces and commonly touched objects regularly.

Impetigo

Impetigo is a highly contagious bacterial skin infection most commonly observed in children aged 2 to 5 years. It is caused by *Staphylococcus aureus* or Group A *Streptococcus*. The condition typically presents as a blistering rash localized around the mouth, nose, hands, and feet. The blisters rupture easily, releasing a thick, golden-yellow fluid that dries to form a characteristic crust adhered to the skin. Mild itching and pain often accompany the rash (Paul, 2024).

Transmission occurs through direct contact with discharge from the lesions, making the infection particularly prevalent in crowded environments, such as childcare centers (Department of Health and Social Services Delaware, 2020). Several factors can predispose individuals to impetigo or worsen the infection, including chickenpox, herpes simplex, insect bites, radiation therapy, scabies, burns, and minor trauma (Akiyode, 2013). Treatment typically involves topical or oral antibiotics, depending on the severity and extent of the infection (Paul, 2024).

Preventive measures include:

- Encouraging regular and thorough handwashing in children,
- Cleaning all cuts and abrasions with soap and water,
- Covering wounds with clean gauze or bandages,
- Washing infected children's clothing, towels, and linens daily, and ensuring these items are not shared with others,
- Using disposable gloves when applying prescribed topical antibiotics.

Children diagnosed with impetigo should be excluded from school. They may return to school once treatment has begun and there is visible improvement in the lesions (Johnson, 2020).

Hepatitis A

Hepatitis A is a vaccine-preventable viral infection of the liver caused by the hepatitis A virus (HAV). In children under the age of six, the disease is often asymptomatic or presents with mild symptoms. However, older children and adults are more likely to exhibit classical symptoms, including loss of appetite, fever, nausea, fatigue, abdominal pain, joint pain, dark-colored urine, and jaundice (Kumar et al., 2014). Symptoms usually resolce within two months. In a study by Kumar et al., (2014), the mean age of affected HAV children was 7.85 ± 3.4 years.

All patients presented with jaundice, and common findings included fever (82.1%), hepatomegaly (98.7%), and splenomegaly (39.7%). While most children recovered within two months, prolonged cholestasis was observed in two cases, and the mortality rate was reported as 1.3%.

HAV is transmitted via the fecal-oral route, typically through the ingestion of contaminated food or water, or by touching the mouth with contaminated hands. Infected individuals are most contagious approximately two weeks before symptom onset, and transmission can occur even in the absence of symptoms. Following infection, individuals develop lifelong immunity.

Outbreaks of hepatitis A in schools and childcare settings have been documented since the 1970s (Erdoğan et al., 2004). Some of these outbreaks have been linked to home-prepared snacks and meals brought into the school environment. Because infection among children is often mild or has no symptoms, and people are contagious before they develop symptoms, outbreaks are usually only noticed when adults (usually parents) become ill. Poor hygiene practices among food preparation personnel contribute to the spread of hepatitis A (Sintusek et al., 2019).

Vaccination is the most effective preventive measure. Children should be taught proper hand hygiene, especially before eating and after using the restroom. Educational programs for staff and parents should include guidance on post-exposure prophylaxis, which can help prevent infection if administered within two weeks of exposure. A systematic review conducted by Andani et al., (2022) found that both one-dose and two-dose hepatitis A vaccination programs in children significantly reduced the incidence of hepatitis A across all age groups. Notably, two-dose regimens were associated with reductions in incidence for 14 years or more, while the long-term effectiveness of single-dose regimens beyond six years remains uncertain (Andani et al., 2022).

Diarrhea and Giardiasis

Diarrhea is defined as the passage of frequent, loose, or watery stools. It is one of the most common diseases in childhood, contributing significantly to global health and economic burdens. An estimated 4% of per Gross Domestic Product was spent on diarrhea treatment in 2018 (Hasan et al., 2021). Diarrhea may result from infectious causes, including bacteria, viruses, and parasites (Vecchio et al., 2021). Diarrhea can also be caused by non-infectious processes such as food allergies, dietary changes, excessive fruit juice intake, malabsorption syndromes, and the use of certain medications such as antibiotics. Among infectious agents, rotavirus is the most common cause in children (Florez et al., 2020).

Symptoms accompanying diarrhea may include nausea, vomiting, abdominal cramps, headache, fever, and signs of dehydration. Transmission occurs primarily via the fecal-oral route, typically through contact with contaminated hands, surfaces, water, or food. Other modes of transmission include raw or undercooked poultry, contaminated drinking water, swimming in fecally contaminated pools, and contact with infected animals (Ashkenazi and Schwartz, 2020).

A key priority in the clinical management of pediatric diarrhea is the assessment of hydration status, which guides fluid therapy. Laboratory testing is generally not routinely indicated, except in selected cases. Therapeutic strategies to reduce the duration and severity of diarrhea have been widely studied. High-quality evidence supports the effectiveness and safety of zinc supplementation and synbiotics. Ondansetron is currently the only effective and safe antiemetic recommended to control vomiting in children with diarrhea (Florez et al., 2020).

Giardiasis is a diarrheal disease caused by the *Giardia lamblia* (also known as *Giardia intestinalis* or *Giardia duodenalis*). It is recognized as the most common parasitic cause of diarrhea worldwide. Many infected children are asymptomatic. When symptoms occur, they include fatty diarrhea, abdominal cramps, flatulence, nausea, vomiting, dehydration, fatigue, and weight loss. Like other diarrheal diseases, giardiasis spreads via the oral-fecal route. Notably, Giardia is resistant to chlorine, it is most commonly spread through contaminated drinking water, swimming pools, fountains, and recreational water sources (Olszak et al., 2023).

To prevent the spread of diarrheal diseases in the school environment, hygiene practices must be enforced. Children should be taught and routinely prompted to wash their hands upon arriving at school, after using the toilet, and before eating. All food should be stored and cooked safely, and infected food-handling personnel should be excluded until cleared. Toys, toilets, surfaces, and food preparation areas should be disinfected daily and when visibly dirty. School-age children may return to school when symptoms completely resolve, or 48 hours after fever and diarrhea subside, in accordance with public health guidance (Hajare et al., 2022).

Pediculosis Capitis

Pediculosis capitis, or head lice infestation, is caused by small parasitic insects (*Pediculus humanus capitis*) that reside primarily on the human scalp, and less commonly on the eyebrows or eyelashes. It is distinct from body lice, pubic lice, and fleas. According to a systematic review analyzing data from over 1.2 million individuals, the global prevalence of pediculosis capitis among schoolchildren was estimated at 19%, with a significantly higher rate in girls (19%) compared to boys (7%). The highest prevalence was observed in Central and South America (33%), while the lowest was reported in Europe (5%) (Hatam Nahavandi et al., 2020).

Pediculosis capitis infestation is not related to poor hygiene or environmental cleanliness. Although small, adult head lice can be seen with the naked eye. Due to their mobility, they are often difficult to detect, making magnification tools (e.g., a hand lens) useful during examinations. Head lice survive by feeding on human blood and attaching their eggs (nits) to the base of hair shafts, especially near the nape of the neck and behind the ears. Nits appear as small white or dark ovals. Adult lice cannot survive more than 48 hours away from a human host. The primary symptom of infestation is itching, typically in the areas where lice feed, such as the scalp, neck, and behind the ears (Trüeb et al., 2023). Children may also report the sensation of lice moving on their scalp. Because lice are more active at night, they may cause sleep disturbances and irritability. Persistent scratching can lead to open sores and secondary infections (Department of Health and Social Services Delaware, 2020; Thompson et al., 2021).

Pediculosis capitis is spread primarily through direct head-to-head contact. This contact may be common among children at school, at home, at sporting events, on playgrounds, in camps, and at sleepovers. Sharing personal items such as hats, brushes, combs, and sheets, or placing them on pillows or other furniture from an infected person, may play a role in spreading among children, but this is less common (Department of Health and Social Services Delaware,

2020). However, lice have difficulty clinging to smooth surfaces such as metal or plastic, and nits must remain close to the scalp for warmth and successful hatching (Karthikeyan et al., 2022). Risk factors for infestation include infrequent hair washing, limited hygiene awareness, low parental education, large family size, and lack of bathing facilities.

Treatment involves the use of medicated shampoos, rinses, or lotions (pediculicides) specifically formulated for head lice. Products containing permethrin are widely used due to their high residual activity, effectively targeting both adult lice and nits. These treatments must be used as directed. Fine-toothed combs can help remove nits (Leung et al., 2022). In a study by Karthikeyan et al., (2022), a single application of ivermectin shampoo was effective in 86.2% of cases, and repeated application achieved 100% efficacy in persistent cases.

In school settings, when a case is identified, all children in the same class or group should be screened the same day for adult lice and nits. The same comb should not be used on more than one child during the scanning process (Leung et al., 2021). Children found to be infested should be excluded and treated. Parents should be educated about the importance of following the same recommendations at home and notifying the facility if any member of the household has head lice. Clothing, bedding, hats, and scarves should be washed in hot water (at least 130˚F). Combs and brushes should be soaked in hot water for 5–10 minutes, and vacuuming carpets and upholstered furniture is advisable. Suspected cases should be sent home at the end of the school day, and children may return once treatment has been initiated (Maryanti and Haslinda, 2022).

Management of Childhood Infectious Diseases

The WHO Child Health and Development Unit strategy in the management of childhood diseases consists of three core components:

- Improving the case management skills of healthcare providers;
- Improving health systems to ensure the provision of high-quality care;
- Improving family and community health practices to support children's health, growth, and development (WHO, 2024).

This integrated approach aims to support and empower healthcare professionals, families, and caregivers, ensuring that childhood illnesses are managed effectively at both the clinical and community levels. Similarly, the U.S. Centers for Disease Control and Prevention (CDC) outlines strategies to promote a healthy school environment, focusing on the following elements (CDC, 2023):

- Provision of healthier nutrition options and nutrition education;
- Implementation of comprehensive physical activity and physical education programs;
- Enhancement of chronic disease management processes and staff training;
- Delivery of health education to build lifelong health literacy and behaviors;
- Strengthening of school health services and connections to clinical and community-based resources.

(CDC, 2023).

The CDC (2024) also provides detailed preventive tools and resources aimed at reducing the transmission of infectious diseases in school settings. These include:

- Personal hygiene education (e.g., handwashing, coughing/sneezing etiquette, nail and oral hygiene, ventilation, and tooth brushing);
- Guidance on animal contact safety;
- Support for vaccination decision-making processes;
- Measures to prevent the spread of COVID-19 and other infections.

In schools with shared living spaces, several factors facilitate the spread of infectious diseases. These include inadequate hygiene practices, overcrowding, limited hygiene awareness among children, and insufficient school sanitation measures (Akçay, 2016). Therefore, school-based interventions must prioritize hygiene education, regular cleaning routines, health screenings, and infection prevention protocols to effectively manage and prevent childhood infectious diseases.

Conclusion

Children are particularly vulnerable to infectious diseases due to their developing immune systems and close social interactions in school and community settings. Preventive strategies, such as routine immunizations, personal hygiene education, and health literacy programs targeting both children and caregivers, are essential for minimizing the spread and impact of these diseases. Early identification and treatment are essential in managing these infections effectively, reducing absenteeism, and supporting the overall well-being of school-aged children. Education for both parents and children about the symptoms, modes of transmission, and prevention strategies enhances community resilience and facilitates a more proactive approach to health. Creating a coordinated effort among families, educational institutions, and healthcare professionals can significantly strengthen disease prevention and management strategies. Coordinated strategies involving school nurses, educators, public health officials, families, and communities are essential to identify, control, and prevent the spread of infectious diseases among school-aged children.

Disclaimer

None.

References

Aasheim, E. T., Inns, T., Trindall, A., Emmett, L., Brown, K. E., Williams, C. J., & Reacher, M. (2014). Outbreak of mumps in a school setting, United Kingdom, 2013. *Human Vaccines & Immunotherapeutics, 10*(8), 2446–2449.

Adler, N. R., Mahony, A., & Friedman, N. D. (2013). Diphtheria: forgotten, but not gone. *Internal Medicine Journal, 43*(2), 206-210.

Akçay, D. (2016). [The Role of the School Nurse of School Environment Protection from Infectious]. *Cumhuriyet Nursing Journal, 5*(2), 84-94.

Akiyode, O. (2013). Impetigo in Children and Adolescents. *US Pharm, 38*(6), 68-71.

Andani, A., van Damme, P., Bunge, E. M., Salgado, F., van Hoorn, R. C., & Hoet, B. (2022). One or two doses of hepatitis A vaccine in universal immunization programs in children in 2020: A systematic review. *Vaccine, 40*(2), 196-205.

Ashkenazi, S., & Schwartz, E. (2020). Traveler's diarrhea in children: New insights and existing gaps. *Travel Medicine and Infectious Disease, 34*, 101503.

Bou, R., Dominguez, A., Fontanals, D., Sanfeliu, I., Pons, I., Renau, J., & Salleras, L. (2000). Prevalence of Haemophilus influenzae pharyngeal carriers in the school population of Catalonia. *European Journal of Epidemiology, 16*, 521-526.

Cameron, J. C., Allan, G., Johnston, F., Finn, A., Heath, P. T., & Booy, R. (2007). Severe complications of chickenpox in hospitalised children in the UK and Ireland. *Archives of Disease in Childhood, 92*(12), 1062-1066.

CDC. (2023). Centers for Disease Control and Prevention. About CDC Healthy Schools. https://www.cdc.gov/healthyschools/about.htm.

CDC. (2024). Early Care and Education Portal. Prevention and control of infectious diseases. https://www.cdc.gov/earlycare/infectious-diseases/index.html.

Clarke, K. E. (2017). Review of the epidemiology of diphtheria 2000-2016.

Coelingh, K., Olajide, I. R., MacDonald, P., & Yogev, R. (2015). Efficacy and effectiveness of live attenuated influenza vaccine in school-age children. *Expert Review of Vaccines, 14*(10), 1331-1346.

Defay, F., De Serres, G., Skowronski, D. M., Boulianne, N., Ouakki, M., Landry, M., & Ward, B. J. (2013). Measles in children vaccinated with 2 doses of MMR. *Pediatrics, 132*(5), e1126-e1133.

Department of Health and Social Services Delaware. (2020). Managing Infectious Disease In Childcare Settings Informational Guidelines for Directors, Caregivers, and Parents 4th Edition. Department of Health and Social Services Delaware Division of Public Health Office of Infectious Disease Epidemiology Revised 2020. https://dhss.delaware.gov/dhss/dph/epi/files/ChildCareManual2021.pdf.

Erdoğan, M. S., Otkun, M., Tatman-Otkun, M., Akata, F., & Türe, M. (2004). The epidemiology of hepatitis A virus infection in children, in Edirne, Turkey. *European Journal of Epidemiology, 19*, 267-273.

Fashner, J., Ericson, K., & Werner, S. (2012). Treatment of the common cold in children and adults. *American Family Physician, 86*(2), 153-159.

Florez, I. D., Nino-Serna, L. F., & Beltran-Arroyave, C. P. (2020). Acute infectious diarrhea and gastroenteritis in children. *Current Infectious Disease Reports, 22*, 1-12.

Gould, D. (2014). Varicella zoster virus: chickenpox and shingles. *Nursing Standard, 28*(33), 52.

Hajare, S. T., Chekol, Y., & Chauhan, N. M. (2022). Assessment of prevalence of Giardia lamblia infection and its associated factors among government elementary school children from Sidama zone, SNNPR, Ethiopia. *PLoS One, 17*(3), e0264812.

Harling, R., White, J. M., Ramsay, M. E., Macsween, K. F., & van den Bosch, C. (2005). The effectiveness of the mumps component of the MMR vaccine: A case control study. *Vaccine, 23*, 4070-4074.

Hasan, M. Z., Mehdi, G. G., De Broucker, G., Ahmed, S., Ali, M. W., Del Campo, J. M., & Uddin, M. J. (2021). The economic burden of diarrhea in children under 5 years in Bangladesh. *International Journal of Infectious Diseases, 107*, 37-46.

Hatam-Nahavandi, K., Ahmadpour, E., Pashazadeh, F., Dezhkam, A., Zarean, M., Rafiei-Sefiddashti, R., & Otranto, D. (2020). Pediculosis capitis among school-age students worldwide as an emerging public health concern: A systematic review and meta-analysis of past five decades. *Parasitology Research, 119*, 3125-3143.

Healthy People. (2020). Office of Disease Prevention and Health Promotion. Topic Areas at a Glance. https://www.cdc.gov/nchs/healthy_people/hp2020/hp2020_topic_areas.

Healthy People. (2030). Office of Disease Prevention and Health Promotion. Objectives and Data. https://health.gov/healthypeople/objectives-and-data/browse-objectives/infectious-disease/maintain-elimination-measles-rubella-congenital-rubella-syndrome-and-polio-iid-01.

Jaber, S. M. (2006). A serological survey of measles, mumps, and rubella immunity among school-aged children in Western Saudi Arabia. *Saudi Medical Journal, 27*(1), 63.

Johnson, M. K. (2020). Impetigo. *Advanced Emergency Nursing Journal, 42*(4), 262-269.

Karthikeyan, K., Aishwarya, M., & Elayaperumal, S. (2022). Effectiveness of topical 0.5% ivermectin shampoo in the treatment of pediculosis capitis among school-going female children. *International Journal of Trichology, 14*(2), 55-59.

Kauffmann, F., Heffernan, C., Meurice, F., Ota, M. O., Vetter, V., & Casabona, G. (2021). Measles, mumps, rubella prevention: How can we do better? *Expert Review of Vaccines, 20*(7), 811-826.

Kildegaard, H., Lund, L. C., Pottegård, A., & Stensballe, L. G. (2023). Effectiveness of the quadrivalent live attenuated influenza vaccine against influenza-related hospitalisations and morbidity among children aged 2 to 6 years in Denmark: A nationwide cohort study emulating a target trial. *The Lancet Child & Adolescent Health, 7*(12), 852-862.

Kumar, K. J., Kumar, H. K., Manjunath, V. G., Anitha, C., & Mamatha, S. (2014). Hepatitis A in children-clinical course, complications, and laboratory profile. *The Indian Journal of Pediatrics, 81*, 15-19.

Lee, K. Y., Lee, H. S., Hur, J. K., Kang, J. H., & Lee, B. C. (2005). Clinical features of measles according to age in a measles epidemic. *Scandinavian Journal of Infectious Diseases, 37*(6-7), 471-475.

Leung, A. K., Lam, J. M., Leong, K. F., Barankin, B., & Hon, K. L. (2022). Paediatrics: How to manage pediculosis capitis. *Drugs in Context, 11*.

Maryanti, E., & Haslinda, L. (2022). Treatment and education on prevention of capitis pediculosis in female student Pesantren Al-Muslimun at Village Muda Setia, Bandar Seikijang, Pelalawan Regency, Riau. *Engagement: Jurnal Pengabdian Kepada Masyarakat, 6*(1), 107-115.

Ministry of Health. (2025). Childhood Vaccination Schedule. https://asi.saglik.gov.tr/bagisiklama-programi-ve-asi-takvimi/asi-takvimi.html.

Molinari, N. A., Ortega-Sanchez, I. R., Messonnier, M. L., et al., (2007). The annual impact of seasonal influenza in the US: Measuring disease burden and costs. *Vaccine, 25*, 5086-5096.

Jones, N. (2020). How COVID-19 is changing the cold and flu season. *Nature, 588*(7838), 388-390.

Oh, S. Y., Griffiths, D., John, T., Lee, Y. C., Yu, L. M., McCarthy, N., & Pollard, A. J. (2008). School-aged children: A reservoir for continued circulation of Haemophilus influenzae type b in the United Kingdom. *The Journal of Infectious Diseases, 197*(9), 1275-1281.

Olszak, J., Kapłan, W., Rachwał, D., Piątek, E., Zalewa, K., Bartoszek, L., & Rogowska, M. (2023). Giardia intestinalis-atypical symptoms of infection in the daily practice of various specialists. *Journal of Education, Health and Sport, 26*(1), 31-36.

Ortiz-Romero, M. D. M., Espejo-García, M. P., Alfayate-Miguelez, S., Ruiz-López, F. J., Zapata-Hernandez, D., & Gonzalez-Pacanowska, A. J. (2017). Epidemiology of nasopharyngeal carriage by Haemophilus influenzae in healthy children. *The Pediatric Infectious Disease Journal, 36*(10), 919-923.

Paul, J. (2024). *Skin Infections*. In *Disease Causing Microbes* (pp. 65-98). Cham: Springer International Publishing.

Principi, N., Esposito, S., Gasparini, R., Marchisio, P., & Crovari, P. (2004). Burden of influenza in healthy children and their households. *Archives of Disease in Childhood, 89*(11), 1002-1007.

Pappas, D. E., Hendley, J. O., Hayden, F. G., & Winther, B. (2008). Symptom profile of common colds in school-aged children. *The Pediatric Infectious Disease Journal, 27*(1), 862-868.

Sintusek, P., Sa-nguanmoo, P., & Poovorawan, Y. (2019). Viral Hepatitis A in Children: Detection and Management. *Viral Hepatitis in Children: Prevention and Management*, 71-89.

Taylor, H. G., Schatschneider, C., & Minich, N. M. (2000). Longitudinal outcomes of Haemophilus influenzae meningitis in school-age children. *Neuropsychology, 14*(4), 509.

Thompson, R., Westbury, S., & Slape, D. (2021). Paediatrics: How to manage scabies. *Drugs in Context, 10*.

Troullos, E., Baird, L., & Jayawardena, S. (2014). Common cold symptoms in children: Results of an internet-based surveillance program. *Journal of Medical Internet Research, 16*(6), e2.

Trüeb, R. M., Gavazzoni Dias, M. F. R., & Dutra Rezende, H. (2023). *Parasitic Diseases and Infestations of the Hair and Scalp*. In *Hair in Infectious Disease: Recognition, Treatment, and Prevention* (pp. 261-290). Cham: Springer International Publishing.

Vecchio, A. L., Conelli, M. L., & Guarino, A. (2021). Infections and chronic diarrhea in children. *The Pediatric Infectious Disease Journal, 40*(7), e255-e258.

Wan, H. (2024). Research on the influencing factors of the spread of chickenpox. *Highlights in Science, Engineering and Technology, 88*, 988-995.

Wang, S., Zheng, Y., Jin, X., Gan, Z., Shao, Y., Zhu, C., & Xu, N. (2020). Efficacy and safety of a live attenuated influenza vaccine in Chinese healthy children aged 3–17 years in one study center of a randomized, double-blind, placebo-controlled phase 3 clinical trial, 2016/17 season. *Vaccine, 38*(38), 5979-5986.

WHO. (2021). *WHO Guideline on School Health Services.* https://www.who.int/publications/i/item/9789240029392.

WHO. (2022). *Older Children and Young Adolescent Mortality (5 to 14 Years).* https://www.who.int/news-room/fact-sheets/detail/older-children-and-young-adolescent-mortality-(5-to-14-years).

WHO. (2024). *Child Health and Development Unit: Communicable Diseases among Children.* https://www.who.int/teams/maternal-newborn-child-adolescent-health-and-ageing/child-health/communicable-diseases-among-children.

Chapter 23

The Management of Emergency Situations in Schools

Özlem Sinan*, PhD
Department of Midwifery, Marmara University, Faculty of Health Science,, Istanbul, Türkiye

Abstract

Emergency situations are natural events that cannot be predicted, such as earthquakes, floods, landslides, avalanches, tornadoes, and storms, as well as human induced incidents such as fires, accidents, food poisoning, epidemics, violence, and terrorism. When such emergencies occur in schools, the safety of children and school staff depends on rapid intervention and the implementation of effective emergency management strategies. Emergency management is a comprehensive process that involves phases occurring before, during, and after the emergency. These processes include preparedness, risk mitigation, emergency response, and post-emergency recovery. Effective management of emergencies in schools requires proactive measures such as identifying potential hazards and risks, taking necessary precautions, educating students and staff, developing emergency plans, and ensuring their implementation.

Keywords: emergency, school, management

Introduction

Emergency refers to situations and events that require rapid intervention and emergency aid activities. It is a temporary situation necessitating timely precautions and coordinated actions before, during, and after the event. The emergency phase begins with the occurrence of an urgent incident and ends when its underlying causes are resolved. Emergency management defined as a process that starts with taking necessary precautions before an emergency occurs, aims to meet the needs of the affected group quickly and effectively during the event, and includes activities for the post-emergency period aftermath (Bilgin, 2023; Özmen, 2023; AFAD, 2013). In emergencies, the primary responsibility of schools is to ensure student safety. The concept of a "safe school" involves creating an environment where students can develop

* Corresponding Author's Email: ozlemozdemir310@gmail.com

In: Health Promotion and Prevention
Editor: Eda Kılınç İşleyen
ISBN: 979-8-89530-758-8

social skills, manage anger, solve problems, and show respect for others and their surroundings (Pollack and Sundermann, 2001). Schools may face various emergencies, such as fires, violence, earthquakes, severe weather conditions, or poisoning. In such situations, prompt intervention is essential. Therefore, it is crucial for schools to develop comprehensive plans to respond to emergencies and ensure school safety (Çelik, 2007).

The objective of emergency management at school is to establish, in collaboration with provincial/district authorities, school administrators, teachers, students, school staff, and parents, a coordinated response plan for potential emergencies. This also includes planning preventive measures and appropriate responses before, during, and after such events (Özmen et al., 2015).

To ensure effective emergency management, school curricula at all educational levels should include both theoretical knowledge and practical education on first aid, fire safety, appropriate emergency behaviors, and natural disaster preparedness (Widana et al., 2021; Baysal, 2023).

Stages of Emergency Management at School

Preparation Phase

The preparation phase involves determining the necessary actions in the event of an emergency, in coordination with the school and relevant institutions, prior to the occurrence of such events. To effectively prevent and respond to emergencies, school staff, students, and parents must be adequately prepared. Natural disasters and emergencies such as earthquakes, floods, storms, fires, poisoning, bomb threats, chemical spills, and violent incidents cannot be avoided merely by addressing risks. Therefore, it is essential to prepare for emergencies in schools through teamwork and updated knowledge (Çelik, 2007).

Key activities during the preparation phase include:

- Conducting drills to promote appropriate behaviors during emergencies,
- Developing and updating family communication plans,
- Coordinating with relevant institutions and involving in all planning processes,
- Preparing a school emergency plan and informing all stakeholders,
- Supplying necessary emergency materials and providing education on their use (Özmen, 2023; Çelik, 2007).

Harm Reduction Phase

The harm reduction phase aims to minimize loss of life and property by reducing risks and hazards associated with school emergencies. This stage is applicable before, during, and after the emergency.

Main actions during this phase include:

- Identifying, analyzing, and evaluating hazards in and around the school,
- Determination the school's population, physical structure, infrastructure, and human activity inventory,
- Assessing the physical, social, economic, and environmental vulnerabilities,
- Identifying potential secondary risks,
- Evaluating injury and fatality risks,
- Assessing physical risks (e.g., building structure, equipment, installations),
- Determining environmental threats,
- Developing and implementing risk reduction strategies,
- Conducting cost analyses,
- Identifying institutional, legal, and financial capacities,
- Preparing emergency response scenarios.

These proactive efforts form the foundation of the entire emergency management process. Conducting hazard and risk analyses and applying mitigation strategies are vital for the successful implementation of intervention and recovery activities (Sakuraia et al., 2018; Çelik, 2005; Özmen, 2023).

Intervention Phase

The intervention phase encompasses the actions taken immediately after an emergency occurs at school. During this phase, response protocols are activated to ensure the safety and well-being of all individuals on campus. For example, in the case of a school fire, the designated response team is responsible for containing the situation and protecting lives until professional assistance arrives (Baysal, 2023).

Emergency response steps include:

- Assessing the type and impact of the emergency,
- Determining the appropriate course of action,
- Requesting support from relevant agencies,
- Notifying families and authorities,
- Administering first aid to injured students or staff.

Response procedures vary by emergency type, and standard protocols include:

- If the school building is safe: implement shelter-in-place or lockdown procedures,
- If the school building is unsafe: initiate evacuation,
- If the school building is unsafe but the schoolyard is safe: gather outdoors in a designated safe area,
- If both the school building and yard are unsafe: evacuate to a predetermined off-site location,
- Initiate communication with families and deliver students to authorized persons based on the student release protocol (Ronan et al., 2008; Baysal, 2023; Çelik, 2007).

Healing Phase

The healing or recovery phase focuses on restoring the physical, psychological, and social environment of the school following an emergency. This includes repairing damage, ensuring the continuity of education, restoring safety, and providing psychosocial support (Kılınç, 2023; Özmen, 2023).

Emergencies can cause lasting emotional and psychological harm, particularly to school-age children. Therefore, targeted, timely interventions that address children's specific needs during and after the emergency are critical (Çelik, 2007; Chemtob et al., 2002).

Emergency Management Planning at School

The emergency management planning process offers schools a valuable opportunity to assess risks in and around the school environment, identify available resources, and clearly define roles and procedures (Federal Emergency Management Agency, 2013; Çelik, 2007).

Effective school emergency management plans should have the following criteria;

- Clearly outline how hazards and risks within and around the school will be managed.
- Be developed through a team-based approach, ensuring collaboration and coordination with children, families, teachers, and relevant external institutions.
- Consider the gender, age, and cultural backgrounds of the students.
- Identify potential challenges that may affect children and establish preventive measures.
- Incorporate children's perspectives, including their suggestions and preferences related to emergency management.
- Integrate students' roles in the emergency management process into the school curriculum, and ensure families are informed about these roles.
- Be reviewed, updated, and improved at least annually, and revised based on the outcomes and lessons learned from any emergency incidents (Bilgin, 2023; Özmen et al., 2015).

To implement the emergency management process effectively, a school emergency team can be established. This team may include the school principal and assistants, teachers, the school nurse, student representatives, and school personnel (Özmen et al., 2015).

A recommended framework for emergency response is the Incident Command System (ICS), which is adaptable to different types and scales of emergencies. This model, widely used in the United States, ensures structured coordination (Barclay, 2004).

- For smaller-scale emergencies, the school principal can manage the system directly.
- For larger incidents, the principal coordinates with designated staff to manage emergency functions effectively.

To enable a rapid and organized response:

- Specific units should be formed, and responsible personnel should be appointed and trained annually.
- The roles and responsibilities of those involved in emergency planning and drills should be clearly defined and communicated to all school staff and students.
- In schools with limited staff, the ICS should be structured based on the available personnel's knowledge and competencies (Alexander, 2005).

Emergency departments under the ICS structure address all types of emergencies and operate within a well-defined organizational hierarchy. These departments include:

- Planning Department: Responsible for gathering information about emergencies, preparing emergency plans based on the incident manager's priorities, maintaining records, and producing reports (Barclay, 2004).
- Operations Department: Ensures the safety of students and staff during emergencies. Duties include extinguishing minor fires, managing utility systems (gas, electricity, water), conducting search and rescue, performing headcounts, documenting individuals' locations and conditions, administering first aid, and assessing building damage and risks (Alexander, 2005).
- Logistics Department: Provides the essential equipment, communication tools, and other resources needed during emergencies. Responsibilities include ensuring the availability of materials, food, water, personnel, and energy supplies (Akpınar and Köksalan, 2003).
- Finance Department: Manages financial operations during emergencies. This includes maintaining financial records and ensuring timely payments for emergency-related expenses (Akpınar and Köksalan, 2003).

Finally, behavioral guidelines for responding to specific school emergencies—such as earthquakes, fires, or chemical spills—should be defined and practiced regularly (Table 1) (AFAD, 2013).

Table 1. Behaviors related to emergencies at school

Emergencies	Behavior
Earthquake	Drop – Cover – Hold The school should be evacuated when the earthquake is over.
Fire	The school must be evacuated by sounding the fire alarm. If people's clothes catch fire: Stop - Down - Roll
Smoke	If you are stranded, take shelter in place. If not, the school is evacuated. One has to crawl to stay under the smoke layer.
Hazardous substance leak	Shelter in place or evacuate to a safe place
Bomb or Bomb threat	Collapse – Trap – Hold or Evacuate
Violent incidents	Lockdown / Isolation
Explosion	Collapse – Cover – Hold
Flood	Safe evacuation or shelter in place (upper floor of buildings)
Suspicious or unknown persons	Threatening people are evaluated, and the police are called.
Storm	Shelter in place if students are on school grounds, evacuate inside.

Drill

Drills are essential activities conducted to evaluate the appropriateness, adequacy, and timeliness of planned emergency activities under realistic conditions, following a set scenario. The main purpose of drills is to prepare for unforeseen situations, identify potential risks and deficiencies, and enhance readiness through practical experience. Each school should plan and implement drills tailored to the types of emergencies most likely to occur in their region. Drills should cover various topics such as:

- DROP-COVER-HOLD (for earthquakes),
- EVACUATION (for fires, chemical spills, or structural hazards),
- FIRE (evacuation and extinguisher use).
- For instance:
- Schools in earthquake-prone areas must conduct regular earthquake drills.
- Schools near rivers or in low-lying areas should conduct flood drills.
- In regions prone to storms or heavy rainfall, relevant drills should be carried out.

Providing students and staff with experiences of different hazard-specific drills improves their response capabilities (Bokomi, 2010).

Types of Drills

Tabletop exercise: A discussion-based exercise where emergency plans are reviewed with key personnel (such as school administrators, emergency officials, and local authorities). Scenarios are simulated, and the responses are evaluated to identify gaps and improve coordination.

Emergency drill: A practical exercise involving students and staff that simulates an emergency situation. These drills are critical for ensuring individuals know how to respond correctly, avoid panic, locate safe areas and exits, and protect themselves effectively during real emergencies.

Drills should be:

- Conducted regularly throughout the academic year,
- Aligned with current legislation and scientific knowledge,
- Repeated at scheduled intervals to reinforce learning and familiarity.

When drills are implemented collaboratively with the classroom, school administration, and families, the entire school community becomes better prepared, enabling a more coordinated and effective response during actual emergencies (Özmen, 2023).

Stages of the Exercise Plan

Determining the subject of the drill: Priority emergency scenarios that can be drilled in the school, such as fire, earthquake, flood, severe weather conditions, or terrorist attack, should be determined. Selection should be based on a risk assessment specific to the school's location and context.

Setting the time and location of the drill: The time and location of the drill must be scheduled in a way that minimizes disruption to the academic routine. All stakeholders, including students, teachers, and school staff, should be informed in advance about the date, time, type, and objective of the drill to ensure full participation and awareness.

Preparation for the drill scenario: Scenario preparations for the drills should be made, and the beginning, progress, and what to do should be clarified in writing.

Identifying participants: According to the content of the drill, the participation of all students, teachers, and staff in the school should be ensured.

Preparation of the exercise report: A report containing exercise information should be prepared to eliminate the deficiencies after the exercise and to make the next exercise more successful (Özmen, 2023).

Roles of the School Nurse in Emergency Management

School nurses have responsibilities in schools at all stages of emergencies (before, during, and after the disaster), in the management of emergencies, in the execution of health services, and in protecting the health of students and staff at all stages of emergencies.

Regardless of their area of specialization, nurses must possess the skills necessary to plan for and manage emergency situations. The International Council of Nurses (ICN) has emphasized the importance of all nurses being equipped with knowledge and skills related to disaster and emergency management. To support this, the ICN developed a guideline titled *Disaster Nursing Competencies – ICN Framework*, which outlines the core competencies expected of nurses internationally (Loke and Fung, 2014; Erdoğan, 2018).

According to the ICN, disaster nursing competencies are grouped into four main categories:

- Prevention/mitigation competencies
  - Risk reduction, disease prevention, health promotion,
  - Policy development and planning,

- Preparedness competencies
  - Ethical practice, legal practice, and accountability,
  - Communication and information sharing,
  - Training and preparation,

- Response competencies
  - Care of the community,
  - Care of individuals and their families, psychological care,
  - Care for vulnerable individuals,

- Recovery/rehabilitation competencies

It covers long-term individual, family, and community rehabilitation issues (WHO, 2009).

School nurses play an important role in the management of emergencies in schools in all processes of emergency situations. To enable school nurses to take a more active role in managing emergencies, it is essential to expand school nursing education programs and develop national guidelines specifically outlining school nurses' responsibilities in this area (Bilgin, 2023; Erdoğan, 2018; Februanti, 2022; Kolbe, 2019). Through the education they provide before emergencies, school nurses help students develop correct behavioral responses to crises. Following emergencies, they assess students' physical, psychological, and social health based on the data they collect and work to ensure the protection and promotion of student well-being.

Research on Emergency Management in School

The education and experience of nurses are very important in the management of emergency situations. It has been noted that nurses' experience and knowledge affect their preparedness for emergency situations and increase their awareness, self-confidence, and skills regarding the process (Hammad, Arbon, and Gebbie, 2011). However, studies show that nurses often do not feel adequately prepared to intervene during emergencies and lack sufficient knowledge and skills to make appropriate decisions in such situations (Fothergill et al., 2005; Fung, Loke, and Lai, 2008; Al Khalaileh, Bond and Alasad, 2012; Diab and Mabrouk, 2015; Seyedin, Dolatabadi and Rajabifard, 2015; Labrague et al., 2016). In a study conducted with nursing students, it was found that their knowledge was particularly insufficient in areas such as disaster triage, decontamination, post-disaster field hospitals, and the materials needed after disasters (Hisar and Yurdakul, 2015).

Research has shown that schools with plans to prevent violence, respond to emergencies, and implement those plans through designated teams experience several positive outcomes. These include increased academic success, reduced disciplinary issues, a safer and more supportive learning environment, and improved staff morale and security (Dwyer et al., 1998; Çelik, 2005).

In a study conducted in the United States on schools' emergency management practices it was found that 85% of schools had a written emergency plan, 66% had staff responsible for emergency management, and 56% coordinated their plans with other institutions. However, only 39% of public schools conducted emergency drills, and just 20% of school staff believed their schools were truly prepared for emergencies (Warlick, 1994).

In another study evaluating emergency management in public schools across three U.S. states, 95% of 258 schools reported having a crisis management plan, and 77% had an emergency planning and intervention team. However, fewer than half of the schools had conducted a full-scale drill in the past year, indicating low overall preparedness (Smith et al., 2001).

In Delibalta's (2005) study conducted in schools in Ankara Keçiören district, school administrators stated that their schools were not prepared for extraordinary situations such as fire and earthquake. In a study conducted in secondary schools in Istanbul, school employees stated that they needed training, especially in first aid, drills, and emergency management (Kökçü et al., 2012).

In the study conducted by Kano and Bourque (2007) in California, it was determined that the school team felt prepared in drill and practice areas. In Altun-Akbaba's (2005) study, it was determined that school administrators were insufficient in terms of drills. In Oral's (2018) study, it was determined that 27.7% of students and parents were on the disaster planning committee, and 31.8% participated in drills.

In the study conducted by Olympia, Wan, and Avner (2005), it was determined that disaster plans were made in 418 of 573 schools. In the study conducted by Graham et al., (2006) in Arkansas, it was determined that more than 95% of schools had evacuation plans, and more than 80% had disaster plans against armed attacks, bombings, or biological attacks, and it was determined that the majority of schools did not conduct drills regarding emergency plans. In the research conducted by Öcal (2007) in primary schools, it was found that 74.1% of the schools had disaster plans, and school administrators were not aware of their responsibilities in disaster situations. It was determined that drills on first aid, damage assessment, and fire extinguishing were conducted in the majority of schools (75.5%).

In the research of Can and Ozan (2022), it was stated that the cooperation of parents, teachers, and administrators in communication was effective in the management of emergency situations. In a study conducted in the USA on the role of schools during the epidemic, the importance of school administrators communicating inside and outside the school and making decisions together was stated (Faherty et al., 2019).

Conclusion

It is very important to carry out emergency management in schools systematically and consciously. Children are particularly vulnerable to emergencies; they may panic during emergencies and may not be able to manage the emergency effectively. Therefore, raising awareness among students about emergency scenarios and developing as well as applying comprehensive emergency management plans in schools is essential. The primary aim of pre-emergency preparation and response practices is to identify potential risks, eliminate or mitigate them, and promote appropriate behavior during emergencies. Every measure taken before a crisis contributes significantly to the effective management of the situation when it occurs. School nurses play a vital role in all stages of emergency management within schools. However, the presence of school nurses and the implementation of emergency plans are not yet widespread. To ensure functional and efficient emergency management in educational settings, it is necessary to adopt and expand the use of national directive models and increase the employment of school nurses across schools.

Disclaimer

None.

References

Akpınar, B., & Köksalan, B. (2003). States of emergency and school. *Fırat University Journal of Social Sciences, 13*(1), 151-158.

Al Khalaileh, M. A., Bond, E., & Alasad, J. A. (2012). Jordanian nurses' perceptions of their preparedness for disaster management. *International Emergency Nursing, 20*(1), 14-23.

Alexander, D. (2005). Towards the development of a standard in emergency planning. *Disaster Prevention and Management, 14*(2).

Altun-Akbaba, S. (2005). Turkish school principals' earthquake experiences and reactions. *International Journal of Educational Management, 19*(4).

Barclay, C. (2004). Crisis management in a primary school. *Teacher Development, 8*(2-3).

Baysal, Y. H. (2023). During a disaster- disaster and emergency management in schools. In Erci B. & Aktürk Ü. (Eds.), *School Health Nurses* (pp. 705-711). Ankara: Nobel Akademik Publishing.

Bilgin, S. (2023). Disaster and emergency management in schools. In Erci B. & Aktürk Ü. (Eds.), *School Health Nurses* (pp. 695-697). Ankara: Nobel Akademik Publishing.

Bokomi. (2010). *Guidebook.* JICA, Sharing lessons learned by the city of Kobe from the great Hanshin-Awaji earthquake, Community emergency drill programs, and school disaster prevention education programs. https://openjicareport.jica.go.jp/pdf/11980877_01.pdf.

Can, E., & Ozan, C. (2022). Reflections of the Covid-19 pandemic on school management. *TEBD, 20*(2), 368-393. https://doi.org/10.37217/tebd.1007527.

Çelik, K. (2005). *Emergency management model proposal in education. Eurasian Journal of Educational Research, 20*, 87-98.

Çelik, K. (2007). *Emergency management in schools*. Ankara: Anı Publishing.

Chemtob, C. M., Joanne, P., Nakashima, J., & Carlson, J. G. (2002). Brief treatment for elementary school children with disaster-related posttraumatic stress disorder: A field study. *Journal of Clinical Psychology, 58*(1), 99-112.

Delibalta, A. F. (2005). *Preparedness levels of school buildings in Keçiören district of Ankara for extraordinary situations.* Unpublished Master's Thesis, Gazi University, Ankara.

Diab, G. M., & Mabrouk, S. M. (2015). The effect of guidance booklet on knowledge and attitudes of nurses regarding disaster preparedness at hospitals. *Journal of Nursing Education and Practice, 5*(9), 17-31.

Disaster and Emergency Management Presidency (AFAD). (2013). *School disaster and emergency management plan preparation guide.* https://canakkale.meb.gov.tr/meb_iys_dosyalar/2015_11/20021132_02afet_plani_hazirlama_kilavuzu.pdf.

Dwyer, K., Osher, D., & Warger, C. (1998). *Early warning, timely response: A guide to safe schools.* Washington, DC: U.S. Department of Education. https://www.ojp.gov/pdffiles1/172854.pdf.

Erdoğan, Ö. (2018). *Disaster nursing education.* In Öztekin, S. D. (Ed.), *Disaster Nursing* (pp. 115-120). Ankara: Türkiye Clinics.

Faherty, L. J., Schwartz, H. L., Ahmed, F., Zheteyeva, Y., Uzicanin, A., & Uscher-Pines, L. (2019). School and preparedness officials' perspectives on social distancing practices to reduce influenza transmission during a pandemic: Considerations to guide future work. *Preventive Medicine Reports, 14.* https://doi.org/10.1016/j.pmedr.2019.100871.

Februanti, S., Cahyati, A., Mariani, D., & Rosuliana, N. E. (2022). Improving child safety through health education underwear rules, growth monitoring, and disaster preparedness. *ABDIMAS: Jurnal Pengabdian Masyarakat, 5*(1), 2182–2187.

Federal Emergency Management Agency (FEMA). (2013). *Guide for Developing High-Quality School Emergency Operations Plans.*

Fothergill, A., Val Palumbo, M., Rambur, B., Reinier, K., & McIntosh, B. (2005). The volunteer potential of inactive nurses for disaster preparedness. *Public Health Nursing, 22*(5), 414-421.

Fung, O. W. M., Loke, A. Y., & Lai, C. K. (2008). Disaster preparedness among Hong Kong nurses. *Journal of Advanced Nursing, 62*(6), 698-703.

Graham, J., Shirm, S., Liggin, R., Aitken, M. R., & Dick, R. (2006). Mass-casualty events at schools: A national preparedness survey. *Pediatrics, 117*, e8-e15.

Hammad, K. S., Arbon, P., & Gebbie, K. M. (2011). Emergency nurses and disaster response: An exploration of South Australian emergency nurses' knowledge and perceptions of their roles in disaster response. *Australasian Emergency Nursing Journal, 14*(2), 87-94.

Hisar, K. M., & Yurdakul, A. (2015). Evaluation of the knowledge of a university's nursing students about health services in disasters. *MAKÜ Health Sciences Institute Journal, 3*(2), 54-65.

Kalanlar, B. (2019). The challenges and opportunities in disaster nursing education in Turkey. *Journal of Trauma Nursing, 26*(3), 164-170.

Kano, M., & Bourque, L. B. (2007). Experiences with and preparedness for emergencies and disasters among public schools in California. *National Association of Secondary School Principals Bulletin, 91*(3), 201.

Kılınç, N. Ö. (2023). Post-disaster. In Erci B. & Aktürk Ü. (Eds.), *School Health Nurses* (pp. 715-723). Ankara: Nobel Akademik Publishing.

Kökcü, A., Kuğuoğlu, S., & Ergün, A. (2012). An assessment of emergency and disaster preparedness in high schools in Istanbul-Turkey. *HEALTHMED, 6*, 2620-2634.

Kolbe, L. J. (2019). School health as a strategy to improve both public health and education. *Annual Review of Public Health, 40*, 443–463. https://doi.org/10.1146/annurev-publhealth-040218-043727.

Labrague, L. J., Yboa, B. C., McEnroe Petitte, D. M., Lobrino, L. R., & Brennan, M. G. B. (2016). Disaster preparedness in Philippine nurses. *Journal of Nursing Scholarship, 48*(1), 98-105.

Loke, A. Y., & Fung, O. W. M. (2014). Nurses' competencies in disaster nursing: Implications for curriculum development and public health. *International Journal of Environmental Research and Public Health, 11*(3), 3289-3303.

Öcal, A. (2007). Earthquake preparedness in primary schools: The case of Kırıkkale. *Kastamonu Education Journal, 15*(1), 1-12.

Olympia, R. P., Wan, E., & Avner, J. R. (2005). The preparedness of schools to respond to emergencies in children: A national survey of school nurses. *Pediatrics, 116*(6).

Oral, V. (2018). *Evaluation of the institutional preparations of the primary schools for disaster and emergency situations (Sample of province Gümüşhane)*. Unpublished Master's Thesis, Gümüşhane University, Gümüşhane.

Özmen, B. (2023). *Disaster and emergency management planning guide for educational institutions. Istanbul seismic risk reduction and emergency preparedness project (ISMEP).* https://www.ipkb.gov.tr/wp-content/uploads/2023/03/EGITIM-KURUMLARI-ICIN-AFET-ACIL-DURUM-YONETIMI-PLANLAMA-REHBERI.pdf.

Özmen, B., Gerdan, S., & Ergünay, O. (2015). Disaster and emergency management plans for schools. *Electronic Journal of Professional Development and Research, 3*(1), 37-52.

Pollack, I., & Sundermann, C. (2001). Creating safe schools: A comprehensive approach. *Juvenile Justice, 8*(1), 13-20.

Ronan, K. R., Crellin, K., Johnston, D. M., Finnis, K., Paton, D., & Becker, J. (2008). Promoting child and family resilience to disasters: Effects, interventions, and prevention effectiveness. *Children, Youth and Environments, 18*(1), 332-353.

Sakurai, A., Bisri, M. B. F., Odac, T., Oktarid, R. S., Murayama, Y., Nizammudin, Affan, M. (2018). A case of elementary schools in Banda Aceh City, Indonesia. *International Journal of Disaster Risk Reduction, 29*, 73–83.

Seyedin, H., Dolatabadi, Z. A., & Rajabifard, F. (2015). Emergency nurses' requirements for disaster preparedness. *Trauma Monthly, 20*(4), e29033.

Smith, S. M., Kress, T. A., Fenstemaker, E., Ballard, M., & Hyder, G. (2001). Crisis management preparedness of school districts in three southern states in the USA. *Safety Science, 39*(1-2), 83-92.

Warlick, J. S. (1994). *The preparedness for emergency conditions of public schools in Texas*. University of North Texas Libraries, UNT Digital Library. https://digital.library.unt.edu/ark:/67531/metadc277810/m1/1/.

Widana, K., Asmaniati, F., Djati, S. P., & Ingkadijava, R. (2021). Analysis of disaster-safe school level in west coast of Pandeglang Regency, Indonesia. *Technium Social Sciences Journal, 20*, 961-969.

World Health Organization. (2009). *ICN framework of disaster nursing competencies. The Southeast Asian Journal of Tropical Medicine and Public Health, 40*, 57-70.

Chapter 24

Basic First Aid Practices in Schools

Bennur Koca[*], **PhD**
First and Emergency Aid Program, Dokuz Eylul University/Vocational School of Health Services, Izmir, Türkiye

Abstract

School life significantly influences students' physical and mental health. Due to their still developing physical and cognitive abilities, students are particularly vulnerable to various risks, including accidents and injuries. Consequently, the need for effective first aid (FA) practices in schools is critical. This study aims to comprehensively explore FA practices within school settings. Timely and appropriate FA can be lifesaving, as minor injuries or illnesses may escalate into serious or life-threatening conditions if left untreated. In developed countries, school health services are typically provided by school nurses and teachers. Moreover, first aid training (FAT) for students in these countries is systematically organized according to age groups. While numerous studies have been conducted on the implementation of FAT in developed nations, such research is scarce in developing and underdeveloped countries, where FAT rates among children remain low. FA interventions by school nurses, teachers, and trained students are not only vital for saving lives but also for preventing further injury or complications. Ensuring that teachers and students receive age-appropriate and continuous FA training is of paramount importance for public health and school safety.

Keywords: first aid, school-age children, school

Introduction

While the correct and timely application of First Aid (FA) can save lives, critical intervention performed incorrectly may lead to irreversible health consequences (The Turkish Red Crescent, 2021; Dandil et al., 2015). Basic FA procedures can often be performed by lay responders at the scene; however, more complex interventions should only be carried out by professional

---

* Corresponding Author's Email: bennur.koca@deu.edu.tr

In: Health Promotion and Prevention
Editor: Eda Kılınç İşleyen
ISBN: 979-8-89530-758-8

healthcare providers, including doctors, nurses, and other qualified personnel (Grimaldi et al., 2020; Costa et al., 2015; Oliveira, 2015).

First Aid Training (FAT) programs for the general public are of vital importance, as they enable individuals to respond promptly to emergencies and potentially save lives (Tse, 2023). Educating and guiding the public in emergency preparedness is crucial (Guimaraes et al., 2018). School-age children, in particular, are at a heightened risk of accidents and injuries. Although most of these injuries are likely to be relatively minor, in some cases, a child or teenager may be exposed to serious or life-threatening injuries in a school building (Omar et al., 2015). Such injuries often occur during physical activities such as sports events or extracurricular activities, including cycling, swimming, and playground games (Al Gharsan and Alarfaj, 2019).

Injuries among child and adolescent are a leading cause of childhood mortality worldwide leading (LMICs) (Al-Hajj et al., 2020). Globally, injuries account for approximately 1,900 child deaths per day (Roth et al., 2018). Children between the ages of 7 and 16 are especially vulnerable due to their high participation in physical and recreational activities (Tse et al., 2023). Unintentional injuries represent about 90% of fatal injuries among children each year, predominantly affecting those under the age of 18 and occurring most frequently in LMICs. These findings underscore the critical role schools play in both the prevention and early response to accidents involving children and adolescents (Tse et al., 2023; Harvey et al., 2009).

The Importance of First Aid Training in Schools

Childhood injuries are a significant cause of child mortality worldwide (Wilks and Pendergast, 2017; Panda et al., 2019). School-age children are particularly vulnerable to various health emergencies, including sprains, strains, fractures, burns, insect stings, drowning, nosebleeds (epistaxis) and epileptic seizures (Abd El-Hay et al., 2015; Mobarak et al., 2015; Dasgupta et al., 2014).

Providing first aid in such situations is critical to minimizing the consequences of injuries and can be life-saving. Immediate intervention by the injured individual or bystanders can significantly reduce the severity of the injury. Equipping students with the skills to provide first aid to themselves or others represents a major step toward building a safer and more resilient society (Abd El-Hay et al., 2015; Reveruzzi et al., 2020). While many studies on first aid education for children focus solely on CPR, it is important to note that first aid encompasses a much broader range of skills (De Buck et al., 2015; Lubrano et al., 2005).

Introducing FAT at an early age is essential (Banfai et al., 2017). Several studies emphasize that basic first aid education should be mandatory in all schools (Panda et al., 2019; Afifi et al., 2015). Acquiring first aid knowledge and skills during the developmental years enables children to protect both themselves and others in emergencies (Bernardo et al., 2002). Research has demonstrated that children aged 5 to 18 can learn a variety of age-appropriate first aid techniques (Cimpoesu et al., 2012; Banfai et al., 2019). There is broad agreement that first aid education should be tailored to the child's developmental level (Bernardo et al., 2002; Frederick et al., 2006; Bollig et al., 2009).

For instance, younger children can be taught how to assess an emergency situation and call for help. As they grow older, students can learn how to manage common injuries such as nosebleeds and minor burns. In secondary school, training can expand to include interventions for drowning and proper bandaging techniques. By high school, students may be capable of managing more complex scenarios, such as assisting an unconscious or non-breathing person (Calandrim, 2017). Learning these skills early in life fosters awareness, builds confidence, and contributes to a sense of social responsibility.

First aid strategies implemented in schools not only benefit students but also support health education efforts among teachers (Oliveira et al., 2015). Moreover, students often share the knowledge they gain with their peers and families, extending the impact of FAT beyond school settings. In this context, schools play a growing role in health promotion and in the prevention of diseases and accidents among children and adolescents (Baser et al., 2007).

In many countries, school health services are provided by doctors, nurses, and trained teachers. However, in Turkey, school nurses are not routinely present in schools. Therefore, it is essential to integrate nurses into school settings and ensure that both teachers and students receive comprehensive FAT. Making first aid education mandatory in schools significantly reduces the severity of injuries and helps prevent medical emergencies from escalating (Grimaldi et al., 2020).

General First Aid Information

FA is refers to non-pharmacological interventions provided to individuals whose lives may be in danger due to illness or injury. It involves using available tools and materials—without professional medical equipment—until qualified medical personnel arrive at the scene. FA practices aim not only to treat injuries but also to maintain vital functions and prevent conditions from deteriorating (Yavuz et al., 2012). A first aider is someone certified in first aid, who administers non-medicated treatments to a person or injured person (P/I) using the resources available at the scene, without relying on medical tools (European Resuscitation Council, 2015).

An effective first aider must prioritize their own safety. They should possess basic knowledge of human anatomy, remain calm and dependable under pressure, be practical and observant, and act quickly to report incidents. Additionally, a good first aider should be capable of organizing bystanders and communicating effectively.

Emergency treatment, in contrast, refers to professional medical care administered by trained medical personnel at emergency treatment facilities after first aid has been given.

The primary objectives of first aid are to preserve life, prevent the condition of the patient or injured person from worsening, and promote recovery until medical assistance becomes available (Grimaldi et al., 2020).

Basic First Aid Practices

Protection: The first step in any FA situation is ensuring the safety of the scene. A secure environment should be established to prevent further harm. If an accident involves a vehicle, the vehicle should be moved to a safe area off the road if possible, and the ignition should be turned off. Smoking must be prohibited in the area. If there is a risk of gas exposure, appropriate precautions should be taken—such as closing gas valves and ventilating the environment.

Devices that may produce sparks, such as certain lighting or paging equipment, must not be used.

If there is no immediate threat (e.g., explosion, fire, or structural collapse), the P/I should not be moved. However, if imminent danger exists, the individual must be relocated to a safer location using proper transportation techniques. After ensuring safety, a quick assessment should be conducted to check for vital signs, bleeding, and possible fractures.

Oral substances should never be given to an unconscious person. Emergency medical services (EMS) must be contacted immediately. To minimize psychological trauma, the P/I should not be allowed to view their injuries, and they should be treated with calm, supportive communication. All observations about the incident and the P/I's condition should be recorded. The responder must remain at the scene until professional help arrives.

To reduce the risk of disease transmission (e.g., Hepatitis B, Hepatitis C, or HIV/AIDS), protective gloves should be worn when managing bleeding. The first aider should approach the situation with calmness, compassion, and effective communication to alleviate fear and provide comfort to the injured individual.

Reporting: Prompt and accurate communication with emergency services is essential. The report—made either personally or through another person—should include the following details:

- Exact location and address of the incident
- Name and contact number of the caller
- Description of the incident (e.g., type of emergency, cause)
- Number of affected individuals and their condition
- First aid measures already performed

Rescue (Intervention): Once the safety of the scene is confirmed, first aid interventions should be initiated promptly, but always with calmness and precision. If the responder does not have first aid training, they should avoid touching or moving the patient/injured person (P/I), as incorrect actions may worsen the situation.

Essential first aid actions during the intervention phase include:

- Assessing and prioritizing the injured individual's needs
- Addressing fear and anxiety of the P/I
- Coordinating assistance from bystanders
- Providing on-site care for conditions such as fractures, dislocations, and sprains
- Keeping the injured individual warm and preventing them from viewing open wounds to reduce psychological stress
- Avoiding unnecessary movement unless relocation is required due to immediate danger
- Referring or transferring the P/I to the appropriate healthcare facility using the safest and most effective method available

Triage—prioritizing care based on the severity of injuries—is a critical component of effective emergency response. According to the European Resuscitation Council (2015), the following priority levels are recommended:

- Primary priority: Individuals who are unconscious, not breathing, or suffering from severe bleeding or extensive burns
- Secondary priority: Individuals with fractures, moderate bleeding, or burns of lesser severity
- Tertiary priority: Individuals with minor injuries, such as abrasions, sprains, or superficial bleeding.

Evaluation of the Patient/Injured (P/I)

The primary aim of evaluating a P/I is to determine the severity of their condition and to establish the priorities for the appropriate FA interventions. A systematic and accurate assessment enables the first aider to quickly identify life-threatening situations, evaluate the urgency of care, and implement effective measures. This evaluation process is critical for ensuring that time and available resources are used efficiently—particularly in situations involving multiple casualties. Early identification of issues such as compromised airway, breathing difficulties, circulation problems, or signs of shock can significantly improve the outcomes for the affected individuals. Additionally, proper evaluation facilitates informed decision-making regarding when and how to transfer the P/I to medical services.

The Primary Evaluation of the P/I

The primary evaluation is conducted to quickly assess vital functions and identify life-threatening conditions requiring immediate intervention. This assessment follows a systematic approach to determine the P/I's level of consciousness, airway patency, respiration, and circulation.

1. Evaluation of consciousness

Assessment of consciousness begins with checking the P/I's responsiveness: (European Resuscitation Council, 2015; First Aid & Emergencies Treatment Guide, 2015; The Turkish Red Crescent, 2021)

- For adults and children: The first aider should gently shake the shoulders and give a verbal stimulus, such as asking, "Are you okay?"
- For infants (0–12 months): The assessment is performed by gently tapping the soles or heels of the feet.

2. Evaluation of airway patency

Airway patency is assessed by visually inspecting the mouth for any obstructions such as vomit, food, or foreign objects. If present, these should be carefully removed using a finger sweep with the index finger (only if clearly visible and accessible). To maintain an open airway:

(European Resuscitation Council, 2015; First Aid & Emergencies Treatment Guide, 2015; The Turkish Red Crescent, 2021)

- One hand is placed on the forehead to tilt the head backward.
- Two fingers of the other hand are positioned under the chin to lift it upward.
- This maneuver is known as the head-tilt, chin-lift technique, which helps lift the tongue away from the airway and improve airflow.

3. Evaluation of respiration

Respiration is assessed over a span of 10 seconds using the Look–Listen–Feel technique: (European Resuscitation Council, 2015; First Aid & Emergencies Treatment Guide, 2015; The Turkish Red Crescent, 2021)

- Look: Observe the chest for visible rise and fall indicating breathing.
- Listen: Place the ear near the P/I's mouth to detect breathing sounds.
- Feel: Sense airflow from the P/I's mouth or nose on the rescuer's cheek.

This triad helps determine whether the P/I is breathing spontaneously and effectively. (See Figure 1).

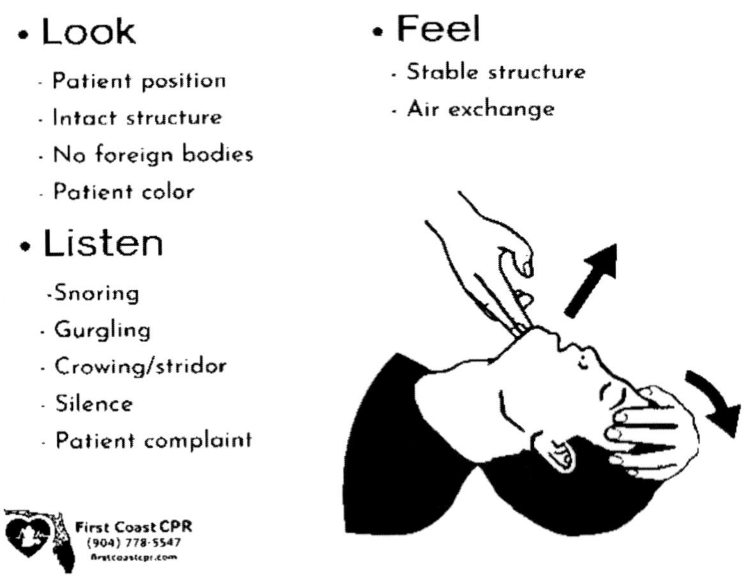

Figure 1. Evaluation of respiration.

4. Evaluation of circulation

Circulation is checked by palpating the appropriate artery to detect a pulse: (European Resuscitation Council, 2015; First Aid & Emergencies Treatment Guide, 2015; The Turkish Red Crescent, 2021)

- Adults and children: The carotid artery in the neck is used.
- Infants: The brachial artery in the upper arm is evaluated.

Three fingers (index, middle, and ring) are used to palpate the pulse for at least five seconds.

Practice of the P/I Recovery Position (RP)

For an unconscious P/I who is breathing and has a detectable pulse, placing them in a supine position is not recommended. In this position, the airway may become obstructed due to the tongue falling back or the accumulation of secretions or stomach contents. Therefore, the Recovery Position (RP) is essential to maintain an open airway and prevent aspiration (European Resuscitation Council, 2015; First Aid & Emergencies Treatment Guide, 2015; The Turkish Red Crescent, 2021).

Steps to Place a P/I in the RP (Figure 2)

- The FAR kneels beside the P/I on the side to which the individual will be turned.
- The FAR extends the P/I person's arm nearest to patient's above the shoulder at head level and rolls the P/I in one move by holding the far shoulder and hip.
- The FAR leg is bent at knee to form a right angle.
- The near arm (closest to the FAR) is positioned outward and straight, extended above the head.
- The FAR gently rolls the P/I towards themselves by holding the far shoulder and hip in a single, smooth motion.
- The upper leg is bent at both the hip and knee to stabilize the body and prevent rolling onto the stomach.

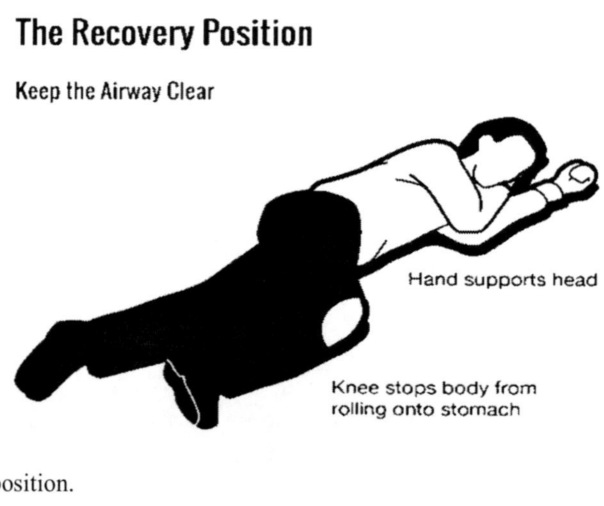

Figure 2. Recovery position.

- The lower leg is slightly flexed for backward support.
- The head is tilted sideways and slightly forward, resting on the extended arm to help keep the airway open.
- The P/I should be maintained in this position until emergency medical services arrive (e.g., 911, 999, or 112).
- The FAR must check breathing every 3 to 5 minutes during this time (European Resuscitation Council, 2015; First Aid & Emergencies Treatment Guide, 2015; The Turkish Red Crescent, 2021).

The Secondary Evaluation of the P/I

The secondary evaluation of the patient or injured person is conducted once vital life-threatening conditions have been ruled out or addressed during the primary assessment. This evaluation involves a more detailed and comprehensive examination, focusing on gathering medical history and identifying injuries that may not be immediately life-threatening but still require attention (European Resuscitation Council, 2015; First Aid & Emergencies Treatment Guide, 2015; The Turkish Red Crescent, 2021).

Obtaining Information by Interviewing the P/I

The FAR should approach the P/I in a calm and respectful manner. Essential interpersonal steps include:

- Introducing themselves and stating their role.
- Using polite language and addressing the P/I by name.
- Establishing trust to encourage cooperation.

Key information should be gathered through brief and focused questioning:

- How the incident occurred
- The individual's personal medical history
- Time and content of the last meal
- Current medication use
- Known allergies

This information helps identify possible internal injuries, complications, or medical conditions that could influence the first aid approach.

General Head–to-Toe Physical Examination

The P/I's level of consciousness is evaluated in terms of ability to understand and perceive. Respiratory rate, rhythm, depth, pulse rate, rhythm, and intensity, as well as body or skin temperature, moisture, and color, are evaluated. The casualty is examined for any signs of trauma during the general examination.

Head: The hair, scalp, head, and face are evaluated for injuries or bruises. The ears or nose are examined for any fluid or blood leak, and the inside of the mouth is checked.

Neck: The neck is examined for pain, tenderness, swelling, and deformity. The possibility of neck injury should not be ignored until proven otherwise.

Rib cage/thorax: The rib cage should be evaluated for stuck objects, open wounds, deformity, bruising, pain with slight pressure, and bleeding. The normality of rib cage expansion should be checked. During chest examination, the back of the patient/injured person should also be checked by moving the hands through the back of the person.

Abdomen: The presence of a stuck object, open wound, deformity, swelling, bruising, pain or sensitivity, and the softness of the abdomen should be evaluated. The hands should be moved through the waist, and the same examination should be done on the hip bones to find out whether there are any fractures or wounds.

Extremities (arms and legs): Strength, loss of sensation, pain, swelling, deformity, loss of function, fractures, and whether the pulse can be taken from the pulse points should be evaluated (European Resuscitation Council, 2015; First Aid & Emergencies Treatment Guide, 2015; The Turkish Red Crescent, 2021).

Basic First-Aid Practices at Schools

Basic Life Support

Basic Life Support (BLS) refers to non-pharmacological emergency interventions administered to individuals whose breathing and/or heartbeat has stopped. These interventions include artificial respiration to deliver oxygen to the lungs and external chest compressions to maintain blood circulation (American Red Cross Standard First Aid & Personal Safety, 1981; Van de Voorde et al., 2021).

BLS Application in Children (Aged 1 to 18 Years)

When providing BLS to a child, the FAR must follow a structured sequence of steps to ensure safety and maximize the chance of survival:

Scene safety and initial assessment

- Ensure the safety of both the FAR and the child.
- Assess the child's consciousness by gently tapping the shoulders and asking, "Are you okay?"
- If the child is unresponsive, shout for help and instruct someone nearby to call 911/999/112.

Positioning and airway management

- Lay the child on their back on a firm surface.
- Kneel beside the child.
- Open the child's mouth and remove any visible foreign objects.
- Perform the head tilt–chin lift maneuver to open the airway.

Breathing and circulation check

- Evaluate for breathing and pulse for up to 10 seconds.
- If there is no breathing and no pulse, proceed with the following BLS steps:

Rescue breaths

- Close the child's nose and seal your mouth over the child's lips.
- Deliver five rescue breaths, each lasting about one second, observing for chest rise.

Chest compressions

- Identify the lower half of the sternum.
- For smaller children, use one hand for compressions; if the child appears adult-sized, use two hands as with adult CPR.
- Position your hand(s) vertically, fingers off the ribcage, and elbows locked.
- Deliver 30 chest compressions, compressing the chest by approximately 5 cm (or 1/3 the depth of the chest).
- Maintain a rate of at least 100 compressions per minute.

Compression-to-breath ratio

- If only one FAR is present, alternate 30 compressions with 2 rescue breaths (30:2).
- If two FARs are available, use a 15:2 compression-to-breath ratio.

Calling for help

- If alone, the FAR should call 911/999/112 after completing five cycles of 30:2 compressions and breaths.
- If a second FAR is present, they should call for help immediately and assist with CPR and AED usage if available.

AED (Automated External Defibrillator) use

- If trained and available, a FAR should use an AED as soon as possible.
- Continue BLS without interruption until:
  - The child begins breathing normally.
  - Medical professionals arrive and take over.

Note: If a FAR is untrained in rescue breathing or unable to provide it, continuous chest compressions should still be administered (American Red Cross Standard First Aid & Personal Safety, 1981; Van de Voorde et al., 2021).

FA for Complete Airway Obstruction in Adults and Children

When a person is experiencing complete airway obstruction due to choking, immediate intervention is critical. The following steps should be followed carefully to dislodge the foreign object and restore breathing:

Step-by-step procedure

(European Resuscitation Council, 2015; First Aid & Emergencies Treatment Guide, 2015; Van de Voorde et al., 2021)

- Positioning
  - The patient may be sitting or standing during the intervention.

- Consciousness Check
  - Quickly assess whether the person is conscious and responsive.

- Back Blows (5–7 times)
  - Stand to the side and slightly behind the choking individual.
  - Using the heel of your hand, deliver 5 to 7 sharp blows between the shoulder blades.
  - After each blow, check to see if the object has been expelled by inspecting the mouth.

- Abdominal Thrusts (Heimlich Maneuver)
  - If the object remains lodged after back blows:
    - Stand behind the person.
    - Form a fist with one hand and place the thumb side of the fist just above the navel (belly button) and below the ribcage.
    - Grasp the fist with your other hand.
    - Deliver quick, forceful thrusts inward and upward.
    - Repeat the thrust 5 to 7 times or until the foreign object is expelled.

- Monitoring
  - Continue alternating back blows and abdominal thrusts until the airway is cleared or the person becomes unconscious.

- If the Person Becomes Unconscious
  - Carefully lower them to the ground.
  - Call emergency services (911/999/112) immediately.
  - Begin BLS procedures, including chest compressions and rescue breaths, checking for and removing the object if visible during breaths.

Important note: Abdominal thrusts should not be used in infants under 1 year old. For infants, a different protocol involving back slaps and chest thrusts must be followed.

FA for Burns

Burns are injuries caused by exposure to physical or chemical agents such as fire, hot objects, radiation, electricity, or corrosive substances. These injuries damage the skin and underlying tissues, and their severity depends on the depth, extent, and cause of the burn. (European Resuscitation Council, 2015; First Aid & Emergencies Treatment Guide, 2015; Van de Voorde et al., 2021).

Burn Types

First-degree burns: They include tissue damage in the form of redness (pink to red) on the lower skin and the surface of the skin. There is pain, edema, and slight swelling in the burn area. It usually heals within 48 hours.

Second-degree burns: They affect the first and second layers of the skin, and water-filled blisters (bullae) form on the skin. They are very painful and heal as the skin renews itself.

Third-degree burns: The entire layer of the skin, including muscles, nerves, and vessels, is affected. The wound goes through color changes from white to black. There is no pain (European Resuscitation Council, 2015; First Aid & Emergencies Treatment Guide, 2015; Van de Voorde et al., 2021).

Systemic Effects of Burns

Depending on their depth, extent, and site of occurrence, they cause dysfunctions in organs and systems. Pain and fluid loss leads to shock. Microbes and toxins present in the P/I person's body cause a risk of infection (European Resuscitation Council, 2015; First Aid & Emergencies Treatment Guide, 2015; Van de Voorde et al., 2021).

FA for Heat Burns

Stop the burning process

- Calm the individual; instruct them not to run if on fire.
- Extinguish flames using a blanket, coat, or by rolling on the ground.

Initial care

- Assess vital signs.
- Cool the burn under cold running water for at least 20 minutes.
- Remove clothing and jewelry carefully, especially if swelling is expected.
- Clean the area gently with soapy water.

Important precautions

- Do not burst blisters or apply any substance (e.g., creams, toothpaste, or oil).
- Do not bandage the burn area tightly.
- Cover the burn loosely with a clean cloth or sterile dressing.
- Keep the patient warm to prevent hypothermia.

Fluid replacement (if needed)

- If the burn is extensive and professional help is delayed, and if the P/I is conscious, not vomiting, and not severely burned:
  - Give oral fluids prepared with:
  - 1 liter of clean water
  - 1 teaspoon of salt
  - 1 teaspoon of baking soda

Call emergency services (911/999/112)

- Always seek professional help for moderate to severe burns (European Resuscitation Council, 2015; First Aid & Emergencies Treatment Guide, 2015; Van de Voorde et al., 2021).

FA for Chemical Burns

Stop exposure immediately

- Remove the chemical from the skin by flushing with large amounts of non-pressurized water for 20–25 minutes.
- Remove contaminated clothing and accessories.

Cover and protect

- Cover the affected area with a clean cloth or dressing.
- Keep the individual warm.

Seek medical help immediately (European Resuscitation Council, 2015; First Aid & Emergencies Treatment Guide, 2015; Van de Voorde et al., 2021).

FA for Electrical Burns

Ensure scene safety

- Do not touch the victim until the power source is turned off.
- If the power cannot be disconnected, use non-conductive material (e.g., wood, rubber) to separate the person from the source.

Initial care

- Do not move the person unless necessary.
- Check vital signs and assess for entry and exit wounds.
- Cover burns with a clean dressing.

Call emergency services ımmediately (European Resuscitation Council, 2015; First Aid & Emergencies Treatment Guide, 2015; Van de Voorde et al., 2021).

FA for Frostbite

Frostbite occurs when prolonged exposure to cold leads to reduced blood flow and tissue damage due to ice crystal formation and blood clotting.

Symptoms by Degre

First-degree frostbite: In the beginning, the skin goes pale, and there is a feeling of coldness, numbness, and weakness. Afterward, the skin turns red, and there is a feeling of tingling.

Second-degree frostbite: A feeling of tension, edema, swelling, pain, and fluid-filled blisters are observed in the damaged area. Over time, as the blisters heal, they turn into black crusts.

Third-degree frostbite: Tissues are irreversibly damaged. A black area that is clearly separated from the live and healthy skin forms (European Resuscitation Council, 2015; First Aid & Emergencies Treatment Guide, 2015; Van de Voorde et al., 2021).

FA Steps

- The P/I is placed in a warm environment, and contact with cold is cut off.
- The person exposed to frostbite is calmed down, rested, and not moved,
- Change into dry clothing. If conscious, offer warm, sugary drinks.
- Areas with blisters are never ruptured. They are covered.
- The frozen area is never rubbed. It is allowed to warm up / dissolve on its own.
- Hands and feet are kept in a natural position.
- If there is still weakness, a cloth bandage is applied.
- Medical assistance is sought (European Resuscitation Council, 2015; First Aid & Emergencies Treatment Guide, 2015; Van de Voorde et al., 2021).

FA for Heat Stroke

Heat stroke is a life-threatening emergency caused by prolonged heat exposure and dehydration.

- First of all, the P/I is placed in a cool and airy place.
- Garments are removed. The person is placed in a supine position, and their arms and legs are elevated.
- If there is no nausea and consciousness is clear, the person is given fluid prepared with water, salt, and baking soda or soda to compensate for water and salt loss (European Resuscitation Council, 2015; First Aid & Emergencies Treatment Guide, 2015; Van de Voorde et al., 2021).

FA for a Foreign Body in the Eye

If it is a substance such as dust or eyelashes:

- The eye is turned toward the light, the lower eyelid is examined, and if necessary, the upper eyelid is also examined,
- The dust or the eyelash in the eye is removed with a damp, clean cloth.
- Encourage blinking.
- Eyes are washed with plenty of water, and they are never rubbed.
- If it does not work, the person is referred to a health institution.

If the object is metallic or embedded:

- The patient should not be moved unless necessary.
- No intervention is applied to the eye; no attempt is made to remove the object.
- Both eyes must be closed.
- Medical help is sought.

The patient is transferred to a healthcare institution that specializes in ophthalmology (European Resuscitation Council, 2015; First Aid & Emergencies Treatment Guide, 2015; Van de Voorde et al., 2021).

FA for a Foreign Body in the Ear

- The ear should never be touched with a sharp or piercing object, nor should it be applied to any water.
- Medical help should be sought (European Resuscitation Council, 2015; First Aid & Emergencies Treatment Guide, 2015; Van de Voorde et al., 2021).

FA for A Foreign Object in the Nose

The object is forced out by pressing on the nasal wall and exhaling strongly. If it does not come off, medical help is sought (European Resuscitation Council, 2015; First Aid & Emergencies Treatment Guide, 2015; Van de Voorde et al., 2021).

FA for Poisoning

Poisoning is the disruption of body functions due to the entry of toxic substances via ingestion, inhalation, or skin contact (European Resuscitation Council, 2015; First Aid & Emergencies Treatment Guide, 2015; Van de Voorde et al., 2021).

Types of Poisoning

Digestive poisoning is caused by chemicals used at home or in the garden, poisonous mushrooms, spoiled foods, excessive medication, and alcohol.

Respiratory poisoning is usually caused by carbon monoxide gas (LPG leaks, water heaters, stoves), carbon dioxide accumulated in the sewage pit, chlorine, adhesives, paints, household cleaners, etc.

Skin poisoning occurs as a result of drug injection, contact with poisonous plants, pesticides, bites and stings of poisonous animals, etc. (European Resuscitation Council, 2015; First Aid & Emergencies Treatment Guide, 2015; Van de Voorde et al., 2021).

Symptoms of Poisoning

Digestive system: Nausea, abdominal pain, vomiting, and diarrhea.

Nervous system: Feeling of discomfort, incompatibility in movements, seizures, loss of consciousness.

Respiratory system: Shortness of breath, cyanosis, respiratory arrest.

Circulatory system: Pulse disorder, cardiac arrest (European Resuscitation Council, 2015; First Aid & Emergencies Treatment Guide, 2015; Van de Voorde et al., 2021).

FA for Digestive Poisoning

Check consciousness and ensure the patient is alert.

If only the mouth has come in contact with poison, rinse thoroughly with water. If hands are contaminated, wash with soapy water.

Evaluate vital signs (breathing, pulse, consciousness).

Do not induce vomiting, especially if the poison is a corrosive chemical.

If unconscious, place in the recovery position and keep warm.

Call emergency services (911/999/112).

Gather and record information:

- Type of poison or substance ingested
- Any medications taken
- Time of exposure or discovery
- Items/medicines found at the scene (European Resuscitation Council, 2015; First Aid & Emergencies Treatment Guide, 2015; Van de Voorde et al., 2021).

FA for Inhalation Poisoning

The safety of the scene is ensured (The environment is ventilated by opening windows, doors, etc. The patient is taken outside to fresh air). Vital signs are evaluated, and the patient is kept in a semi-sitting position to allow him/her to breathe comfortably. If unconscious, a recovery position is given. The FAR calls 911/999/112. (European Resuscitation Council, 2015; First Aid & Emergencies Treatment Guide, 2015; Van de Voorde et al., 2021).

FA for Skin Poisoning

- The safety of the scene is ensured.
- Contact of hands with toxic substances is prevented.
- Vital signs are evaluated.
- Garments contaminated with poison are removed.
- The skin is washed with plenty of water for 15 - 20 minutes.

- The FAR calls 911/999/112. (European Resuscitation Council, 2015; First Aid & Emergencies Treatment Guide, 2015; Van de Voorde et al., 2021).

General FA for Poisoning

- The substance that has caused poisoning is removed (The faster the poisonous substance is removed from the body, the less it will be absorbed).
- Vital functions are maintained.
- The case is reported to a health institution (911/999/112).
- The poison control center is called (European Resuscitation Council, 2015; First Aid & Emergencies Treatment Guide, 2015; Van de Voorde et al., 2021).

FA for Fractures

A fracture is a break or crack in a bone, caused by trauma or force.

Types of Fractures

Closed fractures: Bone integrity has been impaired, but the skin is intact.

Open fractures: Skin integrity has been compromised. Bone ends may protrude, carrying the risk of bleeding and infection.

Comminuted fractures: The bone has been broken in more than one place (European Resuscitation Council, 2015; First Aid & Emergencies Treatment Guide, 2015; Van de Voorde et al., 2021).

Fracture Symptoms

- Intense pain that increases with movement of the area,
- Deformity (compared to other healthy organs),
- Bruising as a result of edema, swelling, and bleeding in the area, and
- Loss of function, limitation in movements (European Resuscitation Council, 2015; First Aid & Emergencies Treatment Guide, 2015; Van de Voorde et al., 2021).

Possible Complications

Injuries and compression of the vessels, nerves, and muscles near the fracture are observed (no pulse, coldness, paleness, and extreme sensitivity in the fracture area). Bleeding in comminuted fractures may lead to the development of shock. There is a risk of infection in open fractures (European Resuscitation Council, 2015; First Aid & Emergencies Treatment Guide, 2015; Van de Voorde et al., 2021).

FA Steps

- The P/I should not be moved.
- Sudden movements should be avoided, and no attempt should be made to replace the fracture.

- If the fracture is in the arm, rings, watches, and similar accessories should be removed as edema will occur.
- It is necessary to restrict movements in the area with a fracture.
- If there is an open fracture, the wound should be covered with a clean cloth before examination.
- The broken area should be fixed using a hard object like cardboard or wood to include the upper and lower joints.
- The fixed area should be kept elevated and rested.
- The pulse and color of the skin should be checked frequently in the area with the fracture.
- The patient should be kept warm.
- Medical assistance should be sought (European Resuscitation Council, 2015; First Aid & Emergencies Treatment Guide, 2015; Van de Voorde et al., 2021).

FA for a Sprain

A sprain is a temporary stretching or tearing of ligaments at a joint.

- The sprained joint is fixed with a compressive bandage in a way that does not obstruct circulation, and the area is elevated to reduce swelling.
- The sprained part should not be moved.
- It is subjected to cold application.
- If it does not recover soon, medical help is sought.

FA for a Dislocation

Dislocation is a permanent displacement of joint surfaces.

- The joint is fixed as it is.
- No attempt is made to fit the dislocation.
- Nothing is given orally to the P/I.
- Pulse, skin color, and temperature are checked in the dislocated area.
- Medical assistance is sought.

FA for Injuries

Types of injuries

Cuts: These are wounds caused by cutting tools such as glass and knives.

Bruises: They result from hitting a hard object, such as a stone or stick.

Piercing wounds: These wounds are caused by long and sharp tools.

Infected wounds: These include deep and dirty wounds and those resulting from biting or stinging (European Resuscitation Council, 2015; First Aid & Emergencies Treatment Guide, 2015; Van de Voorde et al., 2021).

Common Symptoms

Pain, bleeding, and separation of wound edges.

FA Steps

- Bleeding, if any, is stopped.
- Stuck objects, if any, are not removed,
- The injured person is referred to a health institution.
- Tetanus protection should be ensured (European Resuscitation Council, 2015; First Aid & Emergencies Treatment Guide, 2015; Van de Voorde et al., 2021).

In penetrating chest injuries:

- If conscious: Place in a semi-sitting position, support the back, and elevate feet by 30 cm (shock position).
- Call emergency services (911/999/112).

In abdominal injuries:

- Place in a supine position (lying flat on the back).
- Do not press or manipulate the wound.
- Call emergency services immediately.

FA for Skull and Spine Injuries

- Consciousness and other vital signs are evaluated.
- The 911/999/112 is called for medical help.
- If the person is conscious, do not allow movement.
- If environmental danger exists, drag the person by the feet in a straight line without bending the body.
- During transport, ensure the head-neck-body axis is maintained; avoid shock.
- Document all steps taken and report to medical professionals.
- The P/I should never be left alone (European Resuscitation Council, 2015; First Aid & Emergencies Treatment Guide, 2015; Van de Voorde et al., 2021).

FA for Bleeding

The movement of blood out of the vessel (into or out of the body) as a result of disruption of vascular integrity is called bleeding (European Resuscitation Council, 2015; First Aid & Emergencies Treatment Guide, 2015; Van de Voorde et al., 2021).

Types of Bleeding

External bleeding: It is the flow of blood outside the body.

Internal bleeding: It is the flow of blood into the body.

Natural orifice bleeding: Bleeding from the ear, nose, mouth, rectum, or reproductive organs (European Resuscitation Council, 2015; First Aid & Emergencies Treatment Guide, 2015; Van de Voorde et al., 2021).

FA for External Bleeding

- Direct pressure is applied to the wound.
- If the bleeding does not stop, a second cloth is placed, and the pressure is increased.
- If necessary, the pressure is increased by wrapping it with a bandage without removing the bloody cloths.
- Pressure is applied to the pressure point closest to the bleeding area.
- The bleeding area is elevated.
- If bleeding is in the arms or legs and there is no suspicion of fracture, keep the bleeding area above heart level.
- The person is given a shock position,
- Vital signs are checked frequently (every 2-3 minutes). (European Resuscitation Council, 2015; First Aid & Emergencies Treatment Guide, 2015; Van de Voorde et al., 2021).

When to Apply a Tourniquet

Use only when (European Resuscitation Council, 2015; First Aid & Emergencies Treatment Guide, 2015; Van de Voorde et al., 2021):

- A limb is severed.
- All other methods fail to stop bleeding.
- Long-distance transport is required.
- There is only one first aider with many injured persons.

FA for Internal Bleeding

- Consciousness and breathing are evaluated.
- The person is covered with a blanket, and feet are elevated 30 cm (shock position).
- No food or drink is given orally.
- If there is a closed fracture, the person should be kept immobile to prevent injury to the blood vessels and internal bleeding.

- Vital changes of the person are monitored in the shock position.
- The FAR should call 911/999/112 to seek medical help (European Resuscitation Council, 2015; First Aid & Emergencies Treatment Guide, 2015; Van de Voorde et al., 2021).

FA for Nose Bleeding

- First of all, the FAR should stay calm.
- Lean the head forward, not backward.
- The wings of the nose are squeezed with two fingers.
- This process continues for approximately five minutes.
- If the bleeding does not stop, the person must be taken to the nearest health institution (European Resuscitation Council, 2015; First Aid & Emergencies Treatment Guide, 2015; Van de Voorde et al., 2021).

FA for Ear Bleeding

- If it is minor bleeding, it is cleaned with a clean cloth.
- If it is serious, the ear is covered with gauze, paying attention to not obstructing it.
- Keep the person lying on the bleeding side, immobile.
- Medical assistance is sought.
- It should not be forgotten that ear bleeding may be a sign of a possible brain hemorrhage (European Resuscitation Council, 2015; First Aid & Emergencies Treatment Guide, 2015; Van de Voorde et al., 2021).

FA in Convulsions

They are uncontrollable contractions of muscles triggered by electrical discharges that occur in the brain as a result of irritation in the nerve center. They occur due to brain injuries, infections, high fever (>38°C), and some diseases (epileptic seizures). It is usually seen in children between the ages of six months and six years.

- First of all, the patient is wrapped in a towel or sheet soaked in warm water. If the temperature does not go down with this method, the patient is placed in a bathtub at room temperature and given a shower.
- If the temperature still does not go down, medical help is sought (European Resuscitation Council, 2015; First Aid & Emergencies Treatment Guide, 2051; Van de Voorde et al., 2021).

FA for Seizures in Epilepsy

Common Symptoms

The patient may experience early warning signs known as auras, such as an unusual smell (phantosmia) or sudden muscle tension. In some cases, the patient may scream, lose consciousness abruptly, and collapse. This is followed by intense and generalized muscle contractions, during which the person may become short of breath for 10–20 seconds. Bruising of the lips and face, noisy breathing, excessive salivation, incontinence, and brief, repetitive muscle contractions may occur. The patient may also bite their tongue or injure themselves by hitting their head on the ground due to uncontrolled movements. In the final phase, the patient gradually regains consciousness, often appearing confused, disoriented, and drowsy (European Resuscitation Council, 2015; First Aid & Emergencies Treatment Guide, 2015; Van de Voorde et al., 2021).

- Safety measures are taken for the incident, and the seizure is left to its own course.
- The patient should not be tied, and the locked jaw should not be tried to be opened.
- Care is taken not to allow the patient to harm himself/herself. Materials that may cause harm are removed.
- Tight clothes are loosened.
- The FAR should be alert against vomiting.
- If there is an injury as a result of a fall, it is taken care of.
- Medical help is sought (European Resuscitation Council, 2015; First Aid & Emergencies Treatment Guide, 2015; Van de Voorde et al., 2021).

FA for Low Blood Sugar

It is a condition that occurs when blood sugar in the body decreases for some reason. It can be seen due to diabetes, prolonged exercise, fasting, or gastrointestinal surgery.

Symptoms of sudden blood sugar drop: Sweating, rapid pulse, tremors, fatigue, nausea, or sudden feeling of hunger. If it falls slowly and over a long period, then the symptoms may be headaches, difficulty speaking, visual impairment, drowsiness, confusion, or loss of consciousness (European Resuscitation Council, 2015; First Aid & Emergencies Treatment Guide, 2015; Van de Voorde et al., 2021).

- The general condition of the patient is evaluated.
- If person is conscious, sugar water is given. Taking two sugar cubes can be lifesaving whether the blood sugar level is low or high.
- If the symptoms do not disappear within 15-20 minutes, the person should be taken to a healthcare institution.
- If person is unconscious, a recovery position is given, and medical help is sought (European Resuscitation Council, 2015; First Aid & Emergencies Treatment Guide, 2015; Van de Voorde et al., 2021).

Conclusion

In conclusion, teaching schoolchildren first aid is an effective strategy for developing essential life-saving skills and preventing serious injuries resulting from accidents. Therefore, first aid training should be introduced as a mandatory component of the curriculum starting from the first grade of primary school. At this stage, children are capable of learning the fundamental principles of FA. A comprehensive FA curriculum should go beyond knowledge transfer; it should also encourage active participation, foster confidence in administering FA, and focus on the development of practical skills. Age-appropriate educational plans are crucial to ensure the effective delivery of FA education across different developmental stages, and these plans should be fully integrated into the school curriculum.

School nurses play a vital role as educators in this process. Given that timely and correct administration of FA can significantly reduce both morbidity and mortality from injuries, the presence of trained school nurses is essential. In addition, both teachers and students should receive regular training from qualified health professionals to ensure school-wide FA readiness. Currently, FA training is not mandatory in schools, and participation remains limited, despite awareness of its importance. Therefore, it is imperative to provide teachers with adequate training and support, enabling them to effectively assist students in FA-related situations and foster a safety school environment.

Disclaimer

None.

References

Abd El-Hay, S. A., Ibrahim, N. A., & Hassan, L. A. (2015). Effect of training program regarding first aid and basic life support on the management of educational risk injuries among students in industrial secondary schools. *IOSR Journal of Nursing and Health Science, 4*, 32–43.

Afifi, R., Shata, S. Z., Raggal, A., Ayoub, H., & Qulali, A. (2015). Involvement of male youth into accidents in Upper Egypt: Pattern and risk analysis. *Health, 7*, 965–975.

Al Gharsan, M., & Alarfaj, I. (2019). Knowledge and practice of secondary school teachers about first aid. *Journal of Family Medicine and Primary Care, 8*, 1587–1593.

Al-Hajj, S., El Bcheraoui, C., Daoud, F., Khalil, I., Moradi-Lakeh, M., Abu-Raddad, L. J., Hamadeh, R. R., & Mokdad, A. (2020). Child and adolescent injury burden in the Eastern Mediterranean Region: Findings from the Global Burden of Disease 1990–2017. *BMC Public Health, 20*(1), 433.

American Red Cross. (1981). *Standard first aid & personal safety* (2nd ed.). U.S.A.

Bánfai, B., Pandur, A., Schiszler, B., Pek, E., Radnai, B., Csonka, H., & Betlehem, J. (2019). The (second) year of first aid: A 15-month follow-up after a 3-day first aid program. *Emergency Medicine Journal, 36*, 666–669.

Bánfai, B., Pek, E., Pandur, A., Csonka, H., & Betlehem, J. (2017). 'The year of first aid': Effectiveness of a 3-day first aid programme for 7–14-year-old primary school children. *Emergency Medicine Journal, 34*, 526–532.

Baser, M., Coban, S., Tasci, S., Sungur, G., & Bayat, M. (2007). Evaluating first-aid knowledge and attitudes of a sample of Turkish primary school teachers. *Journal of Emergency Nursing, 33*(5), 428–432.

Bernardo, L. M., Doyle, C., & Bryn, S. (2002). Basic emergency lifesaving skills (BELS): A framework for teaching skills to children and adolescents. *International Journal of Trauma Nursing, 8*, 48–50.

Bollig, G., Wahl, H. A., & Svendsen, M. V. (2009). Primary school children are able to perform basic life-saving first aid measures. *Resuscitation, 80*, 689–692.

Calandrim, L. F., Santos, A. B., Oliveira, L. R., Massaro, L. G., Vedovato, C. A., & Boaventura, A. P. (2017). First aid at school: Teacher and staff training. *Rev RENE, 18*(3), 292–299.

Cimpoesu, D., Popa, O., Corlade-Andrei, M., & Petris, A. (2012). Teaching BLS to high school children: When to start? *Resuscitation, 83*, e112.

Costa, C. W. A., Moura, D. L., Costa, F. L. O., Melo, R. S., & Moreira, S. R. (2015). Unidade didática de ensino dos primeiros socorros para escolares: Efeitos do aprendizado. *Pensar Prática, 18*(2), 338–349.

Dandil, E., Öztürk, İ., Ekşi, Z., & Çakıroğlu, M. (2015). First aid guide application for mobile devices. *APJES, 3*(1), 16–20.

Dasgupta, A., Bandyopadhyay, L., & Das, M. (2014). Effectiveness of health education in terms of knowledge acquisition on first-aid measures among school students of a rural area of West Bengal. *Medico Research Chronicles, 1*, 84–91.

De Buck, E., Van Remoortel, H., Dieltjens, T., Verstraeten, H., Clarysse, M., Moens, O., & Vandekerckhove, P. (2015). Evidence-based educational pathway for the integration of first aid training in school curricula. *Resuscitation, 94*, 8–22.

European Resuscitation Council. (2015). *Kids save lives*. Retrieved from https://www.erc.edu/projects/kids-save-lives.

First Aid & Emergencies Treatment Guide. (2015). Retrieved from https://www.bgccentralappalachia.com/wp-content/uploads/2022/06/first_aid_emergencies.pdf.

Frederick, K., Bixby, E., Orzel, M. N., Stewart-Brown, S., & Willett, K. (2006). An evaluation of the effectiveness of the Injury Minimization Program for Schools (IMPS). *Injury Prevention, 6*, 92–95.

Grimaldi, M. R. M., Gonçalves, L. M. S., Melo, A. C. O. S., Melo, F. I., Aguiar, A. S. C., & Lima, M. M. N. (2020). A escola como espaço para aprendizado sobre primeiros socorros. *Revista de Enfermagem da UFSM, 10*, e1–e15.

Guimarães, H. P., Olivato, G. B., & Pispico, A. (2018). Ressuscitação cardíaca pré-hospitalar: Do pré-hospitalar à sala de emergência. *Revista da Sociedade de Cardiologia do Estado de São Paulo, 28*(3), 302–311.

Harvey, A., Towner, E., Peden, M., Soori, H., & Bartolomeos, K. (2009). Injury prevention and the attainment of child and adolescent health. *Bulletin of the World Health Organization, 87*(5), 390–394.

Lubrano, R., Romero, S., Scoppi, P., Cocchi, G., Baroncini, S., Elli, M., Turbacci, M., ... Moscatelli, R. (2005). How to become an under 11 rescuer: A practical method to teach first aid to primary schoolchildren. *Resuscitation, 64*, 303–307.

Mobarak, A. S., Afifi, R. M., & Qulali, A. (2015). First aid knowledge and attitude of secondary school students in Saudi Arabia. *Health, 7*, 1366–1378.

Oliveira, M. R., Leonel, A. R. A., Montezeli, J. H., Gastaldi, A. B., Martins, E. A. P., & Caveião, C. (2015). Conception of undergraduate nursing students on the practice of health education on first aid. *Rev RENE, 16*(2), 150–158.

Omar, N., Khan, R., Farooq, F., Karim, H., Ayoub, M., & Habib, U. (2015). Health care facilities at school: Perception of students. *Professional Medical Journal, 22*(12), 1546–1549.

Panda, P. C., Panda, S. K., Karir, S., & Patra, A. (2019). Effectiveness of first-aid training on school children of urban area of Sambalpur District, Odisha. *International Journal of Medical Science and Public Health, 8*, 838–842.

Reveruzzi, B., Buckley, L., & Sheehan, M. (2020). First aid training in secondary schools: A comparative study and implementation considerations. *Journal of Safety Research, 75*, 32–40.

Roth, G. A., Abate, D., Abate, K. H., Abay, S. M., Abbafati, C., Abbasi, N., ... Geleijnse, J. M. (2018). Global, regional, and national age-sex-specific mortality for 282 causes of death in 195 countries and territories, 1980–2017: A systematic analysis for the Global Burden of Disease Study 2017. *The Lancet, 392*, 1736–1788.

The Turkish Red Crescent. (2021). *Basic first aid information*. Retrieved from http://www.ilkyardim.org.tr/temel-ilk-yardim-bilgileri.html.

Tse, E., Plakitsi, K., Voulgaris, S., & Alexiou, G. A. (2023). The role of a first aid training program for young children: A systematic review. *Children, 10*, 431.

Van de Voorde, P., Turner, N. M., Djakow, J., de Lucas, N., Martinez-Mejias, A., Biarent, D., ... Maconochie, I. (2021). European Resuscitation Council Guidelines 2021: Paediatric life support. *Resuscitation, 161*, 327–387.

Wilks, J., & Pendergast, D. (2017). Skills for life: First aid and cardiopulmonary resuscitation in schools. *Health Education Journal, 76*, 1009–1023.

Yavuz, M., Demir Korkmaz, F., & Özbayır, T. (2012). *Basic first aid.* Meta Basım Printing Services.

Chapter 25

Pandemic (Epidemic Diseases) and Management in Schools

Ebru Öztürk Çopur[1,*], PhD
and Fatma Karasu[2], PhD
[1]Department of Public Health Nursing, Kilis 7 Aralık University,
Yusuf Şerefoğlu Faculty of Health Sciences, Kilis, Turkiye
[2]Department of Public Health Nursing, Kahramanmaras Sütçü İmam University Faculty of Health Sciences, Kahramanmaraş, Turkiye

Abstract

Throughout human history, epidemics have triggered significant changes, often leading to widespread social and individual crises. As with all areas of social life, the continuity of educational activities during pandemics depends on the ability to manage the chaos caused by such events. Understanding the factors contributing to this chaos can support individuals and institutions in adopting more effective strategies to navigate educational disruptions. Schools are an important part of society, as they provide a safe learning environment for students, thus allowing parents or primary caregivers to participate in working life. They are also places where other school staff, especially teachers, are employed. The management of schools during pandemics is a complex, multidimensional process with far-reaching public health implications. In such periods, school administrations must implement evidence-based policies, foster intersectoral collaboration, engage in continuous monitoring, and introduce substantial adaptations to daily school life and the curriculum. At the same time, schools must be prepared for the unpredictable nature of such crises. Consequently, school management practices have become a global priority during pandemics, as they directly impact both educational institutions and their main stakeholders.

Keywords: pandemic, school management, crisis, risk assessment, COVID-19

---

* Corresponding Author's Email: ebruozturkcopur@kilis.edu.tr

In: Health Promotion and Prevention
Editor: Eda Kılınç İşleyen
ISBN: 979-8-89530-758-8

Introduction

It is inevitable that organizations, throughout their life cycle, will be influenced by their external environment and undergo change. This dynamic interaction often brings about uncertainty and chaos. The "butterfly effect," as described in chaos theory-as the metaphor that a butterfly flapping its wings in Beijing can trigger a storm in New York weeks later- illustrates how small changes in interconnected systems can lead to significant consequences (Yeşilorman, 2006). Emerging problems can create a crisis environment for organizations. Such developments can thrust organizations into crisis.

In organizational terms, a crisis is defined as a situation that threatens the goals and survival of the institution, renders existing risk mitigation strategies ineffective, disrupts decision-making and planning processes, and creates considerable tension (Demirtaş, 2000). Epidemic and pandemic diseases are among the most impactful crisis scenarios. These health-related crises can have widespread and profound effects on public health, the economy, national and global security, and social and political stability.

During pandemics, governments and institutions are forced to implement measures aimed at slowing and mitigating the spread of disease (Bozkurt, 2020). Managing how education continues during such times is a complex and multidimensional process with significant public health implications. In response to pandemics, traditional education has largely shifted to remote, screen-based learning environments, often limiting students to digital interactions with their teachers. However, this mode of education disproportionately affects children from lower socioeconomic backgrounds and those with limited internet access, widening educational inequality (Gouëdard et al., 2020).

School leaders play a pivotal role in ensuring that effective and inclusive learning can continue during such crises. They are responsible for implementing strategies that minimize educational disruption and safeguard student well-being. Effective management in this context requires evidence-based planning, cross-sectoral collaboration, ongoing monitoring, and significant adaptations in school operations and curricula. Above all, maintaining health and safety within the school environment becomes top priority (Money and Pacifici, 2020).

Pandemic

An *epidemic* refers to the rapid spread of a disease among a large number of people within a population over a short period. When such an outbreak expands significantly in scope and scale, it may evolve into a pandemic. Etymologically, the term *pandemic* derives from the ancient Greek words *pan* (meaning "all") and *demos* (meaning "people"). A pandemic is characterized by large-scale outbreaks of infectious diseases that spread across countries, continents, or even globally. These outbreaks not only elevate disease and mortality rates but also lead to substantial economic, social, and political disruptions (Jones et al., 2008; Büken, 2010; Porta, 2008).

For an outbreak of a disease to be considered a pandemic, the disease must easily and continuously circulate to people over a widespread area; it must be a novel disease that has not been previously identified; and the emerging disease must be contagious to other people and have dangerous consequences (Tekin, 2021). Numerous factors influence the extent to which an infectious disease can spread. These include increased global travel and mobility, urbanization, environmental degradation, changes in land use, war, and mass displacement of populations (Jones et al., 2008). Collectively, these trends have significantly heightened the risk of pandemics in the modern era.

Unlike in the 19th century—when it could take months for a disease to spread globally—today's interconnected world allows a localized outbreak to escalate into a global health crisis within days, largely due to technological advances and international mobility (Büken, 2010; Tekin, 2021). Historically, several pandemics have had devastating effects on humanity, including the Black Plague, cholera, the Spanish flu, the Hong Kong flu, swine flu, typhoid, and most recently, Coronavirus disease (COVID-19).

The lifestyle of human beings greatly affects the speed and impact of epidemics. Especially today, it is seen that urbanization has spread to a great extent in almost all countries in the world. This lifestyle, where people are lined up on each other, also plays an important role in increasing the rate of infectious diseases. As urban areas grow, natural ecosystems are disrupted, water sources become increasingly polluted, and conditions emerge that support the proliferation of harmful microbes and viruses. Consequently, these environmental disruptions are contributing to climate change, diminishing food security, and increasing the risk of global famine (Tekin, 2021).

Historically, the emergence and recurrence of epidemics have been closely linked to human activities that disrupt the balance of nature. Factors such as environmental pollution, the depletion of clean water resources, and altered patterns of human settlement are often cited as key contributors to the spread of infectious diseases (Tekin, 2021; Öztürk, 2021). Infectious diseases can easily cross borders, posing a serious threat to both economic and regional stability (Verikios et al., 2015). Beyond their health-related consequences, pandemics have widespread social, political, and economic implications (Davies, 2013). For example, the recent COVID-19 pandemic resulted not only in substantial mortality but also in the large-scale disrupted of essential sectors, includings healthcare, education, transportation, agriculture, tourism, and finance.

Crisis Management in Schools during Pandemics

The Turkish Language Association (TLA, 2020) defines a crisis as "a difficult period, depression, or downturn occurring within a country, between countries, or in the life of a society or an organization." One of the most significant vulnerabilities during periods of crisis is the absence of adequate preparedness (Danielsson and Sjöstedt-Landén, 2020; Sarı and Sarı, 2020).

Educational institutions are highly vulnerable to the disruptive consequences of crises such as pandemics (Danielsson and Sjöstedt-Landén, 2020; Sarı and Sarı, 2020). The inability of schools to respond promptly and effectively to crisis situations can lead to far-reaching consequences for students, educators, and society. To mitigate such risks, educational institutions must engage in proactive crisis management planning. This includes developing scenario-based preparedness models, implementing flexible and resilient learning modalities, and establishing comprehensive health and safety protocols. These strategic measures are essential not only for ensuring the continuity of education during health crises but also for protecting the physical and psychological well-being of school communities.

According to Tüz (2004), crisis management involves “the strategic planning and implementation of measures to mitigate the impact of a crisis and to facilitate organizational resilience.” It encompasses three critical phases: pre-crisis (preparation and prevention), crisis response (immediate reaction and containment), and post-crisis (recovery and evaluation) (Tüz, 2004). In the context of educational settings, crisis management includes not only ensuring physical safety but also maintaining the continuity of learning, preserving mental well-being, and restoring a stable educational environment (Sarı and Sarı, 2020; Danielsson and Sjöstedt-Landén, 2020). A collaborative approach involving all school stakeholders is essential to ensure the coherence and effectiveness of crisis management efforts.

The COVID-19 pandemic has highlighted the urgent need for robust crisis management strategies in schools. Schools, as densely populated environments, are particularly vulnerable to the rapid spread of infectious diseases. Effective crisis management during pandemics requires comprehensive planning, clear communication, and coordinated action that prioritizes the safety, health, and educational continuity of all stakeholders (Centers for Disease Control and Prevention, 2016). One of the key components of pandemic crisis management is the development of a school-specific emergency response plan. This plan should include protocols for disease prevention (e.g., hygiene promotion, physical distancing, mask usage), procedures for identifying and responding to suspected cases, and contingency plans for school closures and remote learning.

Communication plays a pivotal role in managing pandemic-related crises. School leaders must ensure transparent, timely, and culturally sensitive communication with students, staff, parents, and health authorities. Establishing a central crisis communication team within the school can help coordinate information flow and counter misinformation that may increase anxiety or resistance. Equally important is the provision of psychosocial support for students and staff. Prolonged school closures, fear of infection, and disruptions to daily routines can significantly affect mental health. Schools should integrate mental health resources into their crisis response, including counseling services and well-being programs (Curran, 2020).

Collaboration with public health agencies is also essential. Schools must align their policies with local and national health guidelines to ensure a coherent and effective response. Building partnerships with health professionals can enhance the school’s capacity to monitor outbreaks, implement vaccinations, and manage health-related data securely. In conclusion, managing pandemics within school settings requires a multi-dimensional approach that combines preparedness, adaptability, and community engagement. By institutionalizing these practices, schools can not only respond more effectively to pandemics but also build resilience against future public health emergencies (Lim, 2023; Rana et al., 2020).

Risk Assessment in Schools During Pandemics

Risk assessment in schools during pandemics is a critical process that enables administrators and stakeholders to identify, evaluate, and respond to potential health threats within the educational environment. As schools are densely populated spaces where close contact is common, they are particularly vulnerable to the rapid transmission of infectious diseases. Therefore, a systematic approach to assessing risks is essential to ensure the safety of students, staff, and the broader community (Center for Disease Control and Prevention, 2016; National Academies of Sciences, Engineering, and Medicine, 2020; Sakarya, 2020).

A comprehensive risk assessment should include both physical and operational aspects of school functioning. This includes evaluating classroom density, ventilation quality, movement patterns within the building, transportation logistics, and the feasibility of hybrid or remote learning models (National Academies of Sciences, Engineering, and Medicine, 2020).

During a pandemic, schools may be required to suspend in-person education and transition to distance learning modalities in order to minimize the risk of disease transmission and safeguard public health. Local situations and conditions must be taken into consideration in the risk assessment when deciding to reopen schools. Since the conditions of schools and the epidemiology of the disease vary by region, it would not be appropriate to make a risk assessment with an approach that does not take into account the local situation (Sakarya, 2020).

In conclusion, risk assessment during pandemics provides a foundation for informed decision-making in schools. By identifying vulnerabilities and planning appropriate mitigation strategies, schools can better protect their communities and sustain educational services throughout public health crises (Center for Disease Control and Prevention, 2012; Sakarya, 2020).

Teaching and Educational Management in Pandemics

Teaching Management

Teaching management refers to the effective planning, execution, and evaluation of lessons. It encompasses organizing the educational environment and learning experiences in alignment with targeted outcomes (Aydın, 2017). To ensure structured and effective education within schools, it is essential to consider teaching principles, strategies, methods, and techniques in detail (Aslan and Eker, 2019) .

Educational management, which includes decision-making, planning, communication, organization, and evaluation, coordinates the human and material resources of educational institutions toward their goals. In times of crisis, this management structure must adapt to changing circumstances. The chaos and uncertainty introduced by crises require educational organizations to be both prepared and flexible in their approaches (Sarı and Sarı, 2020; Sakarya, 2020; Aydın, 2017). A notable example occurred in Turkey during the COVID-19 outbreak. Shortly after the first reported case, the Ministry of National Education announced a transition to distance learning, delivered centrally through television and internet platforms. Despite this swift response, the pandemic disrupted the normal functioning of educational administration in Turkey. Challenges such as unequal access to technology, and the difficulties faced by teachers and students in using digital tools, exposed significant gaps in the system. This situation demonstrated the urgent need for resilient and inclusive education management strategies in times of crisis. It requires collaboration among educators, school leaders, parents, and policymakers to create a supportive and responsive teaching environment that promotes resilience and learning continuity (Sarı and Sarı, 2020).

Distance Education Management

Although the concept of distance education first emerged in the 19th century (Özer, 1990), its development significantly accelerated with the introduction of radio and television technologies (Kahraman, 2020). Although the concept of distance education first emerged in the 19th century (Özer, 1990), its development significantly accelerated with the introduction of radio and television technologies (Kahraman, 2020).

Distance education is the learning and teaching process that is implemented in an organized manner by an organization where the teacher and the learner are not in the same place and communication is provided by technology (Moore and Kearsley, 2012). Distance education is a form of education in which the student and the teacher engage in a learning-teaching interaction without being physically in the same environment. This model enables students to undertake their learning responsibilities and teachers to fulfill their instructional duties without geographical constraints (Kurt et al., 2021).

Mandatory closures and social distancing rules caused by global epidemics have caused significant changes in traditional education methods. Although there have been many epidemics throughout human history, none have spread as quickly and had a wide impact as COVID-19. As a result of the measures taken and the restrictions imposed to reduce the spread of the COVID-19 pandemic, a major change and transformation has begun in the education system, which is one of the areas most affected by the process (OECD, 2020a; Kırmızıgül, 2020). In many parts of the world, face-to-face education has been discontinued, and millions of people have decided to switch to distance education. Although this situation is seen as the right step in terms of crisis management and public health, unprepared training practices have left a question mark in terms of effectiveness, and many problems have been encountered (Daniel, 2020; Erkut, 2020).

The sudden halt in face-to-face education presented complex challenges that impacted not only students but also teachers, administrators, and educational institutions (Daniel, 2020; Allen et al., 2020). It draws attention to the management process of the crisis in terms of education; it states that a successfully managed process can bring opportunities to review and improve existing practices (Zhao, 2020). Among the platforms that can provide distance education, the most common are online teaching methods and television-based courses. While disparities existed in traditional education settings, these became even more pronounced during the distance education process, further highlighting the need for equitable access to digital learning tools and infrastructure.

Global Inequality in Education

The world already faces major challenges in ensuring education as a fundamental human right. The closure of schools and the transition to distance education during pandemics have brought the existing inequality problems in the system to the agenda again. Most distance learning strategies during the COVID-19 pandemic relied heavily on technology-supported platforms (OECD, 2020a). As a result, students' access to technological devices and internet connectivity emerged as crucial factors that directly affected the effectiveness and inclusivity of educational processes.

This technological dependency has deepened existing educational disparities. Students from low-income families, lacking access to adequate digital tools or internet connectivity, have been disproportionately disadvantaged. Consequently, the gap between students with and without access to digital resources has widened, exacerbating existing inequities (World Bank, 2020).

This phenomenon is widely referred to as the "digital divide" (Karp and McGowan, 2020). However, the divide is not limited to device ownership. It also encompasses differences in digital literacy among teachers, students, and parents; internet accessibility; and the quality of digital platforms provided by schools (OECD, 2020b).

Moreover, access to technology alone is not sufficient to ensure effective learning. The suitability of home environments for focused learning — including quiet space, parental support, and overall household stability — plays a significant role in student success.

Pandemics also aggravate the economic challenges faced by many families, further impeding children's access to quality education. Families with already limited means are more severely impacted by economic downturns, which can lead to increased dropout rates or reduced engagement in education. Vulnerable groups such as students with special education needs, refugees, displaced children, and those from impoverished backgrounds face even greater barriers during health crises (OECD, 2020a). As such, pandemic-induced school closures not only disrupted education globally but also intensified long-standing inequalities. These developments highlight the urgent need for inclusive, equitable education policies that prioritize access, adaptability, and support for students.

Precautions to be Taken in Schools

During pandemics, schools must implement a comprehensive set of precautions to ensure the health and safety of students, teachers, and school staff while striving to maintain educational continuity. These measures should be evidence-based, aligned with public health guidelines, and adaptable to the evolving nature of a health crisis (Sakarya, 2020).

1. Hygiene and sanitation measures

Schools must establish strict hygiene protocols, including regular handwashing, the provision of hand sanitizers at key points, and the routine disinfection of frequently touched surfaces such as desks, doorknobs, and learning materials. Students and staff should receive ongoing education about personal hygiene practices.

2. Physical distancing and classroom reorganization

To minimize close contact, class sizes may need to be reduced and physical layouts rearranged. Desks should be spaced according to recommended distances, and one-way corridors or staggered break times can help reduce crowding in common areas such as hallways and cafeterias.

3. Use of personal protective equipment (PPE)

The use of face masks should be encouraged or mandated based on public health advisories, particularly in indoor settings. Staff may also require additional PPE depending on their role and the level of risk.

4. Screening and monitoring

Daily health screenings—such as temperature checks or symptom questionnaires—can help identify potential cases early. Schools should have clear protocols for isolating symptomatic individuals and referring them to healthcare providers.

5. Ventilation and air quality

Improving ventilation in classrooms and other indoor spaces is critical. Whenever possible, windows should be opened, and mechanical ventilation systems should be maintained to ensure proper airflow and air exchange.

6. Continuity of education

To prepare for potential closures or quarantines, schools should have contingency plans for remote or hybrid learning. This includes ensuring access to devices and internet connectivity, providing teacher training for online instruction, and developing digital learning materials.

7. Mental health support

Pandemics can have a profound psychological impact on students and staff. Schools should offer counseling services, create safe spaces for emotional expression, and incorporate social-emotional learning into the curriculum.

8. Communication and community engagement

Transparent and consistent communication with parents, students, and staff is essential. Schools should establish reliable channels to disseminate updates, gather feedback, and coordinate with local health authorities.

It is critical that all stakeholders understand not only what measures are in place but also why they are necessary. This awareness fosters cooperation and compliance. Posters and warning signs should be hung in appropriate places in the school building to remind you of precautions and how to act safely at school, and markings should be made to make it easier to maintain physical distance (Sakarya, 2020). It is very important that students, teachers, school staff, and families understand the need for each measure and how it protects against contamination. The school nurse, if available, and local public health managers, if possible, should also participate in these trainings. A mechanism should also be established to monitor compliance with the rules, and an encouraging approach to complying with the rules should be followed (CDC, 2020a; CDC, 2020b).

Conclusion

Schools are among the most densely populated institutions in society, encompassing individuals from nearly every age group and representing a broad cross-section of the community. As such, major societal disruptions—particularly pandemics—significantly impact school operations. Effective emergency management during pandemics necessitates a systematic and proactive approach to maintain control over the process and ensure a coordinated response.

One of the most important elements in the management of education during pandemics is ensuring continuity in education. Although distance education serves as a temporary substitute, it cannot fully replicate the value of in-person instruction. Prolonged interruptions in education have lasting consequences on student achievement, particularly for vulnerable populations. Therefore, the primary responsibility of school leadership during such crises is to ensure the safety and well-being of students while striving to preserve educational continuity.

The COVID-19 pandemic has underscored the urgent need for adaptive, inclusive, and resilient educational systems. Schools, as critical institutions for societal continuity, must be prepared to respond swiftly and effectively to public health crises. Teaching and educational management during pandemics require a shift from conventional methods toward flexible strategies that prioritize both safety and learning continuity. Risk assessment plays a central role in identifying potential hazards and informing decision-making processes, while comprehensive precautionary measures are essential to protect the health and well-being of all school stakeholders. Ultimately, building institutional capacity for crisis response—through strategic planning, technological investment, and collaborative leadership—will ensure that education systems remain functional, equitable, and responsive in the face of future emergencies.

Disclaimer

None.

References

Açıkgöz, K. Ü. (2005). *Effective learning and teaching.* Izmir: Education World Publications.

Aksoy, H., & Aksoy, N. (2003). Crisis intervention planning in schools. *Ankara University Faculty of Educational Sciences Journal, 36*(1-2), 37-49. https://doi.org/10.1501/Egifak_0000000076.

Allen, J., Rowan, L., & Singh, P. (2020). Teaching and teacher education in the time of COVID-19. *Asia-Pacific Journal of Teacher Education, 48*(3), 233-236. https://doi.org/10.1080/1359866X.2020.1752051.

Aslan, A., & Eker C. (2019). *Teaching principles and methods.* Ankara: Nobel Academic Publishing.

Aydın, A. (2017). *Classroom management.* Ankara: Pegem Akademi Publishing.

Bozkurt, A. (2020). Coronavirus (Covid-19) pandemic process and evaluations regarding education in the post-pandemic world: New normal and new education paradigm. *Journal of Open Education Applications and Research, 6*(3), 112-142.

Büken, N. Ö. (2010). Pandemic influenza and ethics. *Hacettepe Medical Journal, 41*, 62-68.

Center for Disease Control and Prevention. (2012). *Results from the School Health Policies and Practices Study 2012.* https://www.cdc.gov/healthyyouth/data/shpps/pdf/shpps-results_2012.pdf.

Center for Disease Control and Prevention. (2016). *Results from the School Health Policies and Practices Study 2016*. https://www.cdc.gov/healthyyouth/data/shpps/pdf/shpps-results_2016.pdf.
Center for Disease Control and Prevention. (2020 a). Preparing K-12 school administrators for a safe return to school in fall 2020. https://www.cdc.gov/coronavirus/2019-ncov/community/schools-childcare/preparesafe-return.html.
Center for Disease Control and Prevention. (2020b). The Organization for Economic Cooperation and Development. *A framework to guide an education response to the COVID-19 pandemic of 2020*. Paris: OECD Publishing.
Curran, F. C. (2020). School preparedness plans for pandemics and continuity of education. *UF Education Policy Research Center Policy Brief*, University of Florida.
Daniel, S. J. (2020). Education and the COVID-19 pandemic. *Prospects, 49*, 91-96. https://doi.org/10.1007/s11125-020-09464-3.
Danielsson, E., & Sjöstedt-Landén, A. (2020). Leader normativity in crisis management: Tales from a school fire. *Risks, Hazards & Crisis in Public Policy, 11*(2), 139-165. https://doi.org/10.1002/rhc3.12182.
Davies, S. E. (2013). National security and pandemics. *Flour Chronicle, 50*(2), 20-24.
Demirtaş, H. (2000). Crisis management. *Educational Management in Theory and Practice, 6*(23), 353-373.
Erkut, E. (2020). Higher education after Covid-19. *Journal of Higher Education, 10*(2), 125-133. https://doi.org/10.2399/yod.20.002.
Gouedard, P., Pontand, B., & Viennet, R. (2020). Education responses to covid-19: Implementing a way forward. *OECD Working Paper No. 224*. https://www.oecd-ilibrary.org/docserver/8e95f977-en.pdf.
Jones, K. E., Patel, N. G., Levy, M. A., Storeygard, A., Balk, D., Gittleman, J. L., & Daszak, P. (2008). Global trends in emerging infectious diseases. *Nature, 451*(7181), 990–993. https://doi.org/10.1038/nature06536.
Kahraman, M. E. (2020). The impact of the Covid-19 epidemic on applied courses and conducting these courses via distance education: An example of a basic design course. *Istanbul Medeniyet University Medeniyet Art Magazine, 6*(1), 44-56. https://doi.org/10.46641/medeniyetsanat.741737.
Karp, P., & McGowan, M. (2020). Schools ask for online learning help as coronavirus policy confusion persists. *The Guardian*.
Kırık, A. M. (2014). Historical development of distance education and its situation in Turkey. *Marmara Communication Journal, 21*, 73-94.
Kırmızıgül, H. G. (2020). The COVID-19 pandemic and the education process it brought with it. *Eurasian Journal of Social and Economic Research, 7*(5), 283-289.
Kurt, K., Kandemir, M., & Çelik, Y. (2021). Opinions of classroom teachers regarding distance education during the Covid-19 pandemic period. *Turkish Journal of Scientific Research, 6*(1), 88-103.
Lim, W. M., Gunasekara, A., Pallant, J. L., Pallant, J. I., & Pechenkina, E. (2023). Generative AI and the future of education: Ragnarök or reformation? A paradoxical perspective from management educators. *International Journal of Management in Education, 21*(2), 100790. https://doi.org/10.1016/j.ijme.2023.100790.
Money, K. W., & Pacifici, L. C. (2020). Principal candidates' sense of efficacy: Can they lead during a pandemic? *Journal of School Administration Research and Development, 5*(1), 42-48.
Moore, M., & Kearsley, G. (2012). *Distance education: A system view of online learning* (3rd ed.). Wadsworth, Belmont.
OECD. (2020a). Digital Strategies in Education Across OECD Countries: Exploring Education Policies on Digital Technologies. (2020a). OECD. https://www.oecd-ilibrary.org/pub2web/404.jsp.
OECD. (2020b). *Turkey: School Education During Covid-19 Were Teachers and Students Ready?* www.oecd.org/education/Turkey-coronavirus-education-country-note.pdf.
Ozer, B. (1990). The universal structure of the distance education system. *Journal of Fiction, 8*, 569-594.
Ozturk, O. (2021). Pandemic and pandemics in outline. In A. Şen (Ed.), *Corona with Questions*. Academician Online Database.
Porta, M. (2008). *Dictionary of Epidemiology*. Oxford.
Rana, S., Anand, A., Prashar, S., & Haque, M. M. (2020). A perspective on the positioning of Indian business schools post COVID-19 pandemic. *International Journal of Emerging Markets, 17*(2), 353–367.
Sakarya, S. (2020). School health during the pandemic. *Türk Tabipler Birliği Covid-19 Altıncı Değerlendirme Raporu*. https://www.ttb.org.tr/kutuphane/covid19-rapor_6/covid19-rapor_6_Part65.pdf.

Sarı, E., & Sarı, B. (2020). Education management during crises: The case of Covid-19. *International Journal of Leadership Studies: Theory and Practice, 3*(2), 49-63.

Şimşek, Ş. M. (2002). *Management and organization*. Konya: Günay Ofset Matbaacılık.

Tekin, A. (2021). Epidemics and pandemics from history to the present and their economic results. *Süleyman Demirel Üniversitesi Sosyal Bilimler Enstitüsü Dergisi, (40)*, 330-355.

Türk Dil Kurumu. (2020). *Turkish language institution dictionaries*. https://sozluk.gov.tr/.

Tüz, M. V. (2004). *Crisis management*. İstanbul: Alfa Yayıncılık.

Verikios, G., Sullivan, M., Stojanovski, P., Giesecke, J., & Woo, G. (2015). Assessing regional risks from pandemic influenza: A scenario analysis. *The World Economy, 39*(8), 1225-1255. https://doi.org/10.1111/twec.12296.

World Bank. (2020). Rapid Response Briefing Note: Remote Learning and COVID-19 Outbreak. *World Bank Emergency Response Briefing Note*. https://documents1.worldbank.org/curated/en/266811584657843186/pdf/Rapid-Response-Briefing-Note-Remote-Learning-and-COVID-19-Outbreak.pdf.

Yeşilorman, M. (2006). To whom does the butterfly flap its wings? Chaos and social sciences on the edge of unified science. *Journal of Istanbul Kültür University, 3*, 77-86.

Zhao, Y. (2020). COVID-19 as a catalyst for educational change. *Prospects, 49*, 29-33. https://doi.org/10.1007/s11125-020-09477-y.

Index

A

abdominal pain, 33, 208, 271, 275, 310
absenteeism, 5, 7, 29, 30, 33, 94, 102, 104, 107, 108, 112, 182, 223, 226, 227, 229, 263, 270, 279
abuse, 4, 9, 49, 50, 51, 53, 76, 77, 79, 102, 134, 136, 154, 233, 250, 253, 254, 255, 256, 257, 258, 259, 260, 261, 262, 263, 264, 265, 266, 267
abuse and neglect, 254, 255, 256, 258, 260, 261, 262, 265, 266
academic success, v, 7, 8, 9, 10, 27, 30, 36, 49, 55, 59, 62, 87, 106, 179, 181, 185, 218, 223, 234, 239, 246, 247, 290
accident prevention, v, 6, 105, 131, 138
accident-related injuries, 6
accidents, 3, 6, 102, 103, 105, 114, 129, 130, 131, 132, 133, 134, 135, 136, 137, 139, 157, 184, 189, 192, 195, 196, 283, 295, 296, 297, 317
accidents and injuries, 129, 130, 131, 132, 134, 137, 192, 295, 296
acute gastroenteritis, 97
adolescent, 25, 39, 44, 49, 53, 66, 67, 74, 77, 91, 99, 115, 118, 125, 139, 187, 192, 196, 206, 209, 212, 237, 238, 255, 265, 267, 270, 281, 282, 296, 317, 318
adolescents and children, 69, 206
aggressive behavior, 70, 75, 77, 105, 111, 131, 174, 175, 242
air pollution, 107, 112, 113, 226, 227, 236
alcohol, v, 7, 8, 35, 94, 95, 102, 136, 156, 157, 182, 184, 192, 193, 200, 201, 220, 226, 256, 258, 272, 309
anger, 3, 69, 70, 71, 72, 73, 74, 75, 76, 77, 78, 79, 80, 82, 87, 233, 256, 284
anger management, 3, 69, 70, 71, 72, 74, 75, 76, 77, 78, 79, 80, 82
anger regulation, 71
anthropometric measurements, 203
anti-bullying policies, 57
anxiety, 2, 20, 33, 35, 48, 57, 58, 59, 60, 61, 66, 67, 70, 72, 74, 78, 79, 86, 87, 88, 104, 123, 127, 155, 183, 202, 233, 256, 266, 298, 324
assessment of health, 153, 155, 195, 199, 201
asthma, 127, 156, 157, 158, 208, 226, 227, 231, 235, 236, 237, 238, 247, 249, 250, 251, 252, 256
autism, 79, 90, 112, 124, 127, 214, 233, 242, 248

B

bedwetting, 31, 33, 34, 86, 210
behavioral assessment, 210
bladder and bowel dysfunction (BBD), 31, 32, 38
body mass index (BMI), 5, 8, 23, 36, 38, 203, 204, 211, 213, 214, 215, 216, 223, 224, 228, 230, 238
bullying, 3, 6, 7, 9, 18, 58, 64, 65, 70, 75, 78, 79, 81, 82, 83, 84, 85, 86, 88, 89, 90, 91, 101, 104, 111, 112, 130, 139, 156, 158, 179, 180, 182, 205, 211, 230, 233, 246

C

cancers, 49, 119, 141, 147, 173, 197, 226, 231, 237
cardiovascular health, 19, 183, 186, 212
chickenpox, 117, 118, 121, 269, 270, 274, 275, 280, 281
child abuse, v, 50, 52, 210, 254, 255, 259, 260, 261, 262, 263, 264, 265, 266, 267
child-centered play therapy, 72, 76
childhood vaccines, 115, 116, 125
children with intellectual disability, 47
children with special needs, 52, 239, 240, 242, 245, 247, 248, 249, 250, 251
chronic diseases, 4, 6, 8, 10, 15, 16, 109, 120, 154, 155, 174, 190, 225, 226, 230, 234, 238, 242, 244, 247, 250, 251
cleanliness, 28, 29, 30, 32, 108, 133, 157, 277
cognitive behavioral therapy (CBT), 55, 60, 73, 79, 228
cognitive development, 16, 17, 24, 73, 103, 170, 176, 191, 204, 227, 256
cognitive-behavioral play therapy, 72
collaborations, 64
collaborative models, 63
common cold, 269, 270, 271, 273, 274, 280, 281
community engagement, 167, 324, 328

community mental health, 69, 233
comprehensive school health program (CSHP), 167, 168, 174, 175
constipation, 31, 33, 34, 37, 38, 208
control, 5, 18, 19, 27, 31, 46, 49, 54, 60, 61, 62, 63, 66, 69, 70, 71, 72, 73, 74, 75, 76, 78, 93, 100, 107, 108, 109, 117, 125, 134, 138, 154, 156, 170, 171, 174, 191, 203, 229, 235, 236, 247, 251, 256, 265, 269, 270, 272, 277, 278, 279, 280, 311, 324, 325, 329, 330
coordinated school health program (CSHP), 166, 167, 168, 169, 176
coping skills, 11, 60, 228
counseling services, 55, 57, 63, 64, 194, 251, 264, 324, 328
COVID-19, 2, 11, 12, 13, 80, 90, 125, 126, 279, 281, 292, 321, 323, 324, 325, 326, 329, 330, 331
crisis management, 58, 290, 292, 293, 323, 324, 326, 330, 331
cultural structure, 43

D

daytime incontinence (DI), 9, 31, 33, 38, 39, 53, 77, 86, 104, 122, 131, 214, 230, 233, 237, 239, 241, 242, 243, 244, 245, 246, 249, 251, 252, 256, 267
dental caries, 30, 208, 219
dental caries prevention, 219
dental health screening, 5, 215, 219, 220
depression, 2, 20, 33, 57, 58, 60, 66, 67, 73, 86, 87, 88, 104, 155, 210, 231, 233, 243, 256, 266, 323
developmental characteristics, 199, 203, 210, 214
developmental disorder, 79, 112, 214, 218
developmental health, 1
developmental skills, 242
developmental stages, 41, 43, 45, 107, 202, 205, 239, 317
diabetes, 3, 8, 10, 15, 16, 17, 23, 104, 155, 173, 214, 226, 227, 228, 231, 235, 236, 243, 247, 249, 256, 316
diarrhea, 29, 108, 120, 208, 276, 277, 280, 281, 310
diphtheria, 115, 116, 117, 118, 119, 121, 273, 274, 279, 280
diphtheria-pertussis and tetanus vaccines (DPT), 118, 119
disability, 9, 53, 86, 104, 122, 131, 214, 230, 233, 237, 239, 241, 242, 243, 244, 245, 246, 249, 251, 252, 256, 267
disaster awareness, v
disaster management, 10, 110, 292
disasters, 9, 110, 113, 131, 133, 284, 290, 292, 293
discrimination, 3, 18, 43, 81, 82, 83, 86, 87, 88, 89, 90, 92, 102, 111, 228, 229, 243
distance education, 2, 326, 329, 330
diversity and equality, 57
drills, 284, 287, 288, 289, 290, 291

E

educational interventions, 30, 36, 50, 52, 66
emergency, 4, v, 10, 101, 103, 113, 130, 132, 136, 139, 155, 156, 166, 180, 189, 190, 194, 227, 228, 237, 249, 262, 281, 283, 284, 285, 286, 287, 288, 289, 290, 291, 292, 293, 295, 296, 297, 298, 302, 303, 305, 307, 308, 310, 313, 317, 318, 324, 329, 331
emergency health care, v
emergency management, 155, 283, 284, 285, 286, 289, 290, 291, 292, 293, 329
emergency management planning, 286, 293
emotional intelligence, 57, 70, 71, 81
emotional learning, 55, 57, 66, 247, 261, 328
emotions, 2, 41, 56, 70, 72, 73, 75, 169, 172, 203, 205, 233, 242, 263
encopresis, 31
environmental cleaning, 93, 95
epilepsy, 155, 226, 229, 230, 235, 236, 237, 238, 316
ethnicity, 83, 163, 183
evidence-based practice, v, 60, 61, 63, 155
examination, 4, 51, 54, 77, 89, 90, 91, 146, 199, 200, 202, 203, 207, 209, 210, 211, 214, 222, 223, 251, 302, 303, 312
exclusion, 83, 87, 88, 111, 236
excretion, 3, 27, 28, 31, 37

F

family participation, 8
family structure, 27, 35, 70, 256
fecal incontinence (FI), 31, 32, 187
first aid, v, 6, 105, 133, 135, 136, 138, 139, 154, 156, 157, 181, 194, 229, 284, 285, 287, 290, 291, 295, 296, 297, 298, 299, 300, 301, 302, 303, 304, 305, 306, 307, 308, 309, 310, 311, 312, 313, 314, 315, 316, 317, 318, 319
first aid training (FAT), 109, 139, 174, 226, 230, 231, 295, 296, 297, 298, 317, 318, 319
food poisoning, 97, 283
foodborne infections, 95
functional abdominal pain (FAP), 33
functional constipation, 31, 32, 38

G

gender, 18, 32, 42, 43, 44, 46, 48, 51, 54, 70, 83, 85, 89, 131, 132, 142, 163, 171, 215, 216, 230, 233, 241, 245, 256, 258, 266, 286

giardiasis, 269, 270, 276, 277
glucose intolerance, 34
growth and development, v, 5, 7, 15, 16, 18, 19, 22, 35, 38, 105, 109, 124, 130, 131, 154, 184, 200, 226

H

Haemophilus influenzae type b (Hib), 115, 117, 118, 119, 121, 122, 273, 281
hand hygiene, 5, 29, 31, 37, 38, 93, 94, 97, 99, 108, 112, 113, 271, 272, 273, 275, 276
handicap, 241
harm reduction phase, 284
head lice screening, 5, 222, 223
healing phase, 286
Health Behavior Interaction Model (HBIM), 169, 174, 175
Health Belief Model (HBM), 112, 138, 163, 164, 176
health care, v, 10, 45, 116, 152, 154, 155, 196, 224, 234, 252, 318
health education, v, 1, 2, 3, 5, 7, 9, 11, 12, 13, 15, 18, 19, 21, 23, 29, 36, 41, 43, 45, 46, 47, 52, 54, 55, 57, 58, 63, 89, 90, 113, 116, 129, 137, 139, 148, 151, 152, 153, 154, 155, 156, 157, 158, 159, 164, 166, 168, 173, 177, 180, 181, 182, 183, 184, 185, 192, 193, 194, 195, 196, 197, 200, 219, 243, 246, 267, 278, 292, 297, 318, 319
health education programs, v, 1, 3, 7, 9, 46, 116, 157, 184, 192, 194, 195
health examination, 4, 5
health history, 199, 200, 201, 202, 210, 211, 212, 215
health interventions, 55, 60, 62, 64, 65, 199, 200
health literacy, 4, 1, 3, 7, 99, 124, 156, 158, 180, 189, 190, 191, 192, 193, 194, 195, 196, 197, 198, 225, 243, 251, 278, 279
health literacy measurement tool, 189, 192, 195
health monitoring, 2
health of students, v, 6, 103, 110, 130, 179, 184, 289
health prevention and promotion, 1, 2, 6, 7, 199
health problems, v, 6, 7, 8, 9, 10, 16, 70, 85, 104, 137, 152, 155, 157, 166, 173, 199, 200, 213, 214, 215, 223, 232, 233, 244, 246, 247, 248, 260
health promotion, v, 1, 2, 3, 9, 10, 11, 12, 17, 18, 21, 29, 39, 52, 57, 63, 67, 93, 111, 151, 152, 154, 155, 156, 158, 159, 161, 162, 163, 166, 173, 174, 175, 176, 179, 180, 181, 182, 183, 184, 185, 186, 193, 197, 199, 212, 223, 224, 231, 237, 239, 248, 252, 269, 270, 280, 289, 297
Health Promotion Model (HPM), 155, 162, 163, 173, 174, 175
health promotion program(s), 4, 155, 173, 174, 175, 179, 180, 181, 182, 183, 184, 185
health screening(s), 4, 5, 8, 10, 12, 184, 213, 214, 215, 219, 223, 224, 264, 279, 328
healthcare providers, 10, 201, 214, 225, 250, 274, 278, 296, 328
health-promoting schools, 1, 29, 153, 173, 182
healthy environment, v, 107, 136, 166, 184
healthy lifestyle, v, 1, 2, 3, 9, 15, 16, 18, 21, 22, 27, 36, 38, 101, 102, 104, 105, 153, 155, 166, 175, 183, 184, 200, 246
healthy nutrition, v, 7, 8, 17, 27, 108, 151, 152, 154, 155, 156, 174, 175, 176
healthy school, 3, 1, 7, 9, 12, 101, 102, 104, 105, 109, 110, 111, 134, 139, 166, 167, 168, 179, 180, 181, 182, 186, 194, 201, 227, 235, 278, 280
hearing loss, 120, 121, 207, 218
hearing screening, 3, 5, 215, 218, 219
Hepatitis A, 117, 118, 120, 275, 281
Hepatitis B, 49, 98, 115, 117, 118, 120, 298
hormones, 34, 42
human papillomavirus (HPV), 49, 51, 97, 99, 115, 116, 117, 119, 125, 126, 156, 158, 183, 185, 187
hygiene, 3, 2, 3, 5, 9, 18, 27, 28, 29, 30, 31, 34, 36, 37, 38, 39, 93, 94, 95, 97, 101, 102, 103, 108, 109, 126, 134, 155, 156, 157, 180, 189, 192, 193, 194, 197, 202, 248, 269, 276, 277, 278, 279, 324, 327
hygiene habits, 5, 27, 28, 29, 30, 31, 34, 36
hygiene practices, 2, 28, 29, 30, 94, 108, 276, 277, 279, 327

I

immunization, 2, 4, 9, 49, 94, 115, 116, 117, 118, 119, 121, 122, 123, 124, 125, 126, 127, 183, 184, 246, 270, 273, 274, 280
immunization program, 94, 116, 117, 273, 280
impairment, 74, 240, 241, 251
impetigo, 98, 99, 269, 270, 275, 280, 281
indoor environment, 103, 107, 108
infection control, 3, 93, 94, 96, 99, 100, 113, 126
infectious diseases, v, 2, 5, 6, 10, 11, 27, 28, 29, 93, 94, 96, 108, 110, 116, 117, 123, 125, 126, 127, 156, 200, 201, 269, 270, 278, 279, 280, 281, 322, 323, 324, 330
influenza, 115, 116, 117, 119, 121, 122, 125, 269, 270, 271, 280, 281, 282, 292, 329, 331
injury, 6, 9, 77, 105, 130, 131, 132, 135, 139, 154, 166, 190, 200, 241, 255, 270, 285, 295, 296, 297, 303, 314, 316, 317, 318
insulin resistance, 19, 34
integrated care models, 63

intellectually disabled children, 47
intervention phase, 285, 298

L

language development, 242
lifestyle-related diseases, 15, 21
literacy skills, 189, 190, 192, 194, 195

M

malignant melanoma (MM), 141, 142, 206, 216
management, v, 1, 6, 9, 10, 16, 17, 22, 24, 37, 58, 70, 74, 77, 78, 79, 89, 90, 93, 99, 110, 126, 154, 155, 156, 158, 166, 167, 174, 176, 180, 183, 190, 194, 197, 211, 212, 223, 224, 225, 226, 227, 228, 229, 231, 232, 233, 234, 235, 236, 237, 239, 247, 248, 249, 251, 253, 255, 256, 259, 260, 262, 264, 265, 266, 269, 270, 276, 278, 279, 281, 283, 286, 289, 290, 291, 292, 303, 317, 321, 322, 324, 325, 326, 329, 330, 331
measles, 115, 116, 117, 120, 121, 123, 126, 269, 270, 272, 280, 281
Measles, Mumps, Rubella (MMR), 115, 117, 120, 121, 122, 272, 280, 281
mental disorders, 58, 232, 233, 236, 265
mental health, v, 1, 2, 3, 5, 6, 8, 10, 12, 13, 20, 23, 55, 56, 57, 58, 59, 60, 61, 62, 63, 64, 65, 66, 67, 69, 71, 75, 77, 79, 85, 88, 90, 91, 102, 103, 104, 106, 107, 109, 110, 111, 112, 151, 152, 154, 155, 156, 172, 182, 183, 184, 185, 186, 187, 199, 200, 203, 210, 226, 233, 235, 236, 237, 238, 244, 256, 259, 260, 270, 295, 324, 328
mental health evaluation, 199
mental health promotion, 57, 59, 67, 183, 187
mental health services, 6, 12, 62, 66, 67, 111, 237
mental health struggles, 58
mental illnesses, 56
mental well-being, 2, 56, 57, 58, 59, 60, 61, 63, 64, 65, 181, 324
metabolism, 24, 25, 34
mobility, 202, 203, 209, 242, 277, 323
morbidity, 8, 115, 131, 137, 184, 215, 230, 281, 317
mortality, 5, 8, 10, 19, 23, 24, 115, 131, 137, 147, 148, 184, 212, 230, 276, 282, 296, 317, 318, 322, 323
multi-tiered systems of support (MTSS), 63
mumps, 115, 117, 118, 121, 123, 126, 269, 270, 272, 279, 280
mumps infection, 121

N

National Association of School Nursing (NASN), v, 9, 13, 16, 19, 24, 53, 58, 66, 153, 213, 214, 215, 219, 222, 223, 224, 226, 237, 266
neglect, 4, 2, 52, 94, 102, 134, 192, 210, 214, 233, 253, 254, 255, 256, 257, 259, 260, 261, 262, 263, 264, 265, 266, 267
neglect and abuse, 2, 192, 214, 253, 255, 256, 257, 259, 261, 262, 263, 264, 265
nocturia, 31
nocturnal enuresis (NE), 31, 32, 33, 39, 90
non-melanoma skin cancers (NMSC), 141
nursing interventions, 33, 155, 199, 223, 239
nutrition, 3, 2, 3, 7, 8, 9, 11, 12, 15, 16, 17, 18, 19, 22, 23, 24, 25, 27, 30, 36, 37, 38, 39, 63, 101, 102, 103, 109, 112, 154, 155, 156, 158, 166, 168, 174, 176, 179, 181, 182, 183, 187, 189, 190, 192, 194, 207, 215, 237, 238, 247, 249, 252, 270, 278
nutrition management, 17, 18, 19
nutrition programs, 2, 8, 19, 63, 101, 252
nutrition-related diseases, 7

O

obesity, 2, 8, 10, 11, 13, 15, 16, 17, 21, 22, 23, 24, 28, 35, 36, 37, 38, 39, 104, 106, 113, 131, 155, 156, 174, 175, 176, 183, 185, 187, 190, 195, 203, 204, 206, 217, 226, 227, 230, 231, 235, 236, 237, 238, 246, 256
online learning, 2, 330
oral health, 3, 156, 183, 186, 190, 195, 196, 208, 219, 224
oral hygiene, 30, 184, 269, 279

P

pandemic, 2, 97, 122, 292, 321, 322, 323, 324, 325, 326, 327, 329, 330, 331
Pediculosis capitis, 269, 277, 280, 281
peer support, 23, 55, 57, 59, 60, 183
peer support groups, 55, 60
peers, 27, 33, 34, 42, 46, 50, 58, 59, 60, 87, 102, 137, 170, 205, 215, 230, 233, 240, 241, 242, 250, 297
pertussis, 115, 116, 117, 118
physical activity, v, 2, 3, 7, 8, 9, 11, 12, 15, 16, 18, 19, 20, 21, 22, 23, 24, 25, 34, 36, 101, 102, 103, 104, 105, 108, 109, 112, 113, 137, 151, 152, 155, 156, 166, 173, 174, 175, 176, 179, 180, 181, 182, 184, 185, 189, 192, 194, 204, 226, 230, 231, 249, 250, 251, 278
physical development, 203, 220
physical examination, 199, 200, 202, 210, 211, 212, 224, 246, 259, 302

physical health examinations, 5
physical school environment, 103, 104
physiological measurements, 205, 210
positive parenting, 35, 37
prejudices, 83, 86
preparation phase, 284
prevention, 1, 2, 3, 4, 6, 9, 10, 11, 43, 49, 50, 51, 52, 53, 60, 63, 64, 65, 66, 67, 81, 82, 83, 84, 85, 86, 89, 90, 91, 94, 99, 104, 108, 112, 113, 114, 117, 125, 129, 130, 133, 134, 138, 139, 145, 146, 147, 148, 151, 152, 154, 155, 156, 158, 159, 162, 166, 173, 174, 175, 179, 181, 182, 183, 184, 185, 190, 192, 193, 203, 214, 218, 219, 222, 223, 225, 226, 230, 234, 235, 236, 237, 239, 240, 246, 248, 251, 253, 255, 257, 258, 259, 260, 261, 264, 265, 266, 267, 268, 270, 271, 274, 275, 278, 279, 280, 281, 289, 292, 293, 296, 297, 318, 324, 325, 329, 330
prevention levels, 239, 246
preventive health services, 1, 3, 8, 11, 137, 190, 195, 215
psychological factors, 43
psychological support, 259, 260
psychosocial development, 6, 31, 191, 205, 214
psychosocial effects, 2, 11, 232
psychotherapy, 72, 78, 83
public health, v, 6, 9, 11, 12, 13, 15, 16, 20, 23, 24, 27, 30, 38, 39, 52, 53, 54, 69, 76, 90, 92, 93, 94, 95, 96, 100, 102, 112, 113, 114, 115, 116, 121, 123, 124, 126, 127, 129, 130, 131, 138, 139, 141, 147, 151, 154, 158, 159, 161, 163, 167, 175, 176, 179, 181, 183, 184, 186, 187, 189, 190, 195, 196, 197, 199, 213, 214, 223, 224, 225, 230, 237, 239, 251, 252, 253, 254, 257, 264, 265, 266, 267, 269, 270, 277, 279, 280, 292, 293, 295, 317, 318, 321, 322, 324, 325, 326, 327, 328, 329

R

recovery phase, 286
recurrent urinary tract infections (UTIs), 33, 37
rehabilitation, 6, 74, 77, 184, 246, 247, 253, 259, 260, 263, 264, 265, 289
release play therapy, 72
resilience, 2, 56, 59, 60, 61, 65, 102, 104, 182, 226, 240, 246, 257, 279, 293, 324, 325
respiratory etiquette, 93, 94, 100, 269, 271, 275
respiratory infection, 95, 97, 112, 208, 243, 244, 269
respiratory tract infection, 108, 208, 270
risk assessment, 155, 289, 321, 324, 325, 329
risky health behaviors, 102
role-playing, 31, 72, 74, 194
Rubella, 115, 117, 118, 120, 121, 126, 269, 270, 272, 280

S

safe school, 1, 3, 7, 12, 84, 101, 103, 111, 283, 292, 293
safe school environment, 1, 3, 7, 84, 101, 103
safety precautions, 133, 134, 137
sanitary conditions, 29
school accident, 6, 11, 105, 112, 129, 130, 131, 132, 133, 135, 136, 137, 138, 139
school buildings, 103, 104, 131, 134, 292
school community, 3, 1, 2, 3, 4, 5, 6, 7, 8, 9, 10, 11, 18, 59, 81, 109, 124, 129, 153, 155, 179, 180, 181, 182, 185, 194, 248, 250, 261, 288
school environment, 1, 2, 3, 5, 6, 7, 10, 11, 12, 17, 18, 19, 20, 24, 27, 56, 57, 59, 60, 61, 62, 64, 65, 82, 84, 87, 96, 99, 101, 102, 103, 106, 107, 109, 110, 111, 112, 113, 114, 130, 132, 133, 134, 137, 138, 139, 155, 158, 166, 184, 186, 193, 227, 228, 230, 231, 239, 240, 250, 260, 264, 269, 270, 276, 277, 280, 286, 317, 322
school health, v, 1, 2, 3, 4, 5, 6, 8, 9, 10, 11, 12, 13, 18, 21, 25, 29, 38, 46, 48, 49, 52, 53, 55, 61, 63, 66, 89, 93, 94, 99, 100, 102, 104, 105, 112, 113, 130, 137, 138, 139, 141, 151, 153, 154, 155, 156, 158, 159, 161, 165, 167, 168, 174, 175, 176, 177, 179, 180, 181, 182, 183, 184, 185, 186, 187, 196, 197, 212, 213, 214, 219, 223, 224, 225, 235, 240, 247, 251, 252, 270, 274, 278, 282, 292, 293, 295, 297, 329, 330
school health services, v, 2, 4, 5, 6, 9, 10, 11, 12, 13, 21, 25, 66, 99, 100, 130, 155, 181, 184, 212, 240, 251, 278, 282, 295, 297
school management, 49, 101, 111, 138, 263, 292, 321
school nurse(s), v, 1, 3, 6, 8, 9, 10, 11, 12, 13, 15, 16, 17, 18, 19, 21, 22, 24, 28, 36, 41, 46, 49, 50, 51, 52, 55, 56, 58, 59, 60, 63, 65, 66, 70, 71, 75, 88, 95, 97, 101, 102, 111, 129, 135, 136, 137, 139, 141, 146, 151, 153, 154, 155, 156, 157, 158, 161, 174, 175, 179, 184, 185, 189, 194, 195, 199, 200, 201, 202, 210, 213, 214, 218, 219, 220, 223, 224, 225, 226, 227, 228, 234, 235, 236, 237, 239, 240, 246, 247, 248, 249, 250, 251, 253, 264, 265, 266, 270, 279, 280, 286, 289, 290, 291, 293, 295, 297, 317, 328
school nursing, v, 9, 13, 22, 24, 49, 53, 66, 130, 139, 147, 148, 151, 154, 155, 159, 173, 174, 186, 189, 194, 196, 224, 226, 234, 235, 236, 237, 247, 251, 252, 253, 269, 290
school nutrition programs, 8, 12, 17
school personnel, 1, 62, 96, 134, 166, 262, 286
school safety, 65, 110, 129, 134, 138, 184, 284, 295
school staff, 1, 3, 8, 9, 18, 21, 58, 59, 61, 62, 64, 65, 67, 75, 82, 88, 93, 94, 95, 99, 101, 130, 135, 142,

154, 156, 157, 169, 179, 180, 182, 184, 185, 219, 225, 226, 227, 229, 233, 236, 249, 260, 263, 264, 283, 284, 287, 289, 290, 321, 327, 328
school success, v, 238
school-age children, v, 1, 2, 3, 4, 5, 6, 7, 8, 12, 15, 16, 17, 19, 20, 27, 28, 29, 30, 31, 32, 34, 36, 37, 38, 39, 41, 42, 52, 55, 56, 57, 58, 59, 60, 61, 62, 63, 64, 65, 69, 70, 71, 73, 74, 75, 78, 79, 81, 82, 85, 86, 87, 88, 93, 98, 101, 102, 105, 106, 107, 108, 109, 115, 116, 117, 124, 126, 129, 130, 131, 132, 137, 141, 142, 145, 151, 152, 154, 156, 158, 179, 180, 181, 184, 185, 189, 190, 191, 192, 193, 194, 195, 199, 200, 201, 202, 203, 204, 205, 206, 207, 208, 209, 210, 213, 214, 215, 219, 222, 223, 225, 226, 228, 234, 239, 253, 260, 264, 265, 266, 269, 270, 273, 274, 277, 280, 281, 286, 295, 296
school-based health interventions, 55
school-based interventions, 60, 61, 62, 64, 148, 177, 236, 279
school-based program, 12, 67, 146, 253, 261, 262, 267
scoliosis, 5, 10, 213, 214, 215, 219, 221, 223, 224
scoliosis screening, 5, 215, 219, 221, 223, 224
sedentary behaviour, 20, 22, 24, 25
sedentary lifestyles, 15, 21
self-esteem, 8, 20, 30, 31, 33, 43, 44, 57, 74, 75, 76, 78, 86, 87, 88, 92, 104, 111, 182, 231, 256, 262
sexual abuse, 46, 47, 48, 49, 50, 52, 53, 77, 133, 254, 255, 261, 265, 266, 267, 268
sexual behavior(s), 41, 42, 43, 44, 45, 46, 50, 52, 182, 256
sexual development, 41, 43, 45, 47, 48, 51, 53
sexual education, 41, 43, 44, 45, 47, 48, 50, 51, 52, 53, 157, 192
sexual educators, 41, 47
sexual health, 3, 41, 43, 44, 45, 46, 47, 48, 49, 50, 51, 52, 53, 54, 155, 156, 159, 182
sexual health education, 41, 43, 44, 45, 46, 47, 48, 49, 50, 52, 53, 54, 159, 182
sexuality, 41, 42, 43, 44, 45, 47, 48, 50, 52, 53, 54, 97
sexually explicit materials, 49
sexually transmitted diseases (STDs), 42, 46, 49, 97, 99, 151, 152, 156, 183
skin cancers, 141, 144
skin infection, 98, 275, 281
sleep, 3, 7, 8, 9, 20, 22, 23, 25, 27, 28, 34, 35, 36, 37, 38, 39, 58, 86, 104, 106, 155, 208, 210, 222, 230, 277
sleep disorder, 34, 36, 37, 210
sleep disturbances, 34, 58, 86, 106, 222, 277
sleep health, 28, 35, 36
sleep patterns, 27, 28, 35, 36
sleep problems, 34, 35, 36, 37
sleep quality, 28, 35, 104
smoking, v, 3, 7, 8, 9, 136, 156, 157, 173, 182, 183, 184, 192, 195, 232, 256, 297
Social Cognitive Learning Theory (SCLT), 171, 172, 174
social health, 3, 4, 7, 75, 152, 194, 290
social interaction, 2, 55, 105, 111, 279
social pain, 83
social well-being, v, 43, 101, 111, 172
socialization, 41, 42, 191, 205
socioeconomic factors, 27
socioeconomic status, 16, 30, 34, 35, 132, 183, 191, 256
special needs, 4, 114, 180, 239, 240, 241, 242, 243, 244, 246, 247, 248, 251, 255
spiritual development, 205, 212
stereotypes, 83, 86
stigmatization, 81, 82, 83, 86, 87, 88, 225, 227, 231, 233
stress management, 36, 58, 59, 60, 155, 228, 229
student health, v, 43, 44, 49, 51, 54, 112, 155, 159, 166
substance abuse, v, 64, 65, 66, 70, 79, 134, 189, 194, 210, 233, 256
substance use prevention, 151
sun exposure, 141, 142, 145, 146, 147
sun protection, 3, 141, 142, 143, 145, 146, 147, 148, 174, 176
sun protection behaviors, 141, 142, 146, 148, 174
sun protection factor (SPF), 143, 144, 147, 148
sunburn, 141, 142
sunglasses, 142, 144, 145, 146, 174
sunscreen products, 142, 143, 144, 174
system evaluation, 199

T

tertiary prevention, v, 184, 225, 234, 239, 240, 246, 247, 248, 250, 258
tetanus, 115, 116, 117, 118, 121, 313
theories and models, 161, 162, 173, 174, 176
three-component model, 165
Transtheoretical Model (TTM), 164, 165, 174, 176

U

ultraviolet (UV) radiation, 141, 142, 143, 144, 145, 146, 147, 148, 149, 232
ultraviolet protection factor (UPF), 143, 144
unhealthy behaviors, 7, 15, 21
urine incontinence, 31

V

vaccination, 2, 5, 49, 93, 94, 98, 115, 116, 117, 118, 119, 120, 121, 122, 123, 124, 125, 126, 127, 155, 183, 184, 185, 187, 270, 271, 272, 273, 274, 276, 279, 281
vaccination policy, 117
vaccine hesitancy, 123, 124, 125, 126, 127
vaccines, 5, 51, 94, 115, 116, 117, 118, 119, 121, 122, 123, 124, 125, 126, 127, 274, 279, 280, 281
victimization, 47, 78, 112
violence, v, 3, 6, 7, 9, 35, 43, 44, 53, 65, 69, 71, 75, 76, 80, 81, 82, 83, 85, 88, 89, 90, 91, 102, 111, 130, 131, 133, 134, 136, 139, 177, 184, 200, 233, 250, 251, 254, 256, 258, 259, 266, 267, 270, 283, 284, 290
viral infections, 97
vision screening, 181, 217, 218
visual impairment(s), 2, 10, 218, 251, 316
vital signs, 135, 136, 205, 211, 212, 213, 214, 298, 306, 307, 310, 313, 314

W

waste management, 95, 102, 109, 113
well-being, v, 2, 5, 7, 8, 9, 10, 11, 13, 15, 16, 17, 19, 20, 21, 27, 29, 30, 32, 33, 36, 46, 55, 56, 57, 58, 59, 60, 61, 62, 63, 64, 65, 66, 69, 70, 71, 73, 75, 77, 82, 83, 84, 85, 87, 88, 93, 99, 101, 102, 103, 104, 105, 108, 109, 110, 111, 138, 152, 158, 166, 167, 169, 172, 173, 176, 179, 180, 181, 182, 185, 186, 190, 191, 201, 210, 212, 213, 218, 225, 230, 235, 240, 249, 250, 256, 262, 279, 285, 290, 322, 323, 324, 329
World Health Organization (WHO), v, 1, 3, 6, 7, 8, 9, 10, 13, 15, 16, 17, 19, 20, 23, 24, 25, 28, 29, 30, 33, 39, 43, 45, 47, 49, 53, 54, 61, 64, 70, 71, 73, 74, 78, 80, 82, 83, 85, 86, 87, 91, 94, 95, 97, 100, 101, 102, 103, 105, 109, 114, 115, 116, 117, 118, 119, 120, 121, 122, 123, 124, 127, 129, 130, 133, 139, 142, 145, 149, 152, 153, 156, 157, 159, 161, 163, 167, 172, 173, 177, 179, 181, 185, 187, 189, 194, 197, 200, 205, 212, 214, 215, 216, 217, 218, 219, 220, 221, 222, 225, 226, 227, 229, 230, 231, 233, 234, 238, 240, 241, 242, 243, 244, 245, 250, 251, 252, 254, 255, 256, 257, 258, 259, 260, 261, 263, 267, 269, 270, 273, 274, 278, 282, 289, 293, 297, 299, 301, 318